Nerve Compression Syndromes of the Upper Limb

Cover illustration
Redrawn with permission from Mackinnon SE, Dellon AL. (1988) Median nerve entrapment in the proximal forearm and brachium. In: Mackinnon SE, Dellon AL, eds. *Surgery of the Peripheral Nerve*. New York: Thieme.

Nerve Compression Syndromes of the Upper Limb

Edited by

Yves Allieu, MD
Centre Hospitalier Universitaire
Hôpital Lapeyronie
Montpellier, France

and

Susan E. Mackinnon, MD
Division of Plastic and Reconstructive Surgery
Washington University School of Medicine
St Louis, Missouri, USA

MARTIN ■ DUNITZ

© 2002 Martin Dunitz Ltd, a member of the Taylor & Francis group

First published in the United Kingdom in 2002
by Martin Dunitz Ltd, The Livery House, 7–9 Pratt Street, London NW1 0AE

Tel.:	+44 (0) 20 74822202
Fax.:	+44 (0) 20 72670159
E-mail:	info.dunitz@tandf.co.uk
Website:	http://www.dunitz.co.uk

Although every effort has been made to ensure that all owners of copyright material have
been acknowledged in this publication, we would be glad to acknowledge in subsequent
reprints or editions any omissions brought to our attention.

A CIP record for this book is available from the British Library.

ISBN 1 85317 609 5

Distributed in the USA by
Fulfilment Center
Taylor & Francis
7625 Empire Drive
Florence, KY 41042, USA

Toll Free Tel.:	+1 800 634 7064
E-mail:	cserve@routledge_ny.com

Distributed in Canada by
Taylor & Francis
74 Rolark Drive
Scarborough, Ontario M1R 4G2, Canada

Toll Free Tel.:	+1 877 226 2237
E-mail:	tal_fran@istar.ca

Distributed in the rest of the world by
ITPS Limited
Cheriton House
North Way
Andover, Hampshire SP10 5BE, UK

Tel.:	+44 (0)1264 332424
E-mail:	reception@itps.co.uk

Composition by Tek-Art, Croydon, Surrey
Printed and bound in Spain by Tallers Gràfics Soler S.A., Barcelona

CONTENTS

LIST OF CONTRIBUTORS

Yves Allieu
Chirurgie Orthopédique et Traumatologique II
Hôpital Lapeyronie
34059 Montpellier Cedex, France

Peter C. Amadio
Hand Surgery
Mayo Clinic
200 First Street, SW
Rochester, MN 55905, USA

Anne Brunon
Functional Rehabilitation Department B
Rehabilitation and Physical Therapy Medicine
Centre Hospitalier Universitaire de Nîmes
30240 Le Grau du Roi, France

Christine J. Cheng
Division of Plastic and Reconstructive Surgery
Washington University School of Medicine
Suite 17424, East Pavilion
One Barnes-Jewish Hospital Plaza
St Louis, MO 63110, USA

Alain Durandeau
Service d'Orthopédie Traumatologique
Centre Hospitalo-Universitaire de Bordeaux
Place Amélie Raba-Léon
33076 Bordeaux Cedex, France

Thierry Fabre
Service d'Orthopédie Traumatologique
Centre Hospitalo-Universitaire de Bordeaux
Place Amélie Raba-Léon
33076 Bordeaux Cedex, France

Guy Foucher
SOS Main
4, boulevard du Président Edwards
67000 Strasbourg, France

Philip E. Higgs
Washington University School of Medicine
Division of Plastic and Reconstructive Surgery
1040 Mason Road, Suite 210
St Louis, MO 63141, USA

Jeanine Laurent
Rehabilitation Medicine
Le Castelet Rehabilitation Centre
34430 St Jean de Védas, France

Carolyn M. Lévis
Division of Plastic Surgery, McMaster University
Hamilton General Hospital, Room 703
237 Barton Street East
Hamilton, Ontario L8L 2X2, Canada

Bruno Lussiez
2, rue Verdi
06000 Nice, France

Susan E. Mackinnon
Division of Plastic and Reconstructive Surgery
Washington University School of Medicine
Suite 17424, East Pavilion
One Barnes-Jewish Hospital Plaza
St Louis, MO 63110, USA

Rahul K. Nath
Department of Plastic Surgery, Baylor University
Texas Children's Hospital
1102 Bates Street, Suite 950
Houston, TX 77030, USA

Christine B. Novak
Division of Plastic and Reconstructive Surgery
Washington University School of Medicine
Suite 17424, East Pavilion
One Barnes-Jewish Hospital Plaza
St Louis, MO 63110, USA

Giorgio Pajardi
Plastic Surgery Institute, University of Milan
Hand Surgery Department, MultiMedica Hospital
Via Milanese 300, 20099 Milan SGG, Italy

Guy Raimbeau
Centre de la Main
2, rue Auguste Gautier
49100 Angers, France

Michel Romain
Functional Rehabilitation Department B
Rehabilitation and Physical Therapy Medicine
Centre Hospitalier Universitaire de Nîmes
30240 Le Grau du Roi, France

Jean-Claude Rouzaud
Chirurgie Orthopédique et Traumatologique II
Hôpital Lapeyronie
34059 Montpellier Cedex, France

Paul Seror
Laboratoire d'electromyographie
146, avenue Ledru-Rollin
75011 Paris, France

Robert J. Spinner
Mayo Clinic
200 First Street, SW
Rochester, MN 55905, USA

Greg Watchmaker
The Milwaukee Hand Center
13133 North Port Washington Road
Mequon, WI 53097, USA

Ian Winspur
Hand Clinic
Devonshire Hospital
29–31 Devonshire Street
London W1N 1RF, UK

Introduction

Nerve compression syndromes comprise, under the term of nerve entrapment, all apparently primitive nerve injuries (excluding secondary compressions caused by adjacent factors such as tumours). They are frequent in the upper limb, and this relatively high frequency, compared to the lower limb, can be explained because of its higher degree of mobility. Injuries in nerve entrapment are caused by both static and dynamic factors: static factors may include an inelastic tunnel or a musculo-tendinous anomaly; dynamic factors, including joint mobility, muscular contraction and nerve mobility during movements of the upper limb, also provoke nerve compression, friction and stretching. This dynamic vision of nerve compression syndromes allows a better understanding of their etiopathogenesis and their treatment.

The dynamic factors are preponderant in the etiopathogenesis of the thoracic outlet syndrome (TOS). Its treatment will hence be mainly medical in the absence of an anatomical anomaly whose responsibility for nerve injury is unquestionable.

The carpal tunnel syndrome (CTS) is by far the most frequent of nerve compressions. The median nerve passes through an fibro-osseous tunnel. The nerve compression is due to the synovium in this inelastic tunnel (hence it is mainly flexor tenosynovitis). Dynamic factors are, however, also present, owing to wrist flexion-extension, and must be taken into account for prevention in professional activities.

After the CTS and the TOS, the most frequent nerve compression syndrome is the ulnar nerve compression at the cubital tunnel of the elbow. In this case static and dynamic factors play an equal role. The static factor (the shape of the cubital tunnel at the elbow) and dynamic factors (during elbow flexion-extension) bring about compression, stretching and friction of the nerve.

The anterior interosseous nerve and the posterior interosseous nerve can be compressed by a musculo-tendinous structure (in particular, the arcade of Frohse for the radial nerve), but these nerve injuries are mainly due to dynamic compressions during prono-supination movements. These movements can affect different levels of the nerve, which explains the hourglass-like fascicular constriction, which can be isolated or at several levels (and which we can also note in the rare proximal compressions of the radial nerve at the arm during flexion-extension moments of the elbow).

Repeated or forced movements of flexion-extension or prono-supination are partly responsible for nerve compressions in athletes and musicians. Conservative treatment, including rest and splinting, will be based on elimination of postural faults, wrong movements and ergonomic hazards.

Ulnar nerve neuropathy at the level of the space of Guyon is classically included in the nerve compression syndromes. However, this compression is much more rare than ulnar nerve compression at the elbow, and is, moreover, always secondary to an adjacent lesion compressing the nerve.

In addition to this dynamic vision of nerve compression syndromes, we must insist on the importance of an electrophysiological evaluation. The present techniques allow us to confirm the diagnosis, and moreover to distinguish between isolated compressions and double crush syndromes (which must always be taken into consideration, since in this case the predominant compression site must be located for treatment).

Recent experimental works clearly explain the different stages of chronic nerve compressions and show the importance of early treatment. Surgical treatment should be indicated only in the case of failure of conservative treatment or in the case of clinical or electrophysiological signs showing important neurological disorders. It should consist in neurolysis which must be complete, taking into account all the possibilities of musculo-tendinous compressions during different movements. Because nerve mobility is important there should be early post-operative mobilization in order to facilitate nerve gliding.

Yves Allieu

Compression neuropathies are being identified with increasing frequency in the upper extremity. Carpal tunnel syndrome, first recognized in 1913 and first treated surgically in 1924, still presents a dilemma in management, especially in the workers' compensation population. The term multi-level nerve compression, or double crush syndrome, was introduced in 1973, yet still remains controversial three decades later. Thus the simplicity of the term nerve compression belies its complexity in evaluation and management.

This text reviews specific compression entrapment syndromes and will allow the surgeon to better evaluate even the most perplexing patient with painful upper extremities and normal electrodiagnostic findings. Where indicated, surgical options are described. Specifics of conservative management are emphasized as modifications in posture and position at home and in the workplace, and personal factors, including improvement in physical fitness, can reduce many symptoms and ensure an overall better result when selective surgical procedures are needed. Chapters in this text from both surgeons and therapists will assist the surgeon in managing compression neuropathies in even the most challenging patient – the worker, the musician, and the athlete.

Susan E. Mackinnon

1
Histopathology of nerve compression and the double crush syndrome

Christine J. Cheng

Introduction

Descriptions of chronic nerve compression syndromes have existed in the medical literature since the middle of the nineteenth century (Mackinnon, 1992). The twentieth century, though, saw a marked increase in the number of described anatomic sites that can be affected. The exhaustive list now includes all of the major peripheral nerves of the upper extremity as well as several in the lower extremity. As can be expected, growing awareness of the entity among patients and its resulting increased diagnosis by physicians has led to an associated rise in its social impact. Some have described the situation as reaching 'near-epidemic proportions' (Mackinnon, 1992). A noteworthy development is the evolution of work-related chronic nerve compression, also termed 'repetitive trauma disorder', which is usually associated with prolonged and/or vigorous upper extremity exertion in the workplace. In 1997, 4% of the 6.1 million injuries and illnesses reported in United States private industry workplaces were attributed to repeated trauma disorders (US Department of Labor, 1998).

A brief chronicle of the history of reported chronic nerve compression syndromes begins in 1821, with Sir Astley Cooper's account of the symptoms of thoracic outlet syndrome (Cooper, 1821; Mackinnon, 1992). Paget reported carpal tunnel syndrome in 1854 (Mackinnon, 1992) and Panas noted three patients with ulnar nerve compression at the elbow in 1878 (Mackinnon, 1992; Panas, 1878). After the turn of the twentieth century, an increased understanding of nerve compression brought Wartenberg's syndrome of radial sensory nerve compression in 1932 (Mackinnon, 1992), which Mackinnon and Dellon characterized histologically (Mackinnon et al., 1986b). Soon it was realized that single nerves could be affected at different sites. Besides being compressed at the elbow, the ulnar nerve could also be affected at Guyon's canal in the wrist, as described by Hunt (Mackinnon, 1992). Different sites of compression along a single nerve were found to produce very specific findings. One such example is pronator syndrome, identified by Seyfarth in 1951, which causes both sensory and motor abnormalities of the median nerve, while anterior interosseous nerve syndrome, described by Kiloh and Nevin in 1952, produces distal median motor dysfunction only, with no sensory deficit (Mackinnon, 1992). Compression syndromes involving the suprascapular, musculocutaneous, axillary, lateral antebrachial cutaneous and tibial nerves have since been reported.

Upton and McComas further advanced the theory of chronic nerve compression with their hypothesis of 'double crush' in 1973 (Upton and McComas, 1973). They proposed that two serial sites of compression along the same nerve would be more deleterious than one, and that the presence of the first lesion would enhance susceptibility to a second, more distal lesion. Despite the logical appeal of this theory, however, controversy still exists regarding its truth. Numerous clinical reports in humans have suggested an association between proximal neural lesions, usually cervical radiculopathy, and distal nerve compression syndromes such as carpal tunnel syndrome and cubital tunnel syndrome (Hurst et al., 1985; Massey et al., 1981; Simpson and Fern, 1996). Animal studies have seemed to demonstrate the phenomenon (Dellon and Mackinnon, 1991; Nemoto et al., 1987; Seiler et al., 1983), but no human studies to date have clearly proven it (Richardson et al., 1999).

Anatomy of the peripheral nerve

The cell body of the motor neuron lies in the anterior horn of the spinal cord. The cell body of the sensory neuron is located in the dorsal root ganglion, just distal to the cord. Axons from each cell body extend peripherally as either myelinated or unmyelinated fibers. A chain of Schwann cells surrounds each myelinated nerve fiber with a multilayered myelin sheath. Groups of unmyelinated fibers are associated with single Schwann cells. Both types of nerve fibers are bound by endoneurium to form bundles, or fascicles. A perineurial membrane surrounds each fascicle, while groups of fascicles are held together by internal and external epineurium, forming the peripheral nerves (Figure 1.1).

Peripheral nerves possess the unique ability to withstand injury and extensive mobilization due to a well-developed intrinsic vascular supply. Regional vessels from surrounding tissues anastomose with longitudinally oriented vessels within the layers of epineurium, perineurium and the endoneurial space. Connections

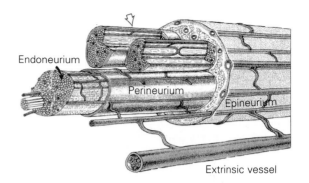

Endoneurium

Perineurium

Epineurium

Extrinsic vessel

Figure 1.2

Graphic representation of peripheral nerve vasculature. Longitudinally-oriented extrinsic vessels supply the intrinsic vessels within the epineurium, perineurium and endoneurium. Note obliquely-oriented vascular connections between the perineurial and endoneurial vascular systems (open arrow). (From Lundborg G, Dahlin LB. The pathophysiology of nerve compression. *Hand Clin* **8**:215–227, 1992; with permission.)

between the perineurial and endoneurial vessels are positioned obliquely and are thought to be vulnerable to compression by external as well as internal forces, such as intrafascicular edema (Lundborg and Dahlin, 1992; Rempel et al., 1999) (Figure 1.2). Within the fascicles, a continuous endoneurial capillary network forms a 'blood–nerve barrier', which, like that in the central nervous system, maintains a highly controlled environment.

The length of an axon may be 10 000 to 15 000 times the diameter of its cell body (Rempel et al., 1999). An extraordinary energy-dependent transport system transfers materials away from (antegrade axonal transport) and toward (retrograde axonal transport) the cell body along the immense span of its axon. Substances needed to maintain the structure and function of the axon are synthesized in the cell body and moved distally, while disposal materials and trophic factors are returned to the cell body to effect necessary metabolic modifications. Axonal transport consists of a fast component (up to 400 mm/day), which moves enzymes, neurotransmitter vesicles and glycoproteins, and a slow component (up to 30 mm/day), which transfers cytoskeletal elements, such as microtubule and neurofilament subunits (Grafstein and Forman, 1980).

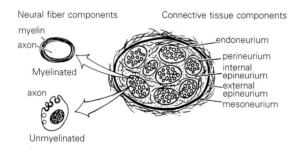

Neural fiber components

Connective tissue components

myelin

axon

Myelinated

axon

Unmyelinated

endoneurium

perineurium

internal epineurium

external epineurium

mesoneurium

Figure 1.1

Schematic of normal peripheral nerve anatomy. (Adapted from Mackinnon SE, Dellon AL. *Surgery of the peripheral nerve*. New York: Thieme Medical Publishers, 1988, p. 42; with permission.)

Acute nerve compression

In experimental animal models, methods of inducing acute peripheral nerve compression have included pressure chambers (Grundfest and Cattell, 1935), synthetic tubing (Weisl and Osborne, 1964), tourniquets (Fowler et al., 1972; Ochoa et al., 1972; Pedowitz et al., 1991), inflatable nerve cuffs (Dahlin et al., 1984; Dyck et al., 1990; Rydevik and Lundborg, 1977), and clamps (Horiuchi, 1983). The first effect of compression is local neural ischemia. Examination of rabbit tibial nerve with a vital microscope showed reduced epineurial venous blood flow at an external compression pressure of 20–30 mmHg. Increasing this compression to 80 mmHg blocked all intraneural blood flow in the segment. Similar results were attained with dog sciatic nerves using the hydrogen washout technique to monitor blood flow (Matsumoto, 1983). In this model, 45–50 mmHg decreased circulation and 120 mmHg completely obstructed flow.

Lundborg and colleagues demonstrated that local nerve ischemia was responsible for early dysfunction in human nerve compression. External median nerve compression of 60 mmHg was applied at the wrist until a sensory conduction block was registered. A tourniquet was then inflated above systolic pressure around the upper arm. Nerve function did not return after release of the local median nerve compression, but immediately recovered after the tourniquet was deflated (Lundborg et al., 1982). The critical pressure threshold for nerve dysfunction due to compression seems to be 30 mmHg below the diastolic pressure. This is usually 40–50 mmHg in normotensive subjects and 60–70 mmHg in hypertensive individuals (Gelberman et al., 1983; Szabo et al., 1983). Accounts of hypertensive patients developing carpal tunnel syndrome following blood pressure correction (Emara and Saadah, 1988) lend further support to the role of acute ischemia in compressive neuropathy.

Anoxic injury to the epineurial and endoneurial vascular endothelium leads to an increase in vascular permeability and loss of the blood–nerve barrier. The resulting intrafascicular edema leads to increased endoneurial fluid pressure (Rydevik and Lundborg, 1977). Experimental compression of rat sciatic nerve at 30 mmHg for 2 hours caused a rapid, three to four-fold increase in the micropipette measurement of endoneurial fluid pressure that persisted for 24 hours after compression ceased (Myers et al., 1978). Persistent edema impedes blood flow through the obliquely oriented transperineurial vessels. Histologically, the endoneurial edema first appears as separated nerve fibers, then progresses to local demyelination at 7 days after compression (Lundborg et al., 1983; Powell and Myers, 1986).

Structural nerve changes as a result of acute compression include distortion and splitting of the myelin sheaths (Dyck et al., 1990) and displacement of the nodes of Ranvier with myelin stretching on one side of the node and invagination on the other (Fowler et al., 1972; Ochoa et al., 1972). Other researchers (Pedowitz et al., 1991) have not noted the latter. In all cases, though, compression has been associated with segmental demyelination and associated conduction block. Local ischemia leading to Schwann cell necrosis is believed to be the cause of this paranodal demyelination (Powell and Myers, 1986).

Acute compression of peripheral nerves interferes with the axonal transport system within neurons. In animal experiments, axonal transport has been demonstrated by radioisotope labeling of intraneural proteins. The slow component (12–30 mm/day) involves cytoskeletal elements such as actin, tubulin, and neurofilament proteins (Black and Lasek, 1980; Grafstein and Forman, 1980; McClean et al., 1983). Compression at 30 mmHg for 8 hours produced proximal and distal accumulations of slow transport components, representing impairment of antegrade and retrograde transport (Dahlin and McLean, 1986). Such impairment could reduce the capacity for repair or regeneration of the distal axon (Dahlin and McLean, 1986; Lundborg and Dahlin, 1992). Similarly, fast axonal transport (34–400 mm/day), which consists of membrane constituents such as proteins, glycoproteins, lipids, neurotransmitters, and other low molecular weight materials such as amino acids (Grafstein and Forman, 1980), is also inhibited by compression. This inhibition seems to be proportional to the degree of compression as well as the duration. Fast transport in animals was not affected by compression at 20 mmHg for 2 hours (Dahlin et al., 1984), but significant accumulation of protein components occurred after 8 hours (Dahlin and McLean, 1986). Increasing the pressure to 30 mmHg produced partial or complete transport blockage after only 2 hours (Dahlin et al., 1984). Presumably, decreased delivery of membrane components and transmitter substances could interfere with synaptic function (Dahlin and McLean, 1986; Lundborg and Dahlin, 1992).

Impaired retrograde axonal transport may alter the presentation of trophic factors from the terminal milieu, such as Schwann cells and target tissues, to the nerve cell body (Dahlin et al., 1986b). Examination of sensory nerve cell bodies one week after peripheral nerve compression showed morphologic changes including decreased nuclear density, eccentric nucleus positioning, and dispersion of the Nissl substance, or chromatolysis (Dahlin et al., 1987; Dahlin et al., 1989a). These morphologic changes may precede functional changes and previously were described after more severe injuries such as nerve crush or transection (Barron, 1983; Lieberman, 1971).

Chronic nerve compression

As with acute nerve compression, many animal models have been developed to study chronic nerve compression. These have included the placement of arterial sleeves (Weiss and Hiscoe, 1948), spring clips (Nemoto, 1983), loose ligatures (Duncan, 1948), and various synthetic tubes (Aguayo et al., 1971; Mackinnon et al., 1984, 1985; Weisl and Osborne, 1964) around peripheral nerves for extended periods of time. Because the amount of extraneural pressure could not be measured or controlled readily, some of the earlier models employing tight bands (Duncan, 1948; Weiss and Hiscoe, 1948) caused severe nerve damage leading to fiber degeneration and regeneration, instead of true chronic compression (Mackinnon et al., 1984). Chronic changes were effectively produced using bands of just slightly greater diameter than that of the peripheral nerve (Mackinnon et al., 1984). The guinea pig has been used as a well-studied model of naturally-occurring nerve compression (Fullerton and Gilliatt, 1965, 1967a,b; Ochoa and Marotte, 1973). These aging animals develop median nerve entrapment from localized compression beneath an ossifying fibrocartilaginous bar at the carpal tunnel. Since the phenomenon is developmental, however, the possibility of central adaptive changes in the animals has been proposed (Mackinnon et al., 1984), which might limit the model's utility. Also, older animals in general have been found to have more pronounced nerve degeneration (Weisl and Osborne, 1964).

Axonal demyelination follows the early changes of perineurial edema, inflammation and fibrin deposition after severe nerve compression (Powell and Myers, 1986). At 1 week, endoneurial fibroblast and capillary endothelial cell proliferation occur. Two weeks after compressive injury, early endoneurial fibrosis, microvessel and perineurial thickening, and nerve fiber remyelination can be seen (Powell and Myers, 1986; Sommer et al., 1993). Larger nerve fibers (Dahlin et al., 1989b; Gasser and Erlanger, 1929) and those located peripherally within fascicles (Powell and Myers, 1986; Spinner and Spencer, 1974) are more vulnerable to compression than smaller, more centrally positioned fibers. These findings have been documented in rat (Mackinnon et al., 1984) and primate (Mackinnon et al., 1985) models of chronic compression (Figures 1.3 and 1.4), as well as human histologic specimens of clinically compressed nerves (Mackinnon et al., 1986a; Neary et al., 1975; Thomas and Fullerton, 1963). This mixed histopathologic pattern could explain the common presentation of the patient with significant symptoms of nerve compression, but relatively normal nerve conduction studies. The most severely affected axons would cause subjective abnormalities, while the unaffected axons would be responsible for the normal conduction parameters (Mackinnon et al., 1986a). In addition, symptoms may vary – sensory versus motor, muscle-to-muscle, or digit-to-digit – depending on the particular fibers involved (Mackinnon et al., 1985).

Increased axon-to-myelin ratios have been consistently demonstrated in areas of compression by morphometric analysis of animal (Mackinnon et al., 1984, 1985) and human (Mackinnon et al., 1986a,b) nerve specimens. Axon size did not change. Large fibers with thin layers of myelin were thought to represent either 'end-stage' demyelination or early remyelination (Figures 1.5 and 1.6). However, in human specimens, new populations of very small unmyelinated fibers were also observed (Mackinnon et al., 1986a,b). Whether these denote degeneration and regeneration of unmyelinated or myelinated fibers remains unclear. Histologic evidence of myelin debris, which would be expected with Wallerian degeneration, was not detected. The presence of regenerating small unmyelinated pain fibers, though, could explain the Tinel's sign and hyperalgesia often associated with compression neuropathy (Mackinnon et al., 1986b). Experimentally, prolonged chronic compression does eventually produce Wallerian degeneration of the myelinated axons (Mackinnon et al., 1984) (Figure 1.7).

Clinical studies of nerve compression in humans are abundant, but histopathologic information is scarce, since nerve biopsy can lead to permanent dysfunction. Past reports have utilized cadaver specimens with obvious muscle wasting or 'subclinical' symptoms of compression to study median (Marie and Foix, 1913; Neary et al., 1975; Thomas and Fullerton, 1963), ulnar (Neary and Eames, 1975; Neary et al., 1975), and lateral femoral cutaneous nerve (Jefferson and Eames, 1979) changes. Mackinnon et al. (1986a) analyzed superficial radial nerve branches in five patients who underwent nerve excision and proximal intramuscular transposition for the treatment of persistent

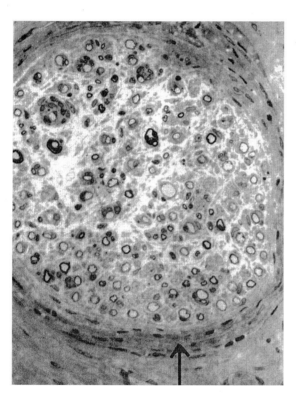

Figure 1.3

Transverse section from primate nerve after five months of compression (toluidine blue stain, × 344). The fascicle is located at the periphery (contrast with Figure 4). The perineurium is markedly thickened (arrow). Damage is characterized by the paucity of large myelinated fibers. (From Mackinnon SE, Dellon AL, Hudson AR, Hunter DA. A primate model for chronic nerve compression. *J Reconstr Microsurg* **1**:185–194, 1985; with permission.)

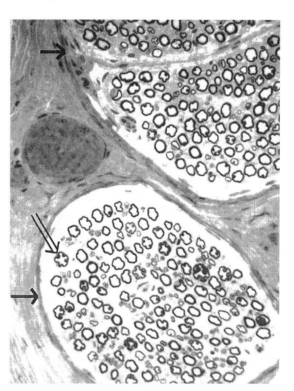

Figure 1.4

Another section from the same compressed primate nerve as in Figure 3 (toluidine blue stain, × 344). These fascicles are located in the center (contrast with Figure 3). The perineurium is not as thickened (solid arrow). The fluted myelin pattern is still present (open arrow). (From Mackinnon SE, Dellon AL, Hudson AR, Hunter DA. A primate model for chronic nerve compression. *J Reconstr Microsurg* **1**:185–194, 1985; with permission.)

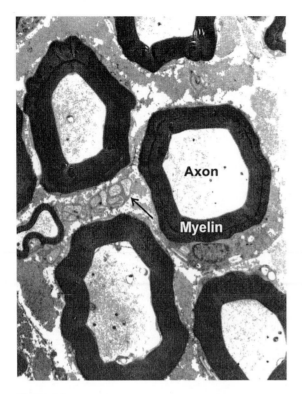

Figure 1.5

Electron micrograph of transverse section from human radial sensory nerve proximal to area of compression demonstrating normal myelinated fibers (uranyl acetate, ×9895). Compare the size of the unmyelinated fibers (arrow) to those in Figure 6. (From Mackinnon SE, Dellon AL, Hudson AR, Hunter DA. Chronic human nerve compression – a histological assessment. *Neuropathol App Neurobiol* **12**:547–565, 1986; with permission.)

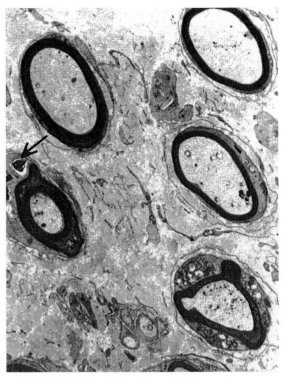

Figure 1.6

Section in the area of compression from the same nerve as in Figure 5 (uranyl acetate, ×9895). Myelin thinning produces obvious increase in the axon-to-myelin ratio. Schwann cell cytoplasm containing myelin debris shows evidence of active Wallerian degeneration (arrow). (From Mackinnon SE, Dellon AL, Hudson AR, Hunter DA. Chronic human nerve compression – a histological assessment. *Neuropathol App Neurobiol* **12**:547–565, 1986; with permission.)

chronic painful compression. The histologic changes described above were noted in all of these specimens, which represented advanced stages of compression (Figures 1.8 and 1.9). Unfortunately, early stages of chronic compressive neuropathy in humans have not been studied histologically. Presumably the same early changes of blood–nerve barrier loss, perineurial and endoneurial edema, and inflammation occur, as in the various animal models. Synovial tissue located adjacent to the median nerve has been biopsied at the time of carpal tunnel release for examination (Fuchs et al., 1991; Kerr et al., 1992; Neal et al., 1987; Phalen, 1972; Scelsi et al., 1989; Schuind et al., 1990).

Like with the experimental findings, edema and thickening of the vascular endothelium were present. Findings of inflammation and fibrosis were more variable.

Clinical scenarios of chronic nerve compression can be related to the various stages of observed histopathologic change. With early or mild compression, symptoms occur only when the extremity is in a provocative position and the nerve is rendered ischemic at the affected site (Lundborg and Dahlin, 1992; Mackinnon and Dellon, 1988; Rempel et al., 1999). Examples include wrist flexion causing median nerve symptoms (Phalen's test) or elbow flexion causing ulnar nerve symptoms. Direct local pressure over the nerve and repetitive or sustained motions can also elicit symptoms. Intraneural microcirculation is restored immediately when the position changes, and the symptoms resolve quickly. If some intraneural edema is present, symptoms may take several days to resolve (Lundborg and Dahlin, 1992). Electrodiagnostic studies and sensory threshold testing will typically be normal. Splinting and avoidance of provocative postures can be effective at this stage.

Constant sensory abnormality or weakness accompanies continued moderate compression. There is segmental demyelination and intraneural edema and fibrosis, but no Wallerian degeneration (Lundborg and Dahlin, 1992; Mackinnon and Dellon, 1988; Rempel et al., 1999). Manual muscle testing or measured strength (e.g. pinch and grip) may demonstrate weakness. Increased vibratory thresholds during tuning fork (Dellon, 1980; Mackinnon and Dellon, 1988) and vibrometer testing (Dellon, 1983; Mackinnon and Dellon, 1988) demonstrate abnormalities in the quickly-adapting sensory receptors of the sensory system. Similarly, Semmes–Weinstein monofilament testing of the

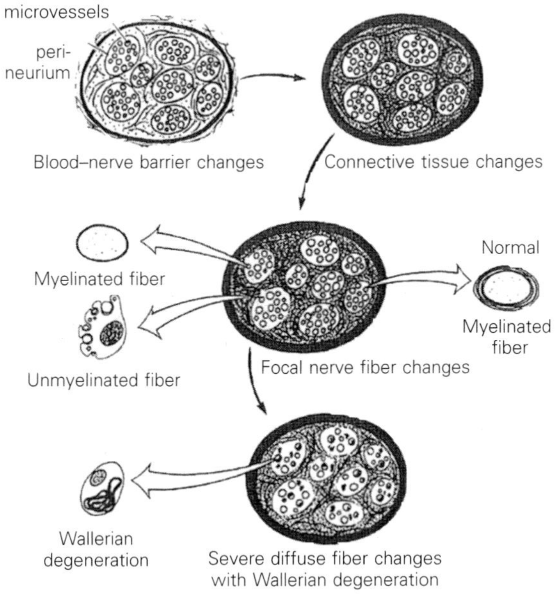

Figure 1.7

Schematic outlining the histologic changes resulting from nerve compression. Initial disruption of the blood–nerve barrier produces subperineurial and endoneurial edema. Next, connective tissue changes cause thickening of the epineurium and perineurium. Local nerve fiber changes follow, with segmental demyelination of large fibers. Other fibers appear entirely normal. Regeneration of unmyelinated fibers is represented by a new population of very small fibers. Continued duration of compression or increased degree of compression leads to severe diffuse fiber changes in both myelinated and unmyelinated fibers. Wallerian degeneration occurs. (Adapted from Mackinnon SE, Dellon AL. *Surgery of the peripheral nerve*. New York: Thieme Medical Publishers, 1988, p. 42; with permission.)

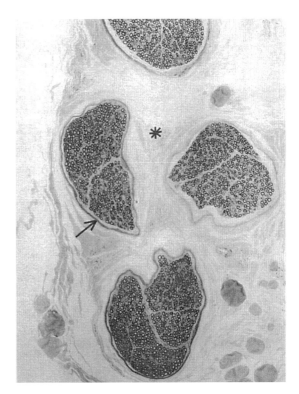

Figure 1.8

Transverse section of normal human radial sensory nerve (toluidine blue stain, ×78). The myelinated fiber population appears uniform. The internal epineurium is loose (*) and the perineurium (arrow) is thin. (Mackinnon SE, Dellon AL, Hudson AR, Hunter DA. Histopathology of compression of the superficial radial nerve in the forearm. *J Hand Surg* **11A**:206–210, 1986; with permission.)

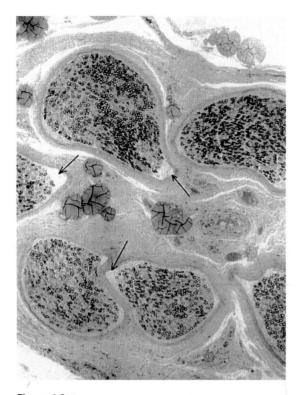

Figure 1.9

Compressed human radial sensory nerve (toluidine blue stain, ×78). The internal epineurium and perineurium are thickened. Fascicles contain nerve fibers with varying degrees of pathology. Renaut's bodies are present (arrows). (Mackinnon SE, Dellon AL, Hudson AR, Hunter DA. Histopathology of compression of the superficial radial nerve in the forearm. *J Hand Surg [Am]* **11A**:206–210, 1986; with permission.)

slowly-adapting sensory fiber system shows increased cutaneous pressure thresholds. Surgical decompression leads to recovery, although usually over a period of weeks.

Numbness and marked muscle weakness or even paralysis is seen with prolonged or severe chronic nerve compression. Constant pain may be present. The advanced morphologic changes include nerve degeneration and regeneration, which manifest clinically as a Tinel's sign. Muscle wasting accompanies motor nerve fiber degeneration. Loss of sensory fibers results in decreased innervation density. This is demonstrated by abnormal static two-point discrimination for the slowly-adapting fiber system and abnormal

moving two-point discrimination for the quickly-adapting system (Dellon et al., 1987). Recovery after decompression is prolonged because it requires axonal regeneration, which occurs at the rate of 1–4 mm/day (Mackinnon and Dellon, 1988) (Figure 1.10).

Double crush syndrome

In 1973, Upton and McComas introduced the concept of 'double crush' in relation to nerve entrapment, or compression syndromes (Upton and McComas, 1973). Their theory stemmed from several intriguing observations regarding patients with carpal tunnel syndrome. First, many people seemed to develop carpal tunnel syndrome without any of the known precipitating factors such as heavy manual labor, obesity, diabetes mellitus or previous wrist injury (Entin, 1968). Second, multiple entrapment neuropathies were noted, even in those without metabolic causes of generalized peripheral neuropathy. Pain from carpal tunnel syndrome was sometimes referred proximally (Crymble, 1968), which was not noted in patients with distal nerve lacerations or crush injuries. Upton and McComas found surprising the phenomenon of incomplete recovery or worsening of symptoms following carpal tunnel surgery, since animal experiments at the time suggested that return of only 10–20% of the original axons was sufficient for recovery of muscle strength (McComas et al., 1971). Finally, median nerve changes observed at the time of surgery that did not always correlate with symptom severity (Tanzer, 1959), and nerve conduction values were sometimes abnormal, even proximal to the carpal tunnel (Cseuz et al., 1966; Thomas, 1960). With these observations in mind, they reviewed 220 patients with upper extremity and neck complaints and found that 115 (70%) of them had cervical root lesions along with carpal tunnel and/or cubital tunnel syndrome. Of note, only some of their patients had electromyographic evidence of cervical root level denervation. In the rest, the diagnosis was inferred by radiographic changes and clinical findings (Wilbourn and Gilliatt, 1997).

To explain these perceived inconsistencies, Upton and McComas developed the 'double

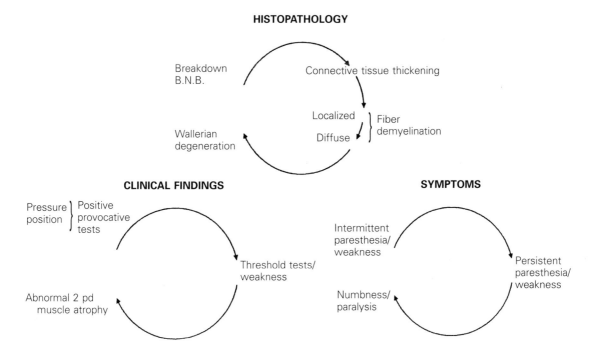

HISTOPATHOLOGY

Figure 1.10

Diagram showing concomitant histopathologic changes and signs and symptoms associated with chronic nerve compression. Histopathology progresses from blood–nerve barrier breakdown to Wallerian degeneration (top circle). Similarly, symptoms are initially transient, but eventually become constant (lower right circle). At first, clinical signs are only present with provocative activities, but ultimately reflect loss of nerve fibers (lower left circle). (From Mackinnon SE. Nerve injuries: primary repair and reconstruction. In *Mastery of plastic and reconstructive surgery*, ed. Cohen, M. Boston: Little, Brown and Co., 1994, p. 1609; with permission.)

crush' hypothesis (Upton and McComas, 1973). Though the nature and function of 'trophic' substances transported through nerves had not yet been defined at the time, the concept of axoplasmic flow was already well accepted (Guth, 1968). 'Double crush' proposed that some instances of nerve compression might be so slight as to produce no symptoms, but still hinder axoplasmic flow. In these situations, a second, more distal, point of compression would reduce trophic factors sufficiently to cause 'denervation'. Thus, a previously subclinical site of nerve compression would become symptomatic. Of course, more than two sites could be involved. In fact, 'triple crush', 'quadruple crush', and finally 'multiple crush' syndromes have been subsequently described (Mackinnon and Dellon, 1988; Wood et al., 1988). Alternatively, the initial

defect could be 'generalised subclinical neuropathy' (Upton and McComas, 1973), presumably of metabolic origin. Again, the addition of an otherwise inconsequential point of compression along the nerve would bring about clinical symptoms. The authors even allowed for the possibility that the proximal lesion might be due to nerve stretch rather than compression, such as at the neck or brachial plexus (Figure 1.11). They recommended that 'all vulnerable points along the course of the nerve' be treated in order to relieve all symptoms of nerve compression effectively (Upton and McComas, 1973).

Though Upton and McComas's theory made logical sense, it required scientific proof for validation. One of the earliest animal experiments attempting to do so was a rat model introduced by Seiler et al. (1983), based on previously

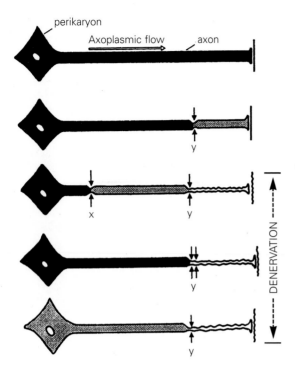

Figure 1.11

Schematic representation of the double crush hypothesis. Mild compression at point Y decreases axoplasmic flow, but does not cause denervation (second from top). Additional point of mild compression at point X combined with point Y causes denervation (third from top). Double arrows represent severe compression. Metabolic neuropathy can also serve as the first lesion, causing denervation with only mild compression (bottom). (From Upton ARM, McComas AJ. The double crush in nerve-entrapment syndromes. *Lancet* **2**:359–362, 1973; with permission.)

established rat and primate models of chronic nerve compression utilizing silastic or polyvinyl bands (Mackinnon et al., 1984, 1985). Single bands placed around rat sciatic nerves for 8 months did not significantly worsen electrical parameters when compared to unbanded controls. In contrast, placement of a second, more distal, band on the tibial nerve worsened electrical parameters significantly after only 4 months. In a more rigorous follow-up study, two simultaneously created sites of nerve compression impeded nerve conduction. However, two successive sites of chronic compression accelerated the deterioration of nerve conduction values

(Dellon and Mackinnon, 1991), whether a proximal first site was followed by a second distal site, or vice versa (Figures 1.12 and 1.13). This model lent credence not only to the double crush hypothesis as originally described by Upton and McComas, but also to the 'reversed double crush' hypothesis proposed later by Lundborg (1986). Analogous to the original theory, Lundborg suggested that distal nerve compression might impair retrograde axonal transport to the nerve cell body. Altered functional and regenerative capabilities of the nerve would then increase its susceptibility to compression at a more proximal site. This was used to explain the clinical situation in which proximal extremity symptoms are sometimes relieved by carpal tunnel release alone (Lundborg and Dahlin, 1992).

The next expected step would be to investigate the treatment of the 'double-crushed' nerve. In a widely referenced experiment performed by

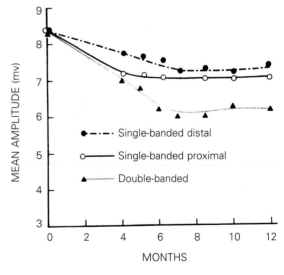

Figure 1.12

Progressive decrease in amplitude of compound action potential due to banding over time. The simultaneously double-banded group of rats becomes significantly worse than either single-banded group by 5 months ($p < 0.0001$). The degree of electrophysiological dysfunction plateaued by 7 months after this degree of minimal chronic pressure. (From Dellon AL, Mackinnon SE. Chronic nerve compression model for the double crush hypothesis. *Ann Plast Surg* **26**:259–264, 1991; with permission.)

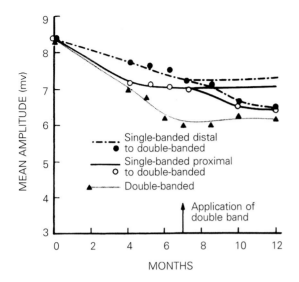

Figure 1.13

Increased effect on amplitude of compound action potential by adding a second band. Note rapid loss of electrophysiologic function, so that within 3 months, the initially single-banded groups of rats reached the level of the simultaneously double-banded group. (From Dellon AL, Mackinnon SE. Chronic nerve compression model for the double crush hypothesis. *Ann Plast Surg* **26**:259–264, 1991; with permission.)

Nemoto and colleagues, specially designed compression clamps were placed on sciatic nerves of dogs to produce mild compression (Nemoto et al., 1987). First, severe macroscopic and microscopic changes resulted from two sequentially applied clamps; motor conduction velocity slowed to 14% of the original value. Half of these double-clamped animals, however, exhibited complete conduction block, with conduction velocity recorded as 0 m/s. Inclusion of these null values has been criticized, as it artificially lowers the mean conduction velocity value (Wilbourn and Gilliatt, 1997). Excluding these animals from the calculations brings the mean conduction velocity to 33% of the original value, which is closer to the value in the single-clamped animals (37% of the original velocity). Despite this shortcoming, the second component of this study is quite significant. Three weeks after the placement of two sequential clamps, one or both were removed. Removal of both clamps allowed the recovery of motor

conduction to 65% of the original velocity. However, removal of only the distal or proximal clamp allowed recovery to just 38%, or 8% of the original conduction velocities, respectively. The authors concluded that a 'good' therapeutic effect was obtained only by removing both clamps, or 'all existing sites of compression', again in keeping with Upton and McComas's hypothesis.

Though the animal studies rather convincingly support the 'double crush' phenomenon, the same cannot be said of human clinical studies. Since the studies of Upton and McComas, others have anecdotally observed the same association between carpal or cubital tunnel syndrome and cervical radiculopathy in their patients (Massey et al., 1981), but likewise could only hypothesize about the cause. Numerous authors have undertaken large retrospective reviews of patients with the appropriate concurrent diagnoses (Hurst et al., 1985; Yu et al., 1979; Osterman, 1988), but most have lacked rigorous criteria for inclusion, diagnosis or follow-up (Morgan and Wilbourn, 1998). Despite the absence of convincing clinical validation, there has been a widespread, almost unquestioning, acceptance of the double crush theory throughout the medical literature.

Critics of the theory have cited methodologic flaws in the published animal and human studies, beginning with the original article by Upton and McComas. As mentioned previously, the diagnosis of cervical radiculopathy in some of their patients was inferred by 'Radiological demonstration of cervical spondylosis or other vertebral abnormality …' 'Complaints of pain and stiffness in the neck …' 'A previous history of neck injury …' and/or 'Clinical evidence of sensory abnormality corresponding to a dermatomal … distribution' (Upton and McComas, 1973), which calls into question the true nature of the proximal lesion (Wilbourn and Gilliatt, 1997). Another criticism has involved the type of electrodiagnostic abnormality demonstrated at the distal site. Upton and McComas described the distal pathology as 'denervation' (Upton and McComas, 1973). If this were interpreted as axonal loss, then electrodiagnostic testing would be expected to show conduction failure in severe cases and low action potential amplitudes in more minor cases. However, most published studies, including Upton and McComas's, have reported slowed conduction velocities or increased terminal latencies, which are more likely to represent demyelination, rather than denervation (Morgan and Wilbourn, 1998; Wilbourn and Gilliatt, 1997).

Recent attention has focused on the anatomic basis of the double crush syndrome. Some contend that double crush syndrome attributed to the combination of spinal radiculopathy and peripheral nerve compression cannot involve sensory fibers (Morgan and Wilbourn, 1998; Richardson et al., 1999; Wilbourn and Gilliatt, 1997). The dorsal spinal root contains only efferent fibers, extending proximally from the cell body in the dorsal root ganglion to the dorsal horn in the cord. Thus, compression on the nerve root outside the spinal column would not interfere with distally directed axoplasmic flow. The basic tenet of the double crush hypothesis would not be met. Additionally, the same authors assert that carpal tunnel syndrome, the most frequently reported peripheral nerve entrapment in double crush cases, is anatomically improbable (Morgan and Wilbourn, 1998; Richardson et al., 1999; Wilbourn and Gilliatt, 1997). The median nerve is derived from multiple spinal roots (C-6, C-7, C-8 and T-1), portions of which pass through all three trunks of the brachial plexus and the medial and lateral cords, before converging distally. A proximal lesion would need to involve multiple nerve roots or most of the brachial plexus in order to compress a significant number of median nerve axons. Double crush, however, may not necessarily be an 'all-or-none' phenomenon. Changes in only some fibers may be sufficient to produce symptoms; just as early chronic nerve compression can be symptomatic, despite the variable involvement of each individual fascicle.

Reviews of electrophysiology patient databases have not shown support for the double crush hypothesis. Morgan and Wilbourn analyzed patients referred for evaluation of cervical radiculopathy, carpal tunnel syndrome, or cubital syndrome, using stringent electrodiagnostic definitions for each diagnosis (Morgan and Wilbourn, 1998). Cases with concomitant cervical radiculopathy, carpal tunnel syndrome or cubital tunnel syndrome were assessed for anatomic correlation of affected axonal fibers. For example, the combination of C-5 radiculopathy and carpal tunnel syndrome was considered 'discordant', since the median nerve derives from the C-6–T-1 nerve roots, while C-7 radiculopathy was classified as 'insufficient', since some, but not all, of the median nerve fibers might be compressed at both sites. A pattern of axonal loss, with or without demyelination, was required as evidence of denervation. Out of 8156 patients, only 69 (0.5%) met the authors' anatomic criteria for double crush syndrome (Morgan and Wilbourn, 1998). Whether the patients in their study were more prone to have combined cervical and distal compression is unclear, since the prevalence of cervical radiculopathy in a control population unaffected by carpal or cubital tunnel syndrome is not available for comparison (Richardson et al., 1999). Interestingly, nearly one-third of the patients with cubital tunnel syndrome also had carpal tunnel syndrome. Anatomically, this situation cannot meet the criteria for double crush. The authors merely propose 'underlying metabolic condition' (Morgan and Wilbourn, 1998) as a possible explanation for this finding.

A related study by Richardson and colleagues identified 154 cases of electrically diagnosed C-6, C-7 and C-8 radiculopathy in patients referred to a tertiary electrophysiology center (Richardson et al., 1999). Again, based on anatomic criteria for double crush syndrome involving the median nerve, these authors sought to test the hypotheses that C-6/7 radiculopathy would more likely be associated with median sensory abnormalities and C-8 radiculopathy would more likely be associated with median motor abnormalities. Nerve conduction latencies and amplitudes were chosen to represent 'denervation'. No significant relationships between either C-6/7 radiculopathy and median sensory neuropathy or C-8 radiculopathy and median motor neuropathy were found. Interestingly, 7–9% of the cervical radiculopathy patients had carpal tunnel syndrome by electrodiagnostic criteria. This is higher than the 0.5–1.5% prevalence reported for the general adult population (Stevens et al., 1998; Tanaka et al., 1995). Of note, neither of the studies discussed above reported the presence or nature of physical findings. Since carpal tunnel syndrome is most accurately diagnosed by a combination of electrodiagnostic abnormalities and symptom characteristics (Rempel et al., 1998), the clinical relevance of studies excluding one or the other is uncertain.

The original description of the double crush syndrome allows for 'generalized subclinical neuropathy' (Upton and McComas, 1973) to be the initial insult to the nerve. Diabetic neuropathy is mentioned specifically. For some time, higher frequencies of mononeuropathies have been reported in diabetic patients (Dahlin et al., 1986a; Mulder et al., 1961). Experimental observations support the belief that peripheral nerves in diabetics are more susceptible to injury (Brown et al., 1980; Moore et al., 1981, 1982). Dahlin et al. (1986a) showed that acute compression on the sciatic nerves of streptozotocin-induced diabetic rats produced greater inhibition of fast axonal transport than in normal rats. Likewise, using their established rat model,

Dellon et al. (1988) found diabetic nerves to be more vulnerable to chronic compression, based on electrodiagnostic parameters. The reasons for this increased susceptibility to compression in diabetic nerves is not known. Possible explanations include structural and rheological microvascular changes in the vasa nervorum, ischemia due to elevated endoneurial fluid pressure, and additional alterations in retrograde axonal transport leading to decreased axon integrity (Dahlin et al., 1986a; Jakobsen and Sidenius, 1980; Myers and Powell, 1984; Powell, 1983). Despite extensive investigation, the underlying pathophysiology of diabetic neuropathy is still unclear. Current theories encompass four general themes: metabolic dysfunction due to

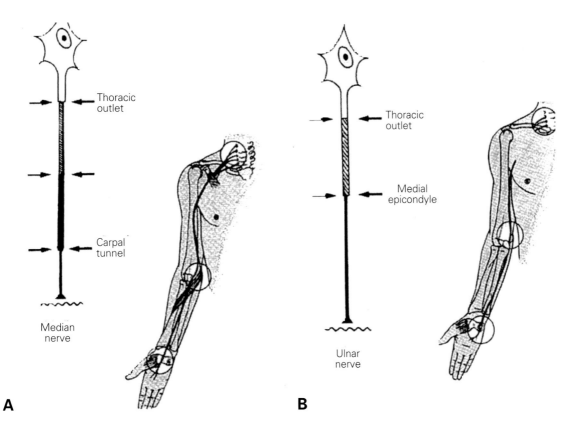

A

B

Figure 1.14

(A) Multiple crush along the median nerve. Mild compression at the brachial plexus, pronator teres, and carpal tunnel levels combine to cause distal symptoms. (B) Double crush along the ulnar nerve. Mild proximal compression at the brachial plexus and cubital tunnel combine to cause distal symptoms. Additional compression can also occur at Guyon's canal. (Adapted from Mackinnon SE. Double and multiple 'crush' syndromes: double and multiple entrapment neuropathies. *Hand Clin* **8**:369–390, 1992; with permission.)

sugar alcohol flux into nerve elements, nerve hypoxia and oxidative stress, glycosylation of structural nerve proteins and neurotrophic or growth factor deficiencies (Zochodne, 1999). Other metabolic causes of peripheral neuropathy such as alcoholism (Mackinnon, 1992; Shields, 1985), uremia (Minami and Ogino 1987; Tegner and Brismar, 1984) and vasculitic diseases (Mackinnon and Dellon, 1988), have also been implicated as possible contributors to double crush situations.

Clinical considerations

Obvious ethical considerations prevent replication of the previously performed double crush animal experiments in humans. As already mentioned, existing clinical studies have contained critical flaws. Nevertheless, even those who refute the theory have noted that patients with nerve compression at one site have an increased occurrence of compression at another site (Richardson et al., 1999). Though this observation cannot be fully explained, it is not unreasonable to regard double crush as a working hypothesis, until convincingly proven otherwise. Mackinnon and Dellon (1988) suggest the broader term 'multiple crush syndrome' which includes, in any combination, compression at 'multiple anatomic regions along a peripheral nerve' (Figure 1.14), 'multiple anatomic structures across a peripheral nerve within an anatomic region' and 'superimposed ... neuropathy'. As initial stages of nerve compression are readily reversible, decompressing one of many 'subclinical' sites in early multiple crush syndromes might be sufficient to relieve symptoms at all of the sites. Similarly, prolonged serial restrictions of axoplasmic flow may eventually cause severe and permanent changes throughout. At this point, decompressing just one location would no longer relieve symptoms at the different sites (Mackinnon and Dellon, 1988). This line of thinking cannot be applied to the distinctly different situation of multiple nerve entrapments, where separate peripheral nerves are concurrently compressed, such as the median nerve (carpal tunnel syndrome) and ulnar nerve (cubital tunnel syndrome) (Mackinnon, 1992; Mackinnon and Dellon, 1988)

(Figure 1.15). When multiple distinct nerves are compressed, each needs to be addressed separately in order to eliminate all symptoms.

In the multiple crush syndrome, each site of compression is 'subclinical', so symptoms typically occur only in response to provocative positions or maneuvers (Mackinnon, 1992; Mackinnon and Dellon, 1988; Novak and Mackinnon, 1999). Pressure on or stretching of a compressed nerve at its entrapment site renders it temporarily ischemic (Lundborg and Dahlin, 1992; Mackinnon and Dellon, 1988; Rempel et al., 1999), producing paresthesia in its distribution (Mackinnon, 1992). This concept is well accepted for carpal tunnel (Durkan, 1997; Paley and McMurtry, 1985; Phalen, 1966; Williams et al., 1992) and cubital tunnel syndromes (Greenwald et al., 1999; Novak et al., 1994), and can be applied to many other peripheral nerves as well (Novak and Mackinnon, 1999) (Table 1.1). Since

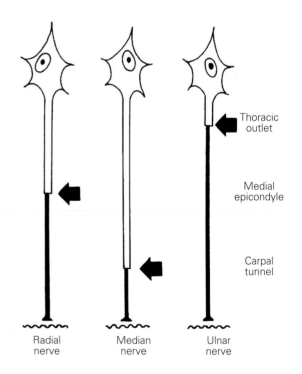

Figure 1.15

Multiple nerve entrapments. Each nerve should be addressed separately. (Adapted from Mackinnon SE. (1992) Double and multiple 'crush' syndromes: double and multiple entrapment neuropathies. *Hard Clinics* **8**:369–90, with permission.)

Table 1.1 Provocative tests for nerve entrapment

Nerve	Entrapment site	Provocative test
Median	Carpal tunnel	Pressure proximal to carpal tunnel, Phalen's/Reverse Phalen's test
Median	Proximal forearm	Pressure over proximal forearm, resisted elbow flexion/pronation /finger flexion
Ulnar	Guyon's canal	Pressure proximal to Guyon's canal
Ulnar	Cubital tunnel	Pressure proximal to cubital tunnel, elbow flexion
Radial (posterior interosseous)	Arcade of Frohse	Pressure over supinator, resisted supination/wrist extension/ long finger extension
Radial (sensory)	Forearm	Pressure over junction of brachioradialis and extensor carpi radialis tendons, forearm pronation
Brachial plexus	Supraclavicular	Elevation of arms overhead, pressure over interscalene area

From Mackinnon SE, Dellon AL. *Surgery of the peripheral nerve.* New York: Thieme Medical Publishers, 1988, p. 79; with permission.

patients tend to avoid the particular positions that bring about their symptoms, nerve compression usually remains in the early stages. Electrodiagnostic studies and clinical measures, such as two-point discrimination, are likely to be normal (Mackinnon, 1992). Because of this, all potential sites of entrapment along the course of a given nerve should be assessed with provocative testing. Treatment should focus on the most severely affected areas, although conservative measures are recommended for all symptomatic sites. Conservative treatment commonly consists of splinting and the correction of muscle imbalance and postural abnormalities. More severely involved sites will exhibit typical signs of advanced nerve compression, such as persistent numbness or weakness and electrodiagnostic changes. Surgery is reserved for these areas, if they do not respond to conservative measures. The distal sites are frequently the most severely affected and decompressing them is usually simpler, with less associated morbidity (Mackinnon, 1992; Mackinnon and Dellon, 1988).

Another variation of the multiple crush scenario is compression of a single peripheral nerve by various structures in an anatomic area. Individually, the degree of compression by each structure may seem trivial, but when combined,

Table 1.2 Multiple crush syndrome due to multiple anatomic structures across the median nerve in the proximal forearm

Tendinous origin of the deep head of the pronator teres

Tendinous origin of the flexor digitorum superficialis

Thrombosis of crossing ulnar collateral vessels

Accessory muscle and tendon from the flexor digitorum superficialis to the flexor pollicis longus

Accessory head of the flexor pollicis longus (Gantzer's muscle)

Aberrant radial artery

Tendinous origin of variant muscles, such as palmaris profundus or flexor carpi radialis brevis

Enlarged bicipital bursa encroaching on median nerve near the region of the origin of the anterior interosseous nerve

High origin of the pronator teres superficial head from the humerus

From Mackinnon SE, Dellon AL. *Surgery of the peripheral nerve.* New York: Thieme Medical Publishers, 1988, p. 359; with permission. Original data from Spinner M. (1978) *Injuries to the major branches of the peripheral nerves of the forearm*, 2nd edn. Philadelphia: WB Saunders.

can cause significant symptoms. This situation has been well described for median nerve compression in the forearm, often diagnosed as pronator syndrome, and for brachial plexus compression, or thoracic outlet syndrome (Tables 1.2 and 1.3). In the upper extremity, the radial nerve can be similarly affected (Mackinnon and Dellon, 1988) (Table 1.4). Structures that can potentially cause nerve compression in each of these regions have been identified. Failure to inspect and release any of these sites may result in recurrence or exacerbation of the patient's original symptoms (Mackinnon, 1992; Mackinnon and Dellon, 1988). It is equally important that the surgeon avoid creating new iatrogenic sites of compression. This situation can be created during anterior transposition of the ulnar nerve for the treatment of cubital tunnel syndrome, either proximally at the triceps fascia and medial intermuscular septum or distally at the flexor carpi ulnaris fascia (Lugnegard et al., 1977; Mackinnon, 1992; Mackinnon and Dellon 1988). Surgical reexploration for recurrent or persistent compression neuropathy should address these problems, if they exist.

histologic changes associated with chronic nerve compression. The application of this knowledge, however, is not always straightforward. Patients with atypical complaints and physical findings present a significant diagnostic challenge to the clinician. Therapeutic success is dependent on meeting this challenge. Upton and McComas's theory that minor, seemingly inconsequential, constraints to axoplasmic flow combine to produce symptomatic nerve dysfunction seems to explain those cases that fail to meet standard criteria. Despite its lack of clinical confirmation, which will be difficult to attain, the concept should be used to aid the management of these difficult cases. Some have charged that the theory provides an excuse to perform multiple surgeries and defends unexpected or unsatisfactory surgical results (Wilbourn and Gilliatt, 1997). On the contrary, it promotes the development of meticulous clinical examination skills, as electrodiagnostic tests are not always helpful. In the treatment of chronic nerve compression, comprehensive diagnosis combined with selective surgery is the key to success with low rates of recurrence.

Conclusion

Extensive research has led to general agreement regarding the etiology, symptomatology, and

Table 1.3 Multiple anatomic structures compressing the brachial plexus in the region of the thoracic outlet

Cervical rib
First rib
Scalene anticus
Pectoralis minor
Omohyoid
Subclavius, scalenus minimus, and scalenus medius muscles
Clavicle
Congenital bands (Roos')
Transverse process of C-7 vertebra
(Sibson's) pleural fascia

From Mackinnon SE. Double and multiple 'crush' syndromes: double and multiple entrapment neuropathies. *Hand Clin* **8**: 369–390, 1992; with permission.

Table 1.4 Potential causes of radial nerve compression by multiple anatomic structures. (Data from MacKinnon and Dillon, 1988.)

Brachioradialis muscle belly at the entrance to the radial tunnel
Shared fibers between the brachioradialis and brachialis muscles
Extensor carpi radialis longus muscle belly in the radial tunnel
Extensor carpi radialis brevis (fascial edge, muscle belly)
Fibrous adhesions at the radial head due to lateral epicondylitis
Recurrent radial artery and vein
Arcade of Frohse
Superficial head of supinator muscle (intramuscular fascial bands, distal fibrous edge)

References

Aguayo A, Nair CPV, Midgely R. (1971) Experimental progressive compression neuropathy in the rabbit. *Arch Neurol* **24**:358–64.

Barron KD. (1983) Comparative observations on the cytologic reactions of central and peripheral nerve cells to axotomy. In: Kau CC, Bunge RP, Reier PJ, eds. *Spinal Cord Reconstruction.* New York: Raven Press: 7–40.

Black MM, Lasek RJ. (1980) Slow components of axonal transport – two cytoskeletal networks. *J Cell Biol* **85**:616–23.

Brown MJ, Sumner AJ, Greene DA, Diamond SM, Asbury AK. (1980) Distal neuropathy in experimental diabetes mellitus. *Ann Neurol* **8**:168–78.

Cooper A. (1821) On exostosis. In: Cooper A, Travers B, eds. *Surgical essays*, 1st edn. Philadelphia, PA: James Webster: 125–63.

Crymble B. (1968) Brachial neuralgia and the carpal tunnel syndrome, *BMJ* **3**:470–1.

Cseuz KA, Thomas JE, Lambert EH, Love JG, Lipscomb PR. (1966) Long-term results of operation for carpal tunnel syndrome. *Mayo Clin Proc* **4**:232–41.

Dahlin LB, Danielsen N, Lundborg G. (1989a) Chronic nerve compression can act as a 'conditioning lesion'. Satellite symposium of the XXXI International Congress of Physiological Sciences: Regulators of Peripheral Nerve Regeneration. Ysta, Sweden, 6–8 July.

Dahlin LB, McLean WG. (1986) Effects of graded experimental compression on slow and fast axonal transport in rabbit vagus nerve. *J Neurol Sci* **72**:19–30.

Dahlin LB, Meiri KF, McLean WG, Rydevik B. Sjöstrand J. (1986a) Effects of nerve compression on fast axonal transport in streptozotocin-induced diabetes mellitus. *Diabetologia* **29**:181–5.

Dahlin LB, Nordborg C, Lundborg G. (1987) Morphological changes in nerve cell bodies induced by experimental graded nerve compression. *Exp Neurol* **95**:611–21.

Dahlin LB, Rydevik B, McLean WG, Sjöstrand J. (1984) Changes in fast axonal transport during experimental nerve compression at low pressures. *Exp Neurol* **84**:29–36.

Dahlin LB, Shyu BC, Danielsen N, Andersson SA. (1989b) Effects of nerve compression or ischemia on conduction properties of myelinated and non-myelinated nerve fibres. An experimental study in the rabbit common peroneal nerve. *Acta Physiol Scand* **136**:97–105.

Dahlin LB, Sjöstrand J, McLean WG. (1986b) Graded inhibition of retrograde axonal transport by compression of rabbit vagus nerve. *J Neurol Sci* **76**:221–30

Dellon AL. (1980) Clinical use of vibratory stimulation to evaluate peripheral nerve compression. *J Hand Surg* **65A**:466–76.

Dellon AL. (1983) The vibrometer. *Plast Reconstr Surg* **71**:427–31.

Dellon AL, Mackinnon SE. (1991) Chronic nerve compression model for the double crush hypothesis. *Ann Plast Surg* **26**:259–64.

Dellon AL, Mackinnon SE, Crosby PM. (1987) Reliability of two-point discrimination measurements. *J Hand Surg* **12A**:693–96.

Dellon AL, Mackinnon SE, Seiler WA. (1988) Susceptibility of the diabetic nerve to chronic compression. *Ann Plast Surg* **20**:117–19.

Duncan D. (1948) Alterations in the structure of nerves caused by restricting their growth with ligatures. *J Neuropathol Exp Neurol* **7**:261–3.

Durkan J. (1997) A new diagnostic test for carpal tunnel syndrome. *J Bone Joint Surg* **73A**:535–8.

Dyck PJ, Lais A, Giannini C, Engelstad JK. (1990) Structural alterations of nerve during cuff compression. *Proc Natl Acad Sci USA*, **87**:9828–32.

Emara M, Saadah AM. (1988) The carpal tunnel syndrome in hypertensive patients treated with beta-blockers. *Postgrad Med J* **64**:191–2.

Entin MA. (1968) Carpal tunnel syndrome and its variants. *Surg Clin N Am* **48**:1097–12.

Fowler TJ, Danta G, Gilliatt RW. (1972) Recovery of nerve conduction after a pneumatic tourniquet: observations on the hind-limb of the baboon. *J Neurol Neurosurg Psychiatry* **35**:638–47.

Fuchs PC, Nathan PA, Myers LD. (1991) Synovial histology and carpal tunnel syndrome. *J Hand Surg* **16A**:753–8.

Fullerton PM, Gilliatt RW. (1965) Changes in nerve conduction in caged guinea pigs. *J Physiol* **178**:47P–48P.

Fullerton PM, Gilliatt RW. (1967a) Pressure neuropathy in the hind foot of the guinea pig. *J Neurol Neurosurg Psychiatry* **30**:18–25.

Fullerton PM, Gilliatt RW. (1967b) Median and ulnar neuropathy in the guinea pig. *J Neurol Neurosurg Psychiatry* **30**:393–402.

Gasser HS, Erlanger J. (1929) The role of fiber size in the establishment of a nerve block by pressure or cocaine. *Am J Physiol* **88**:581–91.

Gelberman RH, Szabo RM, Williamson RV, Dimick MP. (1983) Sensibility testing in peripheral nerve compression syndromes. An experimental study in humans. *J Bone Joint Surg* **65A**:632–8.

Grafstein B, Forman DS. (1980) Intracellular transport in neurons. *Physiol Rev* **60**:1167–83.

Greenwald D, Moffitt M, Cooper B. (1999) Effective surgical treatment of cubital tunnel syndrome based on provocative clinical testing without electrodiagnostics. *Plast Reconstr Surg* **104**:215–18.

Grundfest H, Cattell M. (1935) Some effects of hydrostatic pressure on nerve action potentials. *Am J Physiol* **113**:56–7.

Guth L. (1968) 'Trophic' influences of nerve on muscle. *Physiol Rev* **48**:645–87.

Horiuchi Y. (1983) Experimental study on peripheral nerve lesions – compression neuropathy. *J Jpn Orthop Assoc* **57**:789–803.

Hurst LC, Weissberg D, Carroll RE. (1985) The relationship of the double crush to carpal tunnel syndrome (an analysis of 1,000 cases of carpal tunnel syndrome). *J Hand Surg* **B10**:202–4.

Jakobsen J, Sidenius P. (1980) Decreased axonal transport of structural proteins in streptozotocin diabetic rats. *J Clin Invest* **66**:292–7.

Jefferson D, Eames RA. (1979) Subclinical entrapment of the lateral femoral cutaneous nerve: an autopsy study. *Muscle Nerve* **2**:145–54.

Kerr CD, Sybert DR, Albarracin NS. (1992) An analysis of the flexor synovium in idiopathic carpal tunnel syndrome: a report of 625 cases. *J Hand Surg* **17A**:1028–30.

Kiloh LG, Nerin S. (1952) Isolated neuritis of the anterior interosseus nerve. *Br Med J* **1**: 850.

Lieberman AR. (1971) The axon reaction: a review of the principal features of perikaryal responses to axon injury. *Int Rev Neurobiol* **14**:49–124.

Lugnegard H, Waldhein G, Wenberg G. (1977) Operative treatment of ulnar nerve neuropathy in the elbow region. *Acta Orthop Scand* **48**:168–76.

Lundborg G. (1986) *The reversed double crush lesion.* ASSH Correspondence Newsletter No. 9.

Lundborg G, Dahlin LB. (1992) The pathophysiology of nerve compression. *Hand Clin* **8**:215–27.

Lundborg G, Gelberman RH, Minteer-Convery M, et al. (1982) Median nerve compression in the carpal tunnel – functional response to experimentally induced controlled pressure. *J Hand Surg* **7A**:252–9.

Lundborg G, Myers R, Powell H. (1983) Nerve compression injury and increased endoneurial fluid pressure: a 'miniature compartment syndrome'. *J Neurol Neurosurg Psychiatry* **46**:1119–24.

Mackinnon SE. (1992) Double and multiple 'crush' syndromes: double and multiple entrapment neuropathies. *Hand Clin* **8**:369–90.

Mackinnon SE, Dellon AL. (1988) *Surgery of the peripheral nerve.* New York: Thieme Medical Publishers.

Mackinnon SE, Dellon AL, Hudson AR, Hunter DA. (1984) Chronic nerve compression – an experimental model in the rat. *Ann Plast Surg* **13**:112–20.

Mackinnon SE, Dellon AL, Hudson AR, Hunter DA. (1985) A primate model for chronic nerve compression. *J Reconstr Microsurg* **1**:185–94.

Mackinnon SE, Dellon AL, Hudson AR, Hunter DA. (1986a) Chronic human nerve compression – a histological assessment. *Neuropathol App Neurobiol* **12**:547–65.

Mackinnon SE, Dellon AL, Hudson AR, Hunter DA. (1986b) Histopathology of compression of the superficial radial nerve in the forearm. *J Hand Surg* **11A**:206–10.

Marie P, Foix C. (1913) Atrophie isolee de l'eminence thenar d'origine nevritique. Role du ligament annulaire anterieur de carpe dans la pathogenie de la lesion. *Revue Neurologique* **26**:647–8.

Massey EW, Riley TL, Pleet AB. (1981) Coexistent carpal tunnel syndrome and cervical radiculopathy (double crush syndrome). *South Med J* **74**:956–9.

Matsumoto N. (1983) An experimental study on compression neuropathy – determination of blood flow by a hydrogen washout technique. *J Jpn Orthop Assoc* **57**:805–16.

McClean WG, McKay AL, Sjöstrand J. (1983) Electrophoretic analysis of axonally transported proteins in rabbit vagus nerve. *J Neurobiol* **14**:227–36.

McComas AJ, Sica REP, Campbell MJ, Upton ARM. (1971) Functional compensation in partially denervated muscles. *J Neurol Neurosurg Psychiatry* **34**:453–60.

Minami A, Ogino T. (1987) Carpal tunnel syndrome in patients undergoing chemodialysis. *J Hand Surg* **12A**:93–7.

Moore SA, Peterson RG, Felten DL, O'Connor BL. (1981) Glycogen accumulation in tibial nerves of experimentally diabetic and aging control rats. *J Neurol Sci* **52**:289–303.

Moore SA, Peterson RG, Felten DL, O'Connor BL. (1982) Ultrastructural axonal pathology in experimentally diabetic and aging control rats. *Brain Res Bull* **8**:317–23.

Morgan G, Wilbourn AJ. (1998) Cervical radiculopathy and coexisting distal entrapment neuropathies: double-crush syndromes? *Neurology* **50**:78–83.

Mulder DW, Lambert EH, Bastrom JA, Sprague RG. (1961) The neuropathies associated with diabetes mellitus. *Neurology* **11**:275–84.

Myers RR, Powell HC. (1984) Galactose neuropathy: impact of chronic endoneurial edema on nerve blood flow. *Ann Neurol* **16**:587–94.

Myers RR, Powell HC, Costello ML, et al. (1978) Endoneurial fluid pressure: direct measurement with micropipettes. *Brain Res* **148**:510–15.

Neal NC, McManners, J, Stirling GA. (1987) Pathology of the flexor tendon sheath in the spontaneous carpal tunnel syndrome. *J Hand Surg* **12B**:299–32.

Neary D, Eames RA. (1975) The pathology of ulnar nerve compression in man. *Neuropathol Appl Neurobiol* **1**:69–88.

Neary D, Ochoa J, Gilliatt RW. (1975) Sub-clinical entrapment neuropathy in man. *J Neurol Sci* **24**:283–98.

Nemoto K. (1983) An experimental study on the vulnerability of the peripheral nerve. *J Jpn Orthop Assoc* **57**:1773–86.

Nemoto K, Matsumoto N, Tazaki K-I, et al. (1987) An experimental study on the 'double crush' hypothesis. *J Hand Surg* **12A**:552–9.

Novak CB, Lee GW, Mackinnon SE, Lay L. (1994) Provocative testing for cubital tunnel syndrome. *J Hand Surg* **19A**:817–20.

Novak CB, Mackinnon SE. (1999) Multiple nerve entrapment syndromes in office workers. *Occup Med* **14**:39–59.

Ochoa J, Fowler TJ, Gilliatt RW. (1972) Anatomical changes in peripheral nerves compressed by a pneumatic tourniquet. *J Anat* **113**:433–55.

Ochoa J, Marotte L. (1973) The nature of the nerve lesion caused by chronic entrapment in the guinea-pig. *J Neurol Sci* **19**:491–5.

Osterman AL, (1988) The double crush syndrome: cervical radiculopathy and carpal tunnel syndrome. *Orthop Clin North Am* **19**:147–55.

Paley D, McMurtry RY. (1985) Median nerve compression test on carpal tunnel syndrome diagnosis reproduces signs and symptoms in affected wrist. *Orthop Rev* **14**:41–5.

Panas J. (1878) Sur une cause peu connue de paralysie du nerf cubital. *Arch Gen Med* **2**:5–22.

Pedowitz RA, Nordborg C, Rosenqvist A-L, Rydevik BL, (1991) Nerve function and structure beneath and distal to a pneumatic tourniquet applied to rabbit hindlimbs. *Scand J Plast Reconstr Surg Hand Surg* **25**:109–20.

Phalen GS. (1966) The carpal tunnel syndrome: seventeen years experience in diagnosis and treatment of six hundred and fifty four hands. *J Bone Joint Surg* **48A**:211–28.

Phalen GS. (1972) The carpal-tunnel syndrome. Clinical evaluation of 598 hands. *Clin Orthop* **83**:29–40.

Powell HC. (1983) Pathology of diabetic neuropathy: new observations, new hypotheses. *Lab Invest* **49**:515–18.

Powell HC, Myers RR. (1986) Pathology of experimental nerve compression. *Lab Invest* **55**:91–100.

Rempel D, Dahlin L, Lundborg G. (1999) Pathophysiology of nerve compression syndromes: response of peripheral nerves to loading. *J Bone Joint Surg* **81A**:1600–10.

Rempel D, Evanoff B, Amadio PC, et al. (1998) Consensus criteria for the classification of carpal tunnel syndrome in epidemiologic studies. *Am J Public Health* **88**:1447–51.

Richardson JK, Forman GM, Riley B. (1999) An electrophysiological exploration of the double crush hypothesis. *Muscle Nerve* **22**:71–7.

Rydevik B, Lundborg G. (1977) Permeability of intraneural microvessels and perineurium following acute, graded experimental nerve compression. *Scand J Plast Reconst Surg* **11**:179–87.

Scelsi R, Zanlungo M, Tenti P. (1989) Carpal tunnel syndrome. Anatomical and clinical correlations and morphological and ultrastructural aspects of the tenosynovial sheath. *Ital J Orthop Traumatol* **15**: 75–80.

Schuind F, Ventura M, Pasteels JL. (1990) Idiopathic carpal tunnel syndrome: histologic study of flexor tendon synovium. *J Hand Surg* **15A**:497–503.

Seiler WA, Schelgel R, Mackinnon S, Dellon AL. (1983) Double crush syndrome: experimental model in the rat. *Surg Forum* **34**:596–8.

Seyfarth H. (1951) Primary mycoses of M. pronator teres as cause of lesion of N. medianus (pronator syndrome). *Acta Psychiat et Neurol Scandinav* Suppl **74**:251–4.

Shields RW Jr. (1985) Alcoholic polyneuropathy. *Muscle Nerve* **8**:183–7.

Simpson RL, Fern SA. (1996) Multiple compression neuropathies and the double-crush syndrome. *Orthop Clin North Am* **27**:381–8.

Sommer C, Galbraith JA, Heckman HM, Myers RR. (1993) Pathology of experimental compression neuropathy producing hyperesthesia. *J Neuropathol Exp Neurol* **25**:223–33.

Spinner M. (1978) *Injuries to the major branches of the peripheral nerves of the forearm*, 2nd edn. Philadelphia: WB Saunders.

Spinner M, Spencer PS. (1974) Nerve compression lesions of the upper extremity. A clinical and experimental review. *Clin Orthop* **104**:46–67.

Stevens JC, Sun S, Beard CM, et al. (1988) Carpal tunnel syndrome in Rochester, Minnesota, 1961 to 1980. *Neurology* **38**:134–8.

Szabo RM, Gelberman RH, Williamson RV, Hargens AR. (1983) Effects of increased systemic blood pressure on the tissue fluid pressure threshold of peripheral nerve. *J Orthop Res* **1**: 172–8.

Tanaka S, Wild DK, Seligman PJ, et al. (1995) Prevalence and work-relatedness of self-reported carpal tunnel syndrome among US workers: analysis of the Occupational Health Supplement Data of 1988 National Health Interview Survey. *Am J Ind Med* **27**:451–70.

Tanzer RC. (1959) The carpal tunnel syndrome. *Clin Orthop* **15**:171–9.

Tegner R, Brismar T. (1984) Experimental uremic neuropathy, part I: (decreased nerve conduction velocity in rats). *J Neurol Sci* **65**:29–36.

Thomas PK. (1960) Motor nerve conduction in the carpal tunnel syndrome. *Neurology* **10**:1045–50.

Thomas PK, Fullerton PM. (1963) Nerve fiber size in the carpal tunnel syndrome. *J Neurol Neurosurg Psychiatry* **26**:520–27.

United States Department of Labor. (1998) *News*. Washington, DC: Bureau of Labor Statistics.

Upton ARM, McComas AJ. (1973) The double crush in nerve-entrapment syndromes. *Lancet* **2**:359–62.

Weisl H, Osborne GV. (1964) The pathological changes in rats' nerves subject to moderate compression. *J Bone Joint Surg* **46B**:297–306.

Weiss P, Hiscoe HB. (1948) Experiments on the mechanism of nerve growth. *J Exp Zool* **107**:315–95.

Wilbourn AJ, Gilliatt RW. (1997) Double-crush syndrome: a critical analysis. *Neurology* **49**:21–9.

Williams TM, Mackinnon SE, Novak CB, et al. (1992) Verification of the pressure provocative test in carpal tunnel syndrome. *Ann Plast Surg* **29**:8–11.

Wood VE, Twito R, Verska JM. (1988) Thoracic outlet syndrome. The results of first rib resection in 100 patients. *Orthop Clin North Am* **19**:131–46.

Yu J, Bendler EM, Mentari A. (1979) Neurological disorders associated with carpal tunnel syndrome. *Electromyogr Clin Neurophysiol* **19**:27–32.

Zochodne DW. (1999) Diabetic neuropathies; features and mechanism. *Brain Pathol* **9**:369–91.

2
Electrodiagnosis of the upper limbs

Paul Seror

Introduction

Neurological diseases are frequently encountered in hand surgery. Peripheral neuropathies as nerve compressions are the most frequent; but other pathologies include mononeuritis, multineuritis or polyneuropathies. Anterior horn diseases can also be seen. Rarely, central nervous system diseases may also appear in hand surgery consultation. These disorders have specific clinical signs (Bouche and Vallat, 1992; Chu Andrews and Johnson, 1980; Dawson et al., 1982; Kimura, 1989; Serratrice, 1963; Sunderland, 1978; Swash and Schwartz, 1981) as well as specific electrodiagnostic patterns. A good working knowledge of electrodiagnostic (EDX) methods and results is essential for the hand therapist and hand surgeon if they want to collect optimal information from the EDX examination. It is also important to remember that neuromuscular pathologies are evolving and what cannot be diagnosed at the first investigation may be recognized at a later one.

The first experiments (AAEE, 1969; Bouche and Vallet, 1992; Licht, 1980) using electricity in human beings were performed during the nineteenth century but had no direct consequence in the diagnosis or in the treatment of neuromuscular diseases. In 1869, Baxt and Helmholz (AAEE, 1969) first determined the normal value of motor nerve conduction (64.5 m/s); later Duchenne de Boulogne (1872) used the comparison of electrophysiological findings with anatomo-clinical methods to establish the first steps of clinical EDX. It was only in the 1940s and 1950s that clinical EDX really began, with the use of needle electrodes (1930) and with routine nerve conduction studies (1949) (Simpson, 1956). Since 1970, the personal computer has allowed the routine study of very low amplitude potentials (sensory and somatosensory) with averaging.

EDX equipment

EDX equipment (Figure 2.1) includes three main units: the recording unit, the stimulator and the analysis unit. The *recording unit* is made up of recording electrodes (needle or surface), the preamplifier and the amplifier. The *stimulator*

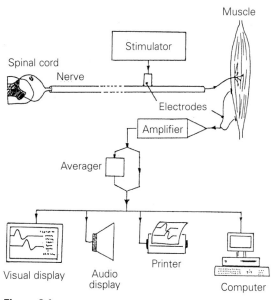

Figure 2.1

EDX equipment.

unit provides electric shocks of variable duration and intensity. The stimulation is delivered by surface electrodes (exceptionally, by needle electrode) and synchronized with the analysis unit. The *analysis unit* displays, after appropriate amplification, the recorded action potentials, both on-screen for visual analysis and through loudspeakers for audio analysis. Electronic cursors allow precise latency and amplitude measurements to be made. The recorded traces are printed and given to the patients with their EDX report and sent to their physician also.

Other units are also of importance. The *averager* system allows the recording of very low action potentials (<5 μV) and also provides better definition of higher amplitude potentials. Averaging is necessary to record some sensory action potentials and all of the somatosensory evoked potentials. The averager adds 2–2000 successive potentials to extract the electrical event linked to the stimulation and to eliminate the background noise or chance electrical phenomena for which the mean is zero. This allows the extraction of potentials of amplitudes as low as 1 μV to 20 nV – the number of stimulations depends on the even/background noise amplitude ratio. A *personal computer* is also useful for data storage and for some special EDX procedures. *External stimulators* (e.g. high voltage, magnetic) are sometimes necessary for special EDX examinations.

EDX methods

There are two principal EDX methods: electromyography (EMG) and the nerve conduction study (Buchtal and Rosenfalk, 1966; Chu Andrews and Johnson, 1980; Dawson et al., 1982; Isch, 1963; Jablecki et al., 1993; Kamp Nielsen, 1973; Kimura, 1989; Mauguiere et al., 1981; Thompson, 1964; Pitres and Testut, 1925; Seror, 1993a; Swash and Schwartz, 1981).

Electromyography

This is also termed 'needle examination' and is performed with coaxial (monofilar/bifilar) or monopolar needle electrodes. Needles are inserted into the muscle and the electrical activity is studied at rest and during voluntary movements until the maximum contraction is obtained. It requires an excellent knowledge of anatomy (Kimura, 1989; Netter, 1991; Pitres and Testut, 1925) and physiology of the different muscles (Lacote et al., 1980), as well as active cooperation of the patient. It provides true muscular testing of strength, which is enhanced with analysis of the number and morphology of motor units. All needle electrodes are sterilized or single use to avoid infectious disease transmission to the patient. However, the electromyographer can prick himself during examination (Seror, 1993a), so it is important that he be informed by the patient of any serious transmissible disease (American Association of Electrodiagnostic Medicine, 1992; Karam, 1986; Seror, 1993a) such as HIV/AIDS or hepatitis.

The *motor unit* (MU) is a functional unit, composed of one motor neuron alpha (cell and axon) and its muscle fibers (Figure 2.2). The MU size varies somewhat in the same muscle and a great deal from one muscle to another. The more precise the movement, the fewer the number of driven muscle fibers, e.g. one motor neuron supplies one muscle fiber in eye muscles but 1000 muscle fibers in the gastrocnemius. The ratio between motor neurons and muscle fibers determines the innervation rate.

The *needle examination at rest* in *normal subjects* does not show activity except at the motor end-plate. The membrane of muscle fibers normally innervated is electrically stable, i.e. there

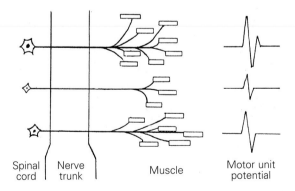

| Spinal cord | Nerve trunk | Muscle | Motor unit potential |

▭ Innervated muscle fibers

Motor unit potential, amplitude and duration depend on the number of muscle fibers

Figure 2.2

The motor unit.

is no spontaneous depolarization. In *pathology* (neurogenic or myogenic) some muscle fibers, or part of them, are not innervated further and can spontaneously depolarize, giving rise to fibrillations and/or positive sharp waves (Figure 2.3) which are the reflection of active and recent denervation. More complex activities reflect chronic denervation or a myogenic disorder. These are pseudomyotonic complex repetitive discharges, or high frequency, very bizarre potentials (see Figure 2.3). Somewhat different is true myotonic discharge, which is characterized by waxing and waning of frequencies and amplitudes (see Figure 2.3). All these repetitive activities can be triggered by needle insertion or by needle mobilization. Myotonia discharge and permanent activity can suggest neuromyotonia or Morvan chorea.

The *needle examination during voluntary contraction* (Figure 2.4) studies the MU potentials: number, morphology, amplitude, turns and firing rate. This semiquantitative study is essential but is the most difficult part of EDX and is linked to examiner experience, with auditory analysis as important as visual analysis. To increase the strength of muscle contractions the normal patient has two possibilities: use of a larger number of MU (spatial recruitment) and/or use of the same MU at a higher frequency (temporal recruitment; normal <20 Hz). In consequence, for minimal effort a single potential pattern is observed; only few MU are recruited and the baseline is clearly seen between each MU potential. When maximum voluntary effort is realized, a full interference pattern is observed; almost all the MU are recruited and beat at their maximal rate, less than 20 Hz; the different MU potentials are superimposed on each other so that neither MU potentials nor the baseline can be distinguished (see Figure 2.4).

Changes in pathologic conditions

In *myogenic disorders* the spatial recruitment is increased as the strength of each MU is decreased by muscle fiber necrosis or degeneration (Figure 2.5). To increase the contraction strength, the patient has to use the full normal MU. The consequence is a full interference pattern with low amplitude polyphasic and short duration MU potentials. The contrast between

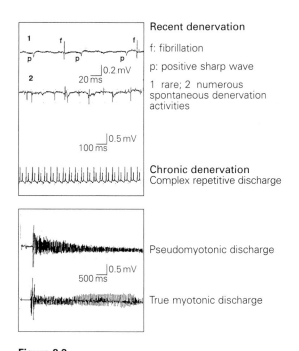

Recent denervation
f: fibrillation
p: positive sharp wave
1 rare; 2 numerous spontaneous denervation activities

Chronic denervation
Complex repetitive discharge

Pseudomyotonic discharge

True myotonic discharge

Figure 2.3

Needle examination at rest in pathological conditions.

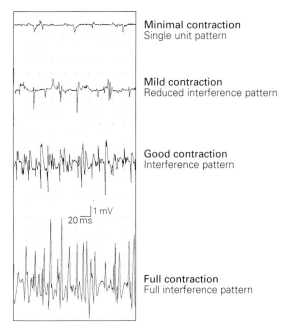

Minimal contraction
Single unit pattern

Mild contraction
Reduced interference pattern

Good contraction
Interference pattern

Full contraction
Full interference pattern

Figure 2.4

Needle examination during normal voluntary contraction.

the muscle weakness and the low amplitude full interference pattern is characteristic of myogenic disorders (see Figure 2.5).

In *neurogenic disorders* the temporal recruitment is increased; in fact, the MU number is reduced, as many axons and/or motoneurons have disappeared (Figure 2.6). To increase the contraction strength, the patient has to increase the firing rate of the remaining MU. The MU are usually polyphasic and can be of high amplitude in chronic disease, since they are enlarged by collateral sprouting which incorporates muscle fibers of denervated MU. The neurogenic pattern (see Figure 2.6) is characterized by a single potential, or a reduced interference pattern with a high firing rate of MU (>20 Hz).

Nerve conduction study

The nerve conduction study is certainly the most reliable and the most sensitive part of EDX. The analysis is quantitative and the actual quasi-systematic use of surface electrodes for recording and for stimulation makes this part of the examination less painful and more reliable. Nerve conduction studies can be undertaken in both motor and sensory fibers. In proximal segments (plexus and in the central nervous system) the study is achieved with *somatosensory evoked potentials* (*SSEP*) or *motor evoked potentials* (*MEP*). It allows precise evaluation of the conduction velocity of large diameter myelinated nervous fibers; the normal velocity in upper limbs varies between 50 and 70 m/s and, in lower limbs, between 40 and 50 m/s. Velocity decreases with age, especially beyond 70 years. Nerve conduction study also estimates the number of nervous fibers through the *compound motor action potential* (*CMAP*) and the *sensory action potential* (*SAP*) amplitudes.

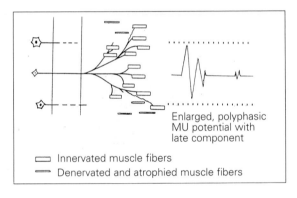

Enlarged, polyphasic MU potential with late component

⊏⊐ Innervated muscle fibers
— Denervated and atrophied muscle fibers

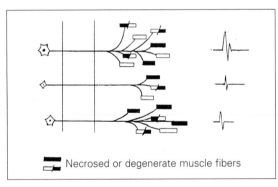

Necrosed or degenerate muscle fibers

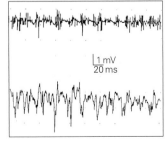

Interference pattern for a weak contraction; potentials are of low amplitude and are polyphasic

1 mV
20 ms

Figure 2.5

Myogenic disorder.

Single unit pattern with high firing rate and low amplitude potentials

Single unit pattern with high firing rate and polyphasic potentials

Reduced interference pattern with high firing rate

Reduced interference pattern with high firing rate and polyphasic potentials of high amplitude (anterior horn disease)

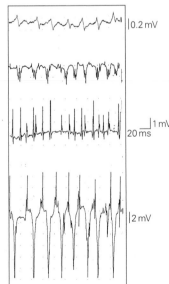

0.2 mV

1 mV
20 ms

2 mV

Figure 2.6

Neurogenic disorder.

Motor conduction velocity (MCV) (Figure 2.7) – the stimulation of a nerve trunk at two levels allows the recording of two CMAP of different latencies. The ratio between the distance (in mm) between the two points of stimulation and the latency difference (in ms) gives the MCV in m/s. The *distal motor latency* (DML) is the latency obtained after stimulation at the most distal point at the wrist for the median nerve, or the Erb point for the suprascapular nerve. It reflects the MCV but it cannot be translated into m/s as this latency reflects not only the time of motor conduction but also the transmission times of the chemical neuromuscular junction and of muscular conduction. The normal CMAP amplitude of hand intrinsic muscles varies from 4 to 15 mV.

Sensory conduction velocity (SCV) (Figure 2.8) – a single stimulation point and a single recording allows measurement of the SCV of the median nerve across the wrist (see Figure 2.8). One stimulation point and two recording points are necessary to calculate the SCV of the ulnar nerve across the elbow (see Figure 2.8). The SAP amplitude usually varies from 10 to 100 μV but an SAP of less than 10 μV (1000 times less than CMAP) is not uncommon in some normal nerves, or in pathological nerves, and averaging is then required (see Figure 2.8). The SAP amplitude is a good indicator of the number of functional sensory axons.

Proximal conduction can be explored by different methods such as the medullar reflexes, the SSEP and MEP (Eisen et al., 1983; Kimura, 1989; Livingstone et al., 1984; Piade et al., 1984; Seror, 1995b; Siivola et al., 1983; Weber and Piero, 1978; Yiannikas and Walsh, 1983; Yiannikas et al., 1983). *Medullar reflexes* (Figure 2.9) are circuit-including sensory 1A fibers and motoneuron alpha (Hoffman reflex), or only motoneuron alpha (F wave). Only F waves are usually studied in the

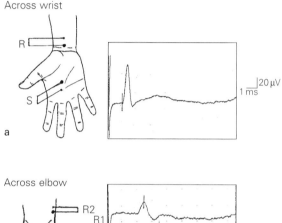
Across wrist

a

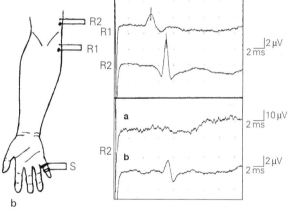
Across elbow

b

Figure 2.8

Orthodromic sensory conduction study. (a) At the wrist, the ratio between the distance (in mm) of the two cathodes (stimulating/recording) and the latency at onset of the potential (in ms) determines the sensory conduction velocity (SCV) (in m/s) across the wrist. (b) At the elbow, the ratio between the distance (100 mm) separating the two recording points (R1/R2) and the two latencies (at peak) of the recorded sensory action potentials (SAP) determines the SCV across the elbow. Normal amplitudes of SAP recorded above the elbow vary from 3 to 10 μV. Averaging is essential to obtain a well-defined SAP which allows both a precise latency measurement and a precise SCV calculation. The direct trace (a) does not give this precision, but the averaged and amplified trace (b) of 35 samples does.

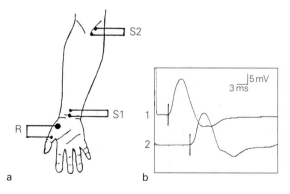
a   b

Figure 2.7

Motor conduction study. The ratio between the distance (in millimeters) between the two points of stimulation and the latency difference (in milliseconds) gives the motor conduction velocity (in m/s). The response recorded after S1 stimulation is also termed the distal motor latency.

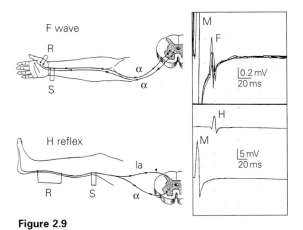

Figure 2.9

H reflex and F wave.

Potentials can be recorded at the axilla, Erb's point, the C-6 cervical spinous process and at the contralateral parietal area (Seror, 1995b). SSEP recording is time consuming and requires the averaging of 200–2000 samples after stimulation of low intensity (two to three times the sensory threshold). Taking multiple recordings in stages allows the study of segments whose normal conduction delay is 3–4 ms (peripheral nerve pathway), where a 2 ms increment of one conduction delay becomes an evident abnormality. MEP (Figure 2.11) correspond to a similar study on motor fibers from proximal to distal points. Recordings are taken from hand intrinsic muscles (abductor digit minimi) and stimulations are performed at the cervical C-7 spinous process, the C-7 transverse process, the supra-clavicular, the axilla and the wrist (Seror, 1995b). The nerve segment conduction delay does not exceed 3–4 ms, allowing the recognition of proximal conduction blocks and nerve velocity slowing. A cerebral stimulation may also be performed with magnetic stimulation to study the central motor pathway.

upper limbs. The nerve length studied is about 150 cm, which corresponds to 25–30 ms latency (two standard deviations = 5 ms). As 95% of carpal tunnel syndromes (CTS) have a DML increment of less than 5 ms, F waves can assess only severe proximal compression. In contrast, F waves are of high diagnostic interest for acute or chronic demyelinating polyneuropathies; in fact, the demyelination involves the nerve over a long distance and in many locations (see Figure 2.13). SSEP (Figure 2.10) can be recorded after nerve stimulation at digits, the wrist or the elbow; it is possible to record the afferent volley through its pathway from stimulation point to the parietal cortex (Mauguière et al., 1981; Chiappa, 1983).

Errors and pitfalls in nerve conduction study

• The nerve conduction velocity decreases with decreasing temperatures, so the electromyographer should warm upper limbs when the

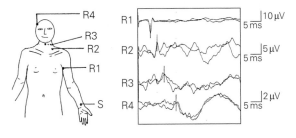

Figure 2.10

Somatosensory evoked potentials (SSEP). The mean latency of cortical potential (R4) after median nerve stimulation at the wrist is 18.2 ms, other latencies are R3=12.7 ms, R2=9.5 ms, R1=6.3 ms. Interpeak mean conduction delays are R1R2=3.2 ms, R2R3=3.2 ms, R3R4=central conduction delay=5.6 ms.

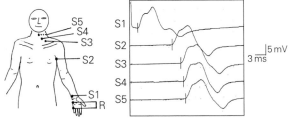

Figure 2.11

Motor evoked potentials (MEP). Abductor digiti minimi mean latency from the cervical spine (S5) is 13.6 ms (50% of F wave latency). Interpeak mean delay values are S1S2=10.5 ms, S2S3=2.6 ms, S3S5=0.6 ms.

cutaneous temperature is less than 31°C. This is essential in diseases of the hand since the conduction velocity slowing of the median nerve across the wrist forms the main data in CTS electrodiagnostic assessment.

- The stimulation must be applied exactly on the studied nerve. An inopportune stimulation increment for a bad response can lead to stimulating the ulnar with the median nerve, leading to erroneous interpretation.
- When nerve stimulation specificity cannot be achieved (e.g. a high level of stimulation, numerous nerves at the brachial plexus) the nerve conduction specificity is only obtained by a coaxial needle electrode recording in a muscle exclusively innervated by the nerve trunk studied.
- When a nerve trunk is deep (brachial plexus) the electromyographer must modify the stimulation mode (e.g. monopolar stimulation, high voltage stimulator) to avoid erroneous conclusions for the conduction block. One can additionally use another technique, e.g. SCV and/or SSEP, to study the nerve conduction in the proximal segment.
- Nerve trunk anastomoses are frequent between median and ulnar nerves in the forearm (Martin–Gruber; Kimura, 1989) and rare in the hand (Riche Cannieu; Pitres and Testut, 1925); they modify the morphology of median and ulnar nerve CMAP.
- The correct orientation of the cathode stimulator is essential, its inversion may lead to abnormal latency and SAP morphology (polyphasic), causing false SAP desynchronization which usually signifies nerve compression or demyelination.

Special stimulo-detection methods

Repetitive stimulations are used specifically to study the neuro-muscular junction. In *myasthenia gravis* (postsynaptic block) the repetitive stimulation at a low rate (3 Hz) can show CMAP amplitude decrements of more than 10% between the first and fifth potentials (Figure 2.12). Ulnar, spinal and facial nerves are usually studied. In *Lambert–Eaton syndrome* (Eaton and Lambert, 1957) (presynaptic block) similar findings occur but the CMAP amplitude is low and increases (100–1000%) after isometric exercise or after 30 Hz repetitive stimulation.

The *sympathetic nervous system* can be investi-gated by the sympathic skin response and heart rate variation after deep breathing or the Valsalva maneuver (McDougall and McLeod, 1996).

High voltage stimulation is frequently necessary to obtain supramaximal stimulation in deep and proximal sites (plexus brachial), and at the cervical spine for MEP study (Seror, 1995b). Patients must be advised before performing such a technique as it is painful, but sometimes it is the only way to assess or eliminate conduction block and abnormal conduction velocity.

Magnetic stimulation is painless and can be applied at the frontoparietal cortex or at the spinal cord. The stimulator electrode (coil) has a large diameter (6–10 cm), preventing the precise determination of the depolarization site and, in turn, that of the conduction delay and of the MCV. Moreover, supramaximal stimulation is never obtained and other nerves can be stimulated at the same time. Also only exceptional study of the motor central pathway requires its use.

Dynamic nerve conduction studies have been proposed (and used) by some authors, especially for thoracic outlet syndrome and posterior interosseous nerve entrapment (Chodoroff et al., 1985; Rainer et al., 1973). The present author's EDX experience does not confirm the usefulness of this method, and experimental studies (Matsen et al., 1977; Seror, 1990) demonstrate, as do others, that no significant nerve conduction changes occur before 15 minutes of 100 mmHg compression. The dynamic maneuver should therefore be maintained for 20–30 minutes, which is quite impractical.

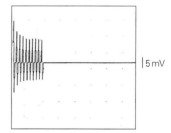

Figure 2.12

Repetitive stimulations in *myasthenia gravis*. The stimulation of the ulnar nerve at the wrist is performed at 3 Hz; the compound motor action potential amplitude decrement is 35%.

Nerve conduction changes in pathologic conditions

In *myogenic disorders*, MCV, SCV and SAP are normal, and only CMAP amplitudes are involved. In *neuromuscular junction diseases* MCV, SCV and SAP are normal, with low CMAP amplitudes, e.g. in Lambert–Eaton syndrome. In *neurogenic disorders*, nerve conduction abnormalities vary with the etiology of nerve impairment.

Polyneuropathies are characterized by diffuse involvement and are usually predominant in lower limbs; a recent study demonstrated that a well-conducted EDX correctly differentiates between axonal and demyelinating polyneuropathies in 90% of cases studied histologically. Conversely, mononeuropathies usually involve one nerve trunk, frequently in the upper limb but also in lower limbs. However, some chronic demyelinating polyneuropathies may mimic, both at their onset and for a long time afterwards, a single trunk involvement of the upper limb and can develop with a mononeuropathy. Polyneuropathies and mononeuropathies will now be considered.

In *axonal polyneuropathy*, MCV and SCV are normal or subnormal, medullar reflexes can be normal or diminished. A decrease in CMAP and SAP amplitudes is usually found in lower limbs since they are nerve-length dependent.

In *demyelinating polyneuropathy* (DPN) *or chronic inflammatory demyelinating polyneuropathy* (CIDP), MSC, SCV, medullar reflexes, CMAP and SAP amplitudes are, or may be, involved. Some findings are specific to CIDP (Figure 2.13), such as motor conduction block, temporal dispersion and delayed DML, and F waves. In CIDP clinical complaints may be mild and very delayed, so sometimes the importance of the EDX findings are surprising (e.g. hereditary neuropathy with liability to pressure palsy). Specific EDX criteria are required to assess CIDP diagnosis (Bouche and Vallat, 1992; Bromberg, 1991; CRITERIA, 1991; Leger et al., 1996; Lewis et al., 1982; Pestronk et al., 1988; Seror, 1996e).

In *anterior horn diseases*, such as amyotrophic lateral sclerosis, monomelic amyotrophy, poliomyelitis, syringomyelia and cervicarthrosis myelopathy, MCV are normal. CMAP amplitudes can be normal or null depending on the local severity of the anterior horn lesions. SCV and SAP amplitudes are always normal.

In *sensory neuropathy*, ganglion, axon or myelin can be involved. Axonal and demyelinating lesions have already been described. In ganglionopathy (Bouche and Vallat, 1992) (Denny Brown neuropathy) SAP are absent or of very low amplitude in upper and lower limbs; the nerve lesion is not length dependent.

Mononeuropathies can involve any sensory and/or motor nerve trunk and can be of viral, immunological or mechanical origin.

The *inflammatory mononeuropathy* (Kiloh and Nevin, 1952; Seror, 1996b, 1996f; Turner and Parsonage, 1957) can be unique or multiple, benign and resolutive (e.g. Parsonage–Turner syndrome) (Turner and Parsonage, 1957; Figure 2.23), or severe with poor recovery when they are due to vasculitis of systemic diseases (e.g. polyarteritis nodosa, necrotizing angiopathy) (Bouche and Vallat, 1992; Seror, 1996f; Swash and Schwartz, 1981). The nerve lesion is axonal, so MCV and SCV are normal when the nerve is still recordable; CMAP and SAP amplitudes are always involved. Sometimes pseudoconduction

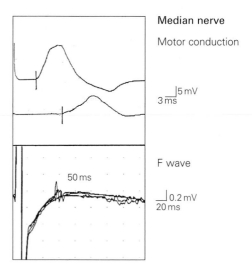

Median nerve

Motor conduction

5 mV
3 ms

F wave

50 ms

0.2 mV
20 ms

Figure 2.13

Demyelinating neuropathy. Motor conduction of the median nerve at the wrist and forearm shows delayed distal motor latency and temporal dispersion of the compound motor action potential recorded at the elbow (decreased amplitude and increased duration). The F wave is delayed (50 ms; NI=27 ms).

block can be observed at the onset of the nerve lesion before the Wallerian degeneration is established.

The *mechanical mononeuropathies* (*traumatic* or *entrapment neuropathy*) are the most frequent nerve lesions encountered by hand surgeons. The main EDX abnormality is focal MCV and SCV, slowing reflecting focal demyelination at the entrapment site; this demyelinated lesion evolves over time (months to years) to progressive axonal loss. In acute compression, motor and sensory conduction blocks can be found (Figures 2.17, 2.18, 2.24 and 2.25). The compression site is usually limited to 1–4 cm, and above and below that nerve conduction is normal. The focal conduction velocity slowing is always diluted in part of the normal velocity. This is why studying conduction on nerve segments of more than 10 cm (especially F waves) is not recommended. The ideal is to study the conduction centimeter by centimeter; this has been performed on median nerves at the wrist (Figure 2.17: mild median nerve lesion) but this method is time consuming (Seror, 1989a) and cannot be used on every nerve. Meanwhile motor and sensory incremental studies every 5 cm can often be performed on the arm or forearm (Figure 2.19). In chronic lesions, CMAP amplitudes remain normal in the severe nerve lesion until axonal loss is less than 90%; in contrast, SAP amplitudes decrease progressively with axonal loss (Figure 2.17: severe median nerve lesion).

Terminology

A thorough knowledge of electrodiagnostic terminology is necessary to understand an EDX report (Chu Andrews and Johnson, 1980; Kimura, 1989; Swash and Schwartz, 1981).

The *nerve conduction block* (CB) is defined by the axon failure to transmit the nerve impulse in myelinated fibers when the axon is not involved. The myelin is altered on at least two to three Ranvier nodes. This phenomenon is reversible and CB is documented on EDX reports when the CMAP or SAP amplitude/area is reduced totally or partially between two near (maximum 10 cm) stimulation or recording points (Figures 2.17, 2.18, 2.24 and 2.25). Supramaximal stimulation above and below the CB site depolarizes all nerve fibers; when stimulated from below only, all of the nerve fibers transmit the nerve impulse to the recording site; when stimulated from above, some of the nerve fibers transmit the nerve impulse while other nerve fibers are blocked. Conduction nerve slowing is usually associated with CB. They can be found in vasculitis, ergotism, hereditary neuropathy with liability to pressure palsy (Case report 1), Guillain Barré syndrome (Case report 5), chronic inflammatory demyelination polyneuropathy and *multifocal motor neuropathy* (*MMN*, Case report 2). The most frequent cause of acute and reversible CB is xylocaine anesthesia. In contrast, MMN is a good example of a long-lasting CB which is potentially reversible with therapy but usually leads to irreversible axon loss over time (years).

The *desynchronization* or *temporal dispersion* can involve both CMAP (Figure 2.13) and SAP (Figure 2.17: severe median nerve lesion; and Figure 2.18). When nerve fibers are homogeneously impaired in the CB, then they are inhomogeneously impaired in desynchronization or temporal dispersion. In fact, each fiber is differently impaired: some have serious slowing while others are slowed only slightly; also, each action potential reaches the recording site at a different time. This temporal dispersion of the action potentials associated with the phase cancellation phenomenon is the basis for the desynchronized traces (Figures 2.17 and 2.18).

The *axonal lesion* is opposite to the myelinated lesion, (e.g. CB, nerve conduction slowing or temporal dispersion). The etiology of axonal lesions end with *Wallerian degeneration*, giving both a very delayed and partial recovery. The EDX performed in the first few days after an acute severe nerve lesion will not always differentiate between a 90% CB and a 90% nerve division, before the Wallerian degeneration is established. A second EDX performed three or four weeks later will give a complete and definitive evaluation of the nerve lesion. Clinical consequences of axonal loss are amyotrophy and hypoesthesiae, but clinical features differ depending on whether the lesion is acute or chronic. In acute lesions, weakness and hypoesthesia are present immediately and amyotrophy occurs a few weeks later. In chronic lesions, amyotrophy is usually tardy, as is hypoesthesiae, which may even be absent when the disease is very slowly progressive. EDX consequences also differ depending on the onset mode. In acute lesions CMAP and SAP amplitudes are immediately (after wallerian degeneration) low or absent. In chronic lesions CMAP amplitude remains normal until the axonal loss is less than 90% (collateral reinnervation); but the SAP amplitude progressively decreases as it is directly linked to axon number (Figure 2.17: severe median nerve lesion).

Mixed lesions (axonal loss and demyelination) are frequent. An important role of EDX is to distinguish each part of the lesion using different EDX tests. This is essential for diagnosis and prognosis and to determine the best treatment.

Reinnervation forms the basis of clinical recovery and it is dependent on both *local conditions* (e.g. nerve lesion severity, length of nerve growing) and *general conditions* (e.g. age, polyneuropathy) (Dawson et al., 1982; Sunderland, 1978). After axon division, axonal regeneration is slow (1–2 mm/day), even under the best conditions. Ages of 70 and over and underlying polyneuropathy are unfavorable factors for recovery. The longer the distance the nerve has to grow, the poorer the reinnervation. In fact, reinnervation of hand intrinsic muscles is obtained after 6–12 months for a nerve lesion at the wrist, whilst this process takes 18–36 months for a nerve lesion at the elbow. Also, for a nerve lesion at Erb's point (e.g. brachial plexus injury, thoracic outlet syndrome) motor axon growth has very little chance of reaching the motor end-plate before motor fibers degenerate. Sensory recovery may be partial even over a long distance of nerve growth. Only CB lesions undergo good, rapid clinical and EDX recovery.

Reinnervation quality differs in function depending on the severity of the nerve lesion. In a *total (100%) nerve division*, immediately after Wallerian degeneration, CMAP and SAP amplitudes are null. After a good maximal recovery the CMAP amplitude will be 50–80% of normal value, whilst the SAP amplitude will rarely reach 10% of normal. In fact, the recovery depends only on axon growth (e.g. direct reinnervation). In a *50% nerve division*, after Wallerian degeneration, CMAP and SAP amplitudes are 50% of normal values. After maximal recovery the CMAP amplitude will usually be 100% of normal values and the SAP amplitude will be around 55% of normal. In these latter cases motor recovery occurs quickly (in a few months) and depends on the collateral reinnervation (Figure 2.6) (i.e. axonal sprouting)

realized by the remaining 50% of axons. The 50% of degenerated axons will grow slowly and provide direct reinnervation months later, when the functional recovery has already been achieved for many months. However, the SAP amplitude increment depends only on axon growth, as it is a direct reflection of axon number.

The difference between neurapraxia (CB) and axonotmesis or neurotmesis (axonal lesions) has already been emphasized, but the difference between axonotmesis and neurotmesis is also very important (Dawson et al., 1982; Seror, 1993a; Sunderland, 1978). In axonotmesis the preservation of the nerve connective tissues (peri-, epi-, and endoneurium) allows axonal regeneration in an orderly manner. This is not the case in neurotmesis.

Practical management of the EDX consultation

A *nerve conduction study* must be performed as part of the examination and is usually performed prior to EMG. Its purpose is to assess diffuse or focal lesions of peripheral nerves. It also determines whether the nerve damage is axonal or demyelination, the precise location site and the severity of the nerve lesion.

If one lesion is found it is certainly an entrapment neuropathy, if multiple lesions are found (median and ulnar nerves) it is useful to study lower limbs and F waves to enable the differences between multiple entrapment neuropathies and demyelinating polyneuropathies to be determined.

If multiple or diffuse lesions are found, EMG will be performed in muscles innervated by damaged nerves, and in muscles innervated by adjacent nerves and myotoma of symptomatic limbs. When generalized involvement is found EMG will be extended to muscles of other limbs and eventually to the neck, the tongue and the face (anterior horn disease) in relation to clinical considerations.

When to use an EDX

EDX is required if acute or progressive *weaknesses, hypoesthesia*, permanent or intermittent *paresthesia*, or *pain* are experienced. In acute nerve lesions (traumatic or non-traumatic), immediate performance of an EDX will determine the exact location of the nerve lesion and provide a good approximation of its severity, thereby determining the therapy given: e.g. the EDX demonstration of a postoperative ulnar nerve lesion at the elbow may benefit from an early nocturnal splintage, thus avoiding recurrence of nocturnal microtraumatism and providing a rapid recovery, especially for an existing CB. In traumatic cases an immediate EDX will not always be able to give an exact evaluation of the severity of the nerve lesion (axon/myelin). An EDX will be necessary three or four weeks later, when a complete evaluation will be established which will in turn determine the prognosis and provide a baseline for further EDX evaluations. The follow-up will be performed at two to three months, six to nine months and 24 months later as necessary.

In *entrapment neuropathies* EDX should be performed in all cases prior to treatment to confirm the nerve lesion and determine its severity, as there is no direct correlation between the clinical complaints, signs (except amyotrophy) and EDX findings (Seror 1989b). This is even more essential prior to surgery, both to prevent unnecessary surgery and to determine the preoperative nerve state, which will be very important if surgery fails to relieve symptoms. When the EDX is normal and symptoms are typical of an entrapment neuropathy it means that the nerve lesion is especially mild and first requires medical care; in fact, the sensitivity of a correct EDX in entrapment neuropathy is at least 90% (except proximal entrapment neuropathy). If it is a true entrapment neuropathy then a new EDX performed some months later, when there is a recurrence of symptoms, will usually confirm the diagnosis. If this new EDX still remains normal, the complaint is a position-related nerve compression, and information should reassure the patient.

Case reports

The following case reports will help in understanding the necessity of never limiting EDX examinations to only the symptomatic territory and extending it as part of the clinical examination. They also demonstrate the importance of a good dialog with the clinician in the most difficult cases.

Case report 1

A 40-year old man had a progressive weakness of the right upper limb. Digit extensors were especially weak and two previous EDX evaluated the right upper limb and concluded that it was C-8 T-1 root disease. Ten years previously he had developed an acute foot drop from which he recovered spontaneously; EDX confirmed the peroneal nerve lesion at the fibula head. The last EDX showed multiple nerve lesions in the upper and lower limbs, and especially in the right posterior interosseous nerve (Seror 1996c) (Figure 2.14). All of these nerve involvements were located in entrapment sites. It was concluded that the patient had demyelinating polyneuropathy, in particular linked to an *hereditary neuropathy with liability to pressure palsy* (Bouche and Vallat, 1992; Serratrice et al., 1985, 1987). Genetic analysis confirmed this diagnosis and found a deletion of the PMP 22 gene (chromosome 17).

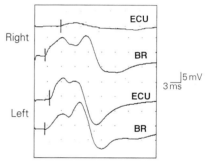

BR: brachioradialis; ECU: extensor carpi ulnaris

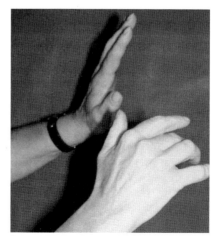

Figure 2.14

Posterior interosseous nerve palsy (Case report 1).

Case report 2

A 64-year old man complained of a progressive weakness of the right hand. There was no sensory complaint but he was not able to hold a pen. A previous EDX had studied nerve conductions in the hand and forearm, and concluded that it was a C-8 T-1 root disease. The last EDX demonstrated motor CB in proximal segments of the right median and ulnar nerves, and also one of the right sciatic nerve trunk (with MEP), F waves were absent. The sensory nerve conductions were normal. It was concluded that the patient had *multifocal motor neuropathy* (Bouche and Vallet, 1992; Pestronk et al., 1988; Seror, 1996e); treatment with intravenous immunoglobulins provided a marked improvement in his condition, whereas corticosteroids had been unsuccessful.

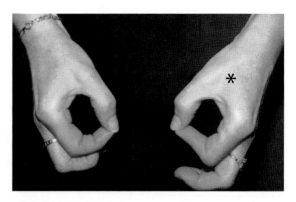

Figure 2.15

Partial anterior interosseous nerve palsy (Case report 4). *, Involved hand.

Case report 3

A 42-year old man complained for three to four years of nocturnal paresthesiae of both upper limbs. Paresthesiae involved digits 4 and 5. Recently, first dorsal interosseous atrophy of the left hand appeared. After many previous clinical and EDX consultations, an ulnar nerve compression at the elbow was diagnosed and surgery was suggested. The last EDX of motor and sensory potentials across the elbow found no ulnar nerve entrapment at either the elbow or the wrist, but did show an important *bilateral C-7 C-8 T-1 root disease* which involved median and ulnar intrinsic muscles, and also involved left wrist/digit extensors and right digitorum flexors. Cervical MRI and scanner confirmed *cervicarthrosis with myelopathy* (Berthier et al., 1996). Six months later a left lower limb clonus appeared and the patient underwent surgical spinal cord decompression.

Case report 4

A 52-year old woman had sudden difficulty in writing as she could no longer flex the distal interphalangeal joint of the second digit (Figure 2.15). A first median and ulnar nerves EDX was normal. The differential diagnosis included a tendon rupture. A second EDX was performed, paying special attention to the *anterior interosseous nerve* (Buchthal et al., 1974; Hill et al., 1985; Kiloh and Nevin, 1952; Seror, 1996b; Spinner, 1970); the latter was partly involved. The diagnosis was a neuralgic amyotrophy of Parsonage and Turner (1948) related to influenza infection.

Case report 5

A 45-year old man complained for three weeks of paresthesiae of the right upper limb, especially in the median digits. The first EDX resulted in a diagnosis of carpal tunnel syndrome and stressed the necessity of surgical release. A later EDX found diffuse motor and sensory demyelinating lesions in the median nerve and also in the ulnar and peroneal nerves; F waves were delayed (Figure 2.13). It was concluded that the patient had *acute or subacute inflammatory demyelinating neuropathy similar to Guillain Barré syndrome* (Bouche and Vallet, 1992; Bromberg, 1991; CRITERIA, 1991; Leger et al., 1996; Swash and Schwartz, 1981). The patient took further clinical advice but no account was taken of the EDX results; it was concluded that the patient had multiple sclerosis. Five solumedrol intravenous perfusions had little effect on the patient's symptoms. The patient was seen again four months later, when he had spontaneously improved. A follow-up EDX then showed a good resolution of demyelinating peripheral nerve lesions, confirming our initial diagnosis.

Care report 6

A 15-year old boy had complained for six months of progressive weakness of the left hand without sensory symptoms. The EDX found an

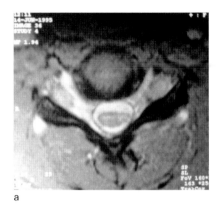 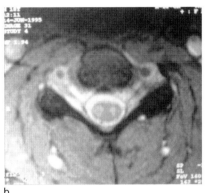

a   b

Figure 2.16

Monomelic anterior horn disease (Case report 6) (also named Hirayama disease). Magnetic resonance imaging of the cervical spinal cord (T2). (a) Atrophy of the left part (arrow) of the spinal cord at C-7/T-1, especially at the anterior horn. (b) Normal finding at C-5/C-6.

important pure motor involvement and it was concluded that the patient had *monomelic anterior horn disease* (Hirayama et al., 1987), but magnetic resonance imaging did not confirm this (Biondi et al., 1991; Seror, 1996a). It was not possible to assess or eliminate thoracic outlet syndrome (TOS) using clinical or paraclinical tests. After discussion with the clinician, a TOS surgical decompression was performed, as there was no alternative treatment. This did not prevent aggravation, as confirmed by a new EDX performed six months later, which also found a benign contralateral involvement. A new MRI found left spinal cord atrophy (Figure 2.16), confirming the initial diagnosis. Two years later clinical and EDX findings have not changed.

EDX in entrapment neuropathy diagnosis

In most upper limb entrapment neuropathies, the EDX performed correctly should be able to assess the nerve lesion and evaluate its severity. *Different conditions* (Dawson et al., 1982; Seror, 1996f, 1997; Stevens et al., 1992) can be associated with entrapment neuropathy and must be investigated before the application of treatment. Most frequent are *injuries* (e.g. Colle's fracture for carpal tunnel syndrome, elbow fracture with tardy ulnar palsy for an ulnar nerve lesion at the elbow), however, *rheumatisms* (e.g. rheumatoid arthritis (Seror, 1994f), osteoarthrosis, chondrocalcinosis), *diabetes mellitus*, *pregnancy* (Ekman et al., 1987; Seror 1987) and *hypothyroidism* are also encountered.

The role of *excessive use* or *cumulative trauma disorder* (Mackinnon and Novak, 1994) must also be considered. Most entrapment neuropathies remain idiopathic, i.e. they exist in a tunnel narrowness or a fibrous band. Sometimes proximal and distal entrapment neuropathies are involved, giving rise to a *double crush syndrome*; two distal entrapment neuropathies may also be implicated. In both conditions a single distal surgical release can be the origin of potential and sometimes total recovery.

Carpal tunnel syndrome

Carpal tunnel syndrome (CTS) is the most common (Phalen, 1966; Seror, 1991; Seze and Dreyfus, 1964; Sunderland, 1976) and best defined entrapment neuropathy and can be considered a model for the development of EDX examination methods (Brown et al., 1976; Buchthal and Rosenfalk, 1966; Jablecki et al., 1993; Kimura, 1979; Marie and Foix, 1913; Nathan et al., 1988; Seror, 1989a, 1994, 1995a; Simpson, 1956; Uncini et al., 1993). The two main purposes of an EDX are to confirm or eliminate a diagnosis and to evaluate the alternative or associated nerve lesions. Two main questions require consideration in unilateral CTS: (1) *which muscles and nerves should be examined?*; (2) *which nerve conduction methods should be used?* (Jablecki et al., 1993; Seror, 1993a).

(1) For completeness, especially in complicated cases with differential diagnosis, needle examination should be performed systematically for abductor pollicis brevis, first dorsal interosseous,

deltoid, biceps brachii, triceps, flexor digitorum superficialis muscles of symptomatic limb and abductor pollicis brevis of the asymptomatic side. Sensory and motor nerve condition should be examined systematically in the median and ulnar nerves at the wrist and forearm of the symptomatic limb and the median nerve at the wrist of the contralateral limb.

(2) Not all nerve conduction methods (Figure 2.17) assess the same proportion of cases. In a recent study (Seror, 1994), it was demonstrated that DML (>4 ms), orthodromic sensory conduction velocity (OSCV) from digit 3 and OSCV from the palm to the wrist (≤45 ms) provided 55, 66 and 76%, respectively, of positive diagnoses. Twenty-four per cent of the CTS were not assessed by these classical tests and special tests were required. The orthodromic medio-ulnar latency difference of the 4th digit (Seror, 1994, 1995a; Uncini et al., 1993) and the orthodromic inching test provided diagnoses of 20/24% and 24/24%, respectively, of the remaining mild cases (Kimura, 1979; Nathan et al., 1988; Seror, 1989a, 1994, 1995a, 2000). The orthodromic inching test was recently improved and

Figure 2.17

Carpal tunnel syndrome: mild median nerve lesion (Seror 2000). The orthodromic sensory inching test (a) provides a very precise anatomo-functional study of sensory conduction across the carpal tunnel, recording the sensory action potential (SAP) every centimeter. This allows recognition of very mild median nerve lesions in which distal motor latency (DML) and orthodromic sensory conduction velocity are normal. In this case the maximal conduction delay per centimeter is 0.52 ms (normal 0.16–0.40 ms). In the orthodromic medio-ulnar latency difference of the 4th digit (b), median and ulnar potentials of the 4th digit are studied separately. The latency difference in these cases is 0.48 ms (normal 0.0–0.40 ms).

Acute median nerve lesion is frequently encountered in pregnancy (Seror, 1997). In motor conduction block (CB) (c) between, above and below wrist the amplitude loss is 80%; sensory CB (d): between palm and above wrist the amplitude loss is 78%.

Severe median nerve lesion (e). Motor conduction shows very delayed DML (7.1 ms) with an amplitude of 8.2 mV due to a good collateral reinnervation (abductor pollicis brevis was not amyotrophied). In contrast, sensory conduction (from the 3rd digit) shows very delayed desynchronized and low amplitude SAP: velocities are 26–11 m/s and the mean amplitude is 1.2 µV versus 26 µV

Mild median nerve lesion

a Orthodromic sensory inching test

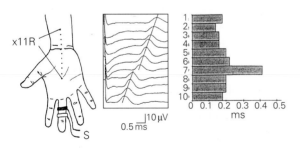

b Orthodromic medio-ulnar sensory latency difference of the 4th digit

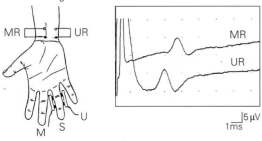

Acute median nerve lesion

c Motor conduction

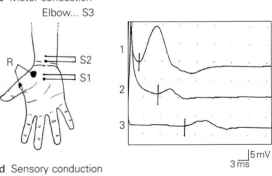

d Sensory conduction

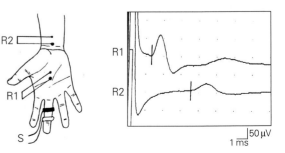

S: Stimulation; R = recording

simplified so that it requires the recording of only three sensory action potentials every 2 cm across the 4 cm of the carpal tunnel (Seror, forthcoming). Some rare typical CTS had normal EDX. In these cases the nerve lesion was especially mild or absent, some were true beginning CTS and others were position-related symptoms (Seror, 1989a); also, to differentiate them, the repetition of EDX 6–12 months later is essential. A special test was developed, called the ultradistal test, which is able to determine exceptional axonal CTS (Seror, 1996d). With good practice, EDX sensitivity and specificity is near 100% for CTS.

---

for the contralateral normal hand. The axonal loss is >90%.

Very severe median nerve lesion (f). No sensory potential can be recorded, motor surface recording is not possible, only needle motor recording is possible and provides DML=-13.1ms with a compound motor action potential (CMAP) amplitude 1 mV. CMAP is polyphasic and of long duration (18ms). Motor conduction velocity at the forearm is also decreased (44m/s) by dying-back neuropathy.

Severe median nerve lesion

e

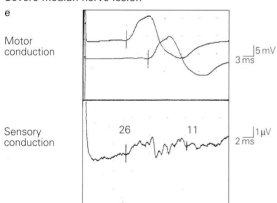

Very severe median nerve lesion

f

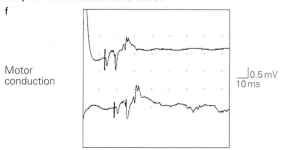

Other median nerve lesions

Anterior interosseous nerve (AIN) *lesions* are the second most frequent median entrapment neuropathy. Partial lesions involving only digit 1 or digit 2 (Figure 2.15) are almost 50% of all cases (Hill et al., 1985; Seror, 1996a; Seror, 1999a). Most of the cases are not entrapment neuropathy but mononeuritis, such as Kiloh–Nevin or Parsonage–Turner syndromes (Kiloh and Nevin, 1952; Parsonage and Turner, 1948; Turner and Parsonage, 1957). EDX assesses 100% of the cases but a thorough knowledge of the clinical pattern and experience of needle examination of muscles innervated by AIN, such as the pronator quadratus, is required. The *teres pronator syndrome* and compression at the *supracondylar process* are rare (Buchthal and Rosenfalk, 1966; Goulin et al., 1963; Mittal and Gupta, 1978; Nigst and Dick, 1979). An inflammatory origin must always be questioned. Motor and sensory conduction studies with needle examination should provide at least 90% of positive diagnoses. In these cases, as in more proximal lesions, recordings and stimulations every 5 cm allow the lesion site to be located precisely (Figure 2.19).

Ulnar nerve lesion (UNL)

A *UNL at the elbow* (UNLE) is the second most common entrapment neuropathy of the upper limb (Eisen, 1974; Gillat and Thomas, 1960; Harding and Halar, 1983; Seror, 1992). Its frequency is certainly underestimated as many nerve conductions are performed without study focussed across the elbow (Figures 2.8 and 2.18), and as many cases are asymptomatic or give symptoms confused with CTS. In a recent study (unpublished data) it was found that 13% of clinical CTS were UNLE. The global motor nerve conduction study from the wrist to the elbow assessed only 45–50% of UNLE determined by studies of MCV and SCV across the elbow (Seror, 1992). Sensory studies provide the most sensitive and reliable results, in particular SAP desynchronization can be the single EDX sign of UNLE (Figure 2.18). A new approach to diagnose UNLE has been described (Merlevede et al., 2000): in our experience this has been shown to be a reliable and simple test to perform, in comparison to MCV and SCV across the elbow. The sensitivity is 90–95%.

UNL at the wrist (UNLW) (Brichet et al., 1980; Gross and Gerlbermann, 1985; Preston and Logigian, 1992; Seror, 1988, 1995b; Wu et al., 1985) are rare (16/312 of UNLE (Seror, 1992). EDX sensitivity is 100% as almost every case had motor deficit. Cases which can escape EDX identification (because of incomplete EDX examination; Seror, 1999b) are due to deep branch lesions of the ulnar nerve. These are 2/3 of UNLW and require DML studies of the first dorsal interosseous or other muscles innervated by the deep branch (Gross and Gerlbermann, 1985; Preston and Logigian, 1992; Seror, 1995a; Seror, 1999b; Wu et al., 1983). In fact, in these cases DML to hypothenar (adductor digiti minimi) and sensory conduction studies (5th digit to wrist) may remain normal.

Ulnar nerve proximal lesions can be found at the arcade of Struther or even more proximal. In these cases, recordings or stimulations every 5 cm (Figure 2.19) are essential to locate the nerve lesion site precisely. These unusual lesions should always lead to consideration of an inflammatory origin: mononeuropathy or demyelinating neuropathy at the onset of the disease (Figure 2.19).

Ulnar postoperative nerve lesions are frequently due to a compression across the elbow, but some exceptional cases do not recognize this etiology and are due to postoperative mononeuritis (Seror and Bouche, 1997), e.g. Parsonage–Turner syndrome.

a Motor conduction

Stimulations at
1: wrist
2: below elbow
3: above elbow
4: 10 cm above elbow
5: ERB point

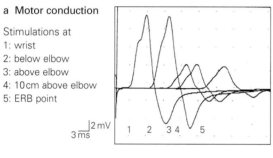

a Motor conduction

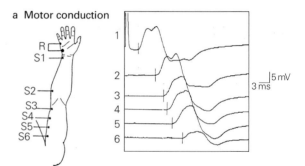

b Sensory conduction

Recording at
1: below elbow
2: above elbow

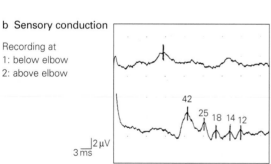

b Sensory conduction

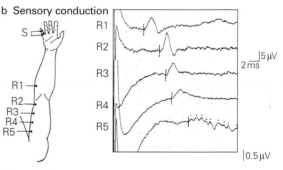

Figure 2.18

Ulnar nerve lesions at the elbow. (a) Motor conduction demonstrated velocity slowing and conduction block across the elbow. Velocity is 32 m/s, the amplitude loss is 68%. Conduction velocity above and below the elbow is normal. (b) Sensory conduction demonstrated sensory action potential desynchronization: velocities ranged from 42 to 12 m/s; in this case the motor conduction was normal.

Figure 2.19

Inching testing in a proximal ulnar nerve lesion (UNL). This patient showed sensory motor impairment in ulnar territory for 4 months. (a) The motor conduction study showed normal conduction in the wrist, forearm, elbow and distal arm. Only axillar stimulation showed a conduction block (65%). More precise study by testing every 5 cm determined that the UNL was located 14–19 cm above the medial epicondyle. (b) A similar sensory conduction study demonstrated similar findings, with conduction slowing and sensory action potential desynchronization at the same site. The diagnosis was a demyelinating neuropathy, Lewis and Sumner type.

Radial nerve lesions

Proximal radial nerve lesions, prior to division into posterior and anterior branches at the elbow, are frequent. Most of them are post-traumatic (e.g. humerus fracture, Saturday night palsy). True chronic entrapments are rare; some rare cases with nerve stenosis (Hoshizume et al., 1993; Lussiez et al., 1993), with or without entrapment were related by some authors to muscular effort and by others to neuralgic amyotrophy (Pou-Serradel et al., 1993).

The *posterior interosseous nerve* (PIN) can be entrapped in a radial tunnel (Guillain and Courtellemont, 1905; Ritts et al., 1987). When there is a clinical weakness EDX sensitivity is 100%; however, with *lateral elbow pain* (Narakas, 1974), classical nerve conduction studies (Jebsen, 1996; Testut et al., 1984) are of little help in detecting mild cases. A new method has been developed (Seror, 1996c; Figure 2.14) which assesses the PIN lesion in each case with extensor digitorum communis motor deficit. This method should provide 90% sensitivity with milder cases, but no satisfactory study can be performed as it is not possible to realize a satisfactory selection of PIN entrapment cases based only on clinical criteria for this disease.

Cheralgia paresthetica is linked to superficial radial nerve lesions at the wrist or the forearm. Involvements are frequently partial, involving one or two digits, and require a strict adaptation of EDX testing to the clinical symptoms. In this condition they are regularly recognized by EDX and the sensitivity is around 90% (Seror, 1993a).

Periscapular nerve entrapments

Suprascapular (Figure 2.20), *long thoracic* (Figure 2.21) and *accessory nerve lesions* (Figure 2.22) entrapments are rare and clinically underrecognized (Alfonsi et al., 1986; Bardot et al., 1985). *Axillary nerve* lesions are rare but easily recognized (Alnot, 1984). These nerve lesions can be due to nerve entrapment and to shoulder girdle or Parsonage and Turner syndrome (neuritis; Figure 2.23). This latter disease, in our experience of non-traumatic referring, is the most frequent etiology of these nerve involvements (Turner and Parsonage, 1957; Case report 4). The place of EDX is essential to differentiate entrapment from neuritis and to determine the severity of the nerve lesion. The sensitivity diagnosis in neuritis is 100%. When dealing with painful entrapment only, DML and needle examination provide only 50–60% sensitivity.

a

b

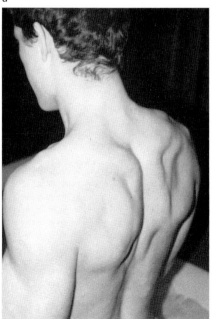
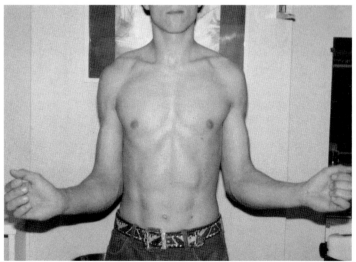

Figure 2.20

Suprascapular nerve palsy. Notice right infraspinatus muscle atrophy (a) and shoulder external rotation weakness (b), sometimes only the last sign is present.

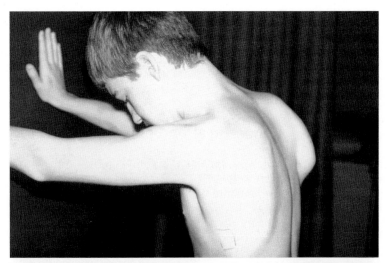

Figure 2.21

A long thoracic nerve palsy (right upper limb) is responsible for a winging scapula.

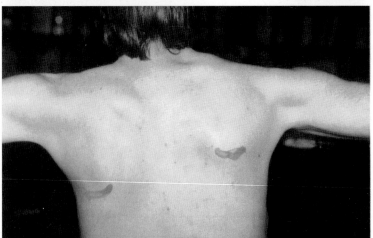

Figure 2.22

An accessory nerve palsy (right upper limb). The superior trapezius muscle is mildly involved and the medial and inferior head are severely impaired. This occurred after knee arthroscopy 6 months previously and was a neuralgic amyotrophy. Notice that the scapula medial margin is too far from the thoracic spinous process and the scapula inferior angle is high.

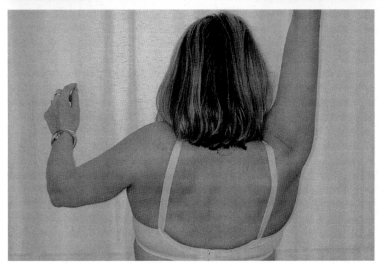

Figure 2.23

Shoulder palsy. This is a false left neuralgic amyotrophy with acute, painful and severe electrodiagnostic involvement (single unit pattern numerous denervation activities) of deltoid and infraspinatus, due to C-5 disk herniation.

Proximal nerve lesions

TOS is certainly the most difficult nerve entrapment to assess, by clinical or paraclinical examinations. The first aim of EDX is to eliminate nerve lesions such as CTS or UNLE. The use of F waves (Livingstone et al., 1984; Weber and Piero, 1978), whose standard deviation is 2.5 ms, can assess no more than 5% of TOS cases. TOS usually involves primarily the lower brachial plexus. We therefore consider that ulnar (Aminoff et al., 1988; Gilliat et al., 1978) and medial antebrachial cutaneous (Reddy, 1983) nerve SAP are the main EDX tools for TOS electrophysiological assessment. In fact, needle examination is of no differential diagnostic interest, since impairment would be similar to C-8–T-1 root disease. One can distinguish two EDX patterns: a classical and a new one. The classical (Gilliat et al., 1998) associates abnormal needle examination in C-8–T-1 innervated muscles, low amplitude of ulnar nerve SAP, low or normal amplitude of median and ulnar nerves CMAP, and normal median nerve SAP. The new pattern, which considers milder TOS cases (or other mild lower brachial plexus lesions: Seror, 2001 and unpublished data), associates normal or mildly impaired needle examination in some C-8–T-1 innervated muscles, low amplitude of medial antebrachial cutaneous nerve SAP, and normal amplitude of median and ulnar nerve SAP and CMAP (Figure 2.24). In the classical pattern medial antebrachial cutaneous nerve SAP is

always involved when it is tested (Le Forestier et al., 1999; Nishida et al., 1993). The first pattern should provide 10–20% diagnostic sensitivity, while the second should provide 50–60% diagnostic sensitivity. SSEP and MEP studied by stages are quite frequently impaired in the first pattern (Chodoroff et al., 1985; Eisen et al., 1983; Livingstone et al., 1984; Seror 1995b; Yiannikas and Walsh, 1983) and may be in some of the new pattern. However, no prospective study has or will be conducted on this subject, as TOS clinical diagnosis is always uncertain and SSEP and MEP are extremely time-consuming.

Postradiation plexopathy is characterized by typical EDX findings (Seror et al., 1999a), which usually allow it to be differentiated from tumoral plexopathy. The lower trunk is usually most

Somatosensory evoked potentials

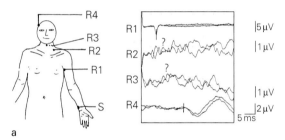

a

Motor evoked potentials

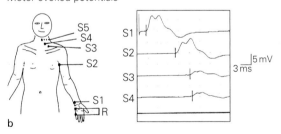

b

Figure 2.25

Postradiation brachial plexus neuropathy. (a) Somatosensory evoked potential (SSEP): stimulation is performed on the ulnar nerve at the wrist. Potentials above the axilla (R2,R3) are not recordable, demonstrating abnormal conduction (slowing and block). Cortical SSEP is slightly delayed (20.8 ms) and of low amplitude. (b) Motor evoked potential (MEP) demonstrated an important conduction block (75%) and velocity slowing (49 m/s; NI=72 m/s) between supraclavicular (S3) and axillar (S2) stimulations.

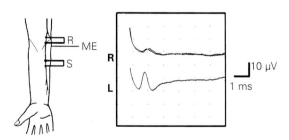

Figure 2.24

Mild thoracic outlet syndrome. The needle examination of the C-8–T-1 innervated muscles and the motor and sensory conduction studies of the ulnar and median nerves gave normal results only when the right medial antebrachial cutaneous nerve was impaired (5μV vs 15μV). ME, medial emicondyle; R, recording; S, stimulation; L, left; R, right.

involved. CMAP and SAP amplitudes are low or very low in some (ulnar and/or medial antebrachial cutaneous) or all nerves of the upper limb. Distal conduction velocities are normal and needle examinations demonstrate neurogenic patterns in some (hand intrinsics) or all muscles. SSEP and MEP studies demonstrate characteristic important and very frequent CB, with significant conduction slowing between axilla and Erb's point (Figure 2.25), which is infrequent in tumoral lesions. Needle examination is also an important tool in these plexopathies: in radiation neuropathy it shows frequent pseudomyotonic discharge and in tumoral neuropathies it shows abundant spontaneous denervation activities (fibrillation, positive sharp waves). The clinical data are also important considerations (Seror, 2001), since a painful brachial plexus lesion occurring less than 5 years after breast cancer treatment will in 90% of cases be a recurrence of the cancer, while a painless brachial plexus lesion occurring under 10 years after cancer treatment will in 90% of cases be a postradiation plexopathy. Naturally, these clinical considerations should not prevent EDX examination. The EDX sensitivity is 100%.

For the clinician or electromyographer recognizing *exceptional entrapment neuropathies* requires two things: one must think of the possible diagnoses; and must have sufficient experience of these particular EDX testings to be able to assess nerve conduction abnormalities. *Ulnar dorsal sensory branch* (Kim et al. 1981) lesions are usually due to extrinsic compression (e.g. cast or bandage) or to laceration. *Lateral* and *medial antebranchial cutaneous nerves* (Foucher, 1996; Seror, 1993b) may also be entrapped by different mechanisms (e.g. fibrous band, lipoma, cast). *Digital nerves* (median or ulnar) can be entrapped against the deep transverse metacarpal ligament (Dawson et al., 1982) or injured by microtraumatisms (Sheilds and Jacobs, 1986).

Differential diagnosis

Polyneuropathies

Only demyelinating neuropathies can perfectly mimic entrapment neuropathies as they can involve a single trunk at the onset of the disease.

In such a case, only an enlarged EDX examination or evolution may confirm the correct diagnosis. Three diseases merit special attention. *Hereditary neuropathy with liability to pressure palsy* (Bouche and Vallat, 1992; Serratrice et al., 1985, 1987) is characterized by focal nerve impairment in entrapment sites. Surgical releases are sometimes required when sensory symptoms are persistent or when weakness is not resolutive. EDX differentiates it easily from entrapment neuropathies, as all the entrapment sites show an abnormal nerve conduction despite there being no clinical complaint. *Chronic inflammatory demyelinating polyneuropathy*, Lewis and Sumner type (Lewis et al., 1982), provides sensory–motor symptoms with focal impairment (CB) on a single nerve trunk at the onset; patients are frequently operated on since medical entrapment neuropathies care remains ineffective. *Motor multifocal neuropathy* (Bouche and Vallat, 1992; Pestronk et al., 1988; Seror, 1996e) with persistent CB can clinically mimic pure motor entrapment neuropathies. Symptoms at onset usually involve the upper limbs in adults. EDX easily differentiates this condition from others as sensory fibers remain normal at the site of the motor CB. Since other nerve lesions are frequently asymptomatic, CB and velocity showing are found only by a large EDX examination.

Parsonage–Turner neuralgic amyotrophy (Turner and Parsonage, 1970) is a frequent and underrecognized cause of mononeuritis or plexitis. Clinical differential diagnosis with some entrapment neuropathies (e.g. suprascapular, axillary, long thoracic, anterior interosseous nerves) is especially difficult and sometimes leads to unnecessary surgical release (Figure 2.23; Case report 4). The opposite is also possible, leading to delayed surgery. The role of EDX is essential to differentiate both neuropathies (entrapment and neuritis).

Brachial plexus injuries can mimic some entrapment neuropathies but onset circumstances usually help to recognize them. Shoulder luxation and motorcycle accidents are frequent causes. EDX is characterized by specific EMG abnormalities depending on the lesion site (e.g. nerves, cords, trunks or roots) and by SAP amplitude changes. The amplitude is low in the correspondent territory when the lesion is postganglionic and remains normal when the lesion is preganglionic. SSEP are sometimes useful in determining the lesion site.

Cervical root disease is an entrapment neuropathy but is usually classified with differential diagnosis. It is not nowadays possible to perform a monoradicular stimulation above and below the root compression to evaluate the nerve conduction slowing. Cervical root disease is indiscernible from, and frequently associated with, cervicarthrosis myelopathy (Berthier et al., 1996). Only needle examination of muscles in the different myotoma is routinely used to assess a root disorder. SSEP (Berthier et al., 1996; Mauguière et al., 1981; Piadé et al., 1984) can sometimes be useful in assessing some purely sensory root diseases. The EDX sensitivity is less than 50%, but EDX is essential to determine precisely the severity and/or extension of the root disorder, and to differentiate multiroot disease from anterior horn disease. Finally, it is essential in any peripheral nerve lesion to evaluate associated root lesions.

Anterior horn disease can be a differential diagnosis of entrapment neuropathies, as it can first involve upper limbs. It usually realizes an Aran Duchenne hand amyotrophy. EDX locates pure motor involvement in the upper limbs and also in the lower limbs, neck and face. When this diffusion is lacking, amyotrophic lateral sclerosis cannot be confirmed, and cervicarthrosis myelopathy and syringomyelia should be considered. Sometimes, especially in young patients (Biondi et al, 1989, Hirayama et al., 1987; Seror, 1996a), anterior horn disease may involve only one upper limb (Figure 2.16) and may lead to the consideration of TOS (Case report 6).

Syringomyelia can realize a typical sensory disease but also an unusual pure "motor" disorder. EDX findings are similar to those encountered in cervicarthrosis myelopathy but magnetic resonance imaging is able to confirm diagnosis.

Cramps and dystonia

Cramps are a rare symptom of the upper limb entrapment neuropathies. Their presence suggests a neurogenic origin of muscle weakness and eliminates myogenic disorders. In contrast, cramps are frequent in *polyneuropathies* (Bouche and Vallat, 1992) as chronic inflammatory demyelination neuropathy, motor multifocal neuropathy, amyotrophic lateral sclerosis etc. *Idiopathic cramps* in the hands during professional

Somatosensory evoked potentials

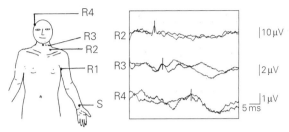

Figure 2.26

Multiple sclerosis. A young woman had been complaining for 20 days about a left upper limb weakness which occurred after a long night of dancing and/or drinking. A brachial plexus injury was diagnosed. Electromyography and nerve conductions were normal. This led to suspicion of a central nervous system lesion. Somatosensory evoked potential (SSEP) study confirmed this hypothesis; it showed a low amplitude and very delayed cortical SSEP (R4=25.2 ms), corresponding to an important central pathway slowing (R3R4=12.3 ms; NI=5.6 ms).

activities are usually caused by *dystonia* and the EDX is normal. When an entrapment neuropathy is demonstrated by EDX, medical treatment (e.g. corticosteroid injection/splintage) should be performed before surgery to evaluate the role of entrapment neuropathy in the symptoms. When dystonia is confirmed, EDX is the first step before treatment with botulinum toxin (Jankovic and Schwartz, 1993). Exceptionally, EDX will suggest a neuromuscular disorder to be myotonia.

Central nervous system diseases

In some cases where central symptoms and their signs are mild or absent, the patient may then logically be referred for an EDX. The needle examination then shows the reduced interference pattern, but never a high firing rate, which is normal, and should lead to an SSEP (Figure 2.26) as visual and audio evoked potentials to assess central pathway involvement (Mauguière et al., 1981). When a central nervous system disease is known, EDX may be useful if a peripheral neuropathy is suspected to be associated with it, such as when central nervous system disease cannot explain all of the symptoms. Sometimes the contrary is the case, i.e. the peripheral neuropathy is known and the central nervous system disease may be identified.

Conclusion

The EDX examination should always be a direct extension of the clinical investigation. In this way it provides a useful quantitative or semiquantitative support to the clinical investigation, e.g. the exact topography, focal or diffuse involvement, the severity of the nerve lesion, the role of axonal loss, and of the CB acute or chronic nerve lesions. EDX has a high sensitivity and specificity in determining nerve lesions, except in proximal segments. In the most difficult cases, the electromyographer's technical experience and a good dialog with the clinician is essential to optimize the interpretation of EDX data. Neuromuscular pathology changes with time and repetition of EDX at the interval of several weeks or months is necessary in the follow-up of recovery, or to assess nerve lesions which were not diagnosed at the first investigation. Finally, EDX evaluation of surgical and non-surgical procedures should be studied more extensively in the clinical evaluation of determining the best treatment for each pathology.

References

Alfonsi E, Moglia A, Sandrini G, Pisoni MR, Arrigo A. (1986) Electrophysiological study of long thoracic nerve conduction in normal subjects. *Electromyogr Clin Neurophysiol* **26**:63–7.

Alnot JY (1984) L'épaule paralytique par l'atteinte des nerfs sus-scapulaire, circonflexe et musculo-cutané. In: Simon, Rodineau, eds. *Epaule et médecine de rééducation*. Paris: Masson, 227–31.

American Association of Electromyography and Electrodiagnosis (1969) One hundred years of research in neuromyography in man 1869–1969. *A historical reprint, 1986*. Rochester: Johnson Printing Company.

American Association of Electrodiagnostic Medicine (1992) Guidelines in electrodiagnostic medicine. *Muscle & Nerve* **15**:229–53.

Aminoff MJ, Olney RK, Parry GJ, Raskin NMH. (1988) Relative utility of different electrophysiologic techniques in the evaluation of brachial plexopathies. *Neurol* **38**:546–50.

Bardot A, Benaim L, Olivares JP, Baetche C, Guillermet AC. (1985) La pathologie du nerf sus scaupaire. In: Simon, ed. *10ème actualité en rééducation fonctionelle et réadaptation*. Paris: Masson, 165–73.

Berthier E, Turjman F, Mauguiere F. (1996) Diagnostic utility of somatosensory evoked potentials (SEPs) in presurgical assessment of cervical spondylotic myelopathy. *Neurophysiol Clin* **26**:300–10.

Biondi A, Dormont D, Weitzner Bouche P, Chaine P, Bories J. (1991) MR imaging of the cervical cord in juvenile amyotrophy of distal upper extremity. *AJNR* **10**:263–8.

Bouche P, Vallat AM. (1992) *Neuropathies périphériques, polyneuropathies et mononeuropathies multiples*. Paris: Doin.

Brichet B, Werner JE, Vespignani H, Weber M. (1980) Apport de l'électromyographie à l'étude des lésions nerveuses du nerf cubital à la main: le syndrome de compression de la branche motrice du nerf cubital. *Rev EEG Neurophysiol* **10**:47–54.

Bromberg MB. (1991) Comparison of electrodiagnostic criteria for primary demyelination in chronic polyneuropathy. *Muscle & Nerve* **14**:968–76.

Brown WF, Ferguson GG, Jones MW, Yates SK. (1976) The location of conduction abnormalities in human entrapment neuropathies. *J Canadian Sci Neurol* **3**:111–22.

Buchthal F, Rosenfalk A. (1966) Evoked action potential and conduction velocity in human. *Brain* **3**:1–122.

Buchthal F, Rosenfalk A, Trojaborg W. (1974) Electrophysiological findings in entrapment of the median nerve at wrist and elbow. *J Neurol Neurosurg Psychiatry* **37**:340–60.

Chiappa KH. (1983) *Evoked potentials in clinical medicine*. New York: Raven Press; 340.

Chodoroff G, Lee DW, Honet JC. (1985) Dynamic approach in the diagnosis of the thoracic outlet syndrome using somatosensory evoked responses. *Arch Phys Med Rehabil* **66**:3–6.

Chu Andrews J, Johnson RJ. (1980) *Electrodiagnosis: an anatomical and clinical approach*. Philadelphia: Lippincott.

CRITERIA (1991) Criteria for diagnostis of chronic inflammatory demyelination of polyneuropathy (CIDP).

Report from an ad hoc subcommittee of the American Academy of Neurology AIDS Task Force. *Neurology* **41**:617–18.

Dawson DM, Hallett M, Millender LH. (1982) *Entrapment neuropathies*. Boston: Little Brown.

Duchenne de Boulogne (1872) *De l'électrisation localisée*, 3rd edn. Paris: Bailliere.

Eaton LLM, Lambert EH. (1957) Electromyography and electric stimulation of nerves in diseases of motor unit. Observations on myasthenic syndrome associated with malignant tumors. *J Am Med Assoc* **163**:1117–24.

Eisen A. (1974) Early diagnosis of ulnar nerve palsy: an electrophysiologic study. *Neurology* **24**:256–62.

Eisen A, Hoirch M, Moll A. (1983) Evaluation of radiculopathies by segmental stimulation and somatosensory evoked potentials. *Canadian J Neurol Sci* **10**:178–82.

Ekman Orderberg GE, Salgeback S, Orderberg G. (1987) Carpal tunnel syndrome in pregnancy. *Acta Obstet Gynecol Scand* **66**:233–5.

Foucher G. (1996) Compression du nerf musculo-cutané. *Rhumatologie* **48**:319–20.

Gilliat RW, Thomas PK. (1960) Changes in nerve conduction with ulnar lesions at elbow. *J Neurol Neurosurg Psychiatry* **23**:312–19.

Gilliat RW, Willison DM, Dietz V, Williams IR. (1978) Peripheral nerve conduction in patients with a cervical rib and band. *Ann Neurol* **4**: 124–9.

Goulon M, Lord G, Bedoiseau M. (1963) L'atteinte du median et du cubital par apophyse sus-épitrochléenne: a propos de 2 observations. *Presse Med* **71**:2355–7.

Gross MS, Gerlbermann RH. (1985) The anatomy of the distal ulnar tunnel. *Clin Orthopaedics and Related Research* **196**:238–47.

Guillain G, Courtellemont H. (1905) L'action du muscle court supinateur dans la paralysie du nerf radial: pathogenie d'une paralysie radial incomplète chez un chef d'orchestre. *Presse Med* **7**:50–2.

Harding C, Halar E. (1983) Motor and sensory ulnar nerve conduction velocities: effect of elbow positon. *Arch Phys Med Rehabil* **64**:227–32.

Hill NA, Howard FM, Huffer BR. (1985) The incomplete anterior interosseous nerve syndrome. *J Hand Surg* **10A**:4–16.

Hirayama K, Tomonaga M, Litano K, Yamada T, Kojima S, Arai K. (1987) Focal cervical poliopathy causing juvenile muscular atrophy of distal upper extremity: a pathological study. *J Neuro Neurosurg Psychiatry* **50**:285–90.

Hoshizume H, Inoue H, Nagashima K, Hamaya K. (1993) Posterior interosseous nerve paralysis related to focal radial nerve constriction secondary to vasculitis. *J Hand Surg* **18B**:757–60.

Isch F. (1963) *Electromyographie*. Paris: Doin.

Jablecki CK, Andary M, So Y, Wilkins D, Williams F. (1993) Literature review of the usefulness of nerve conduction studies and electromyography for the evaluation of patients with carpal tunnel syndrome. *Muscle & Nerve* **16**:1392–414.

Jankovic J, Schwartz KS. (1993) Use of botulinum toxin in the treatment of hand dystonia. *J Hand Surg* **18A**:883–7.

Jebsen RH. (1966) Motor conduction velocity of distal radial nerve. *Arch Phys Med Rehabil* **47**:12–16.

Kamp Nielsen V. (1973) Sensory and motor nerve conduction in the median nerve in normal subjects. *Acta Med Scand* **194**:435–43.

Karam DB. (1986) AIDS and electromyography. *Arch Phys Med Rehabil* **67**:491.

Kiloh LG, Nevin S. (1952) Isolated neuritis of the anterior interosseous nerve. *BMJ* April: 850–1.

Kim DJ, Kalantri A, Guha S, Wainapel F. (1981) Dorsal cutaneous ulnar nerve conduction: diagnostic aid in ulnar neuropathy. *Arch Neurol* **38**:321–2.

Kimura J. (1979) The carpal tunnel syndrome. Localization of conduction abnormalities within the distal segment of median nerve. *Brain* **102**:619–35.

Kimura J. (1989) *Electrodiagnosis in diseases of nerve and muscle. Principles and practice*. Philadelphia: David Co.

Lacote M. Chevalier AM, Miranda A, Bleton JP, Stevenin P. (1980) *Evaluation clinique de la fonction musculaire*. Paris: Maloine.

Le Forestier N, Maisonabe T, Moulonguet A, Leger JM, Bouche P. (1998) True neurogenic outlet syndrome: electrophysiological diagnosis in six cases. *Muscle Nerve* **21**: 1129–34.

Leger JM, Pouget J, Said G, Vallats JM (1996) Neuropathies dysimmunitaires. Réunion internationnale de la Société Français de Neurologie Paris. *Rev Neurol* **152**:307–416.

Lewis RA, Summer AJ, Brown MJ, Asbury AK. (1982) Multiofocal demyelinating neuropathy with persistent conduction block. *Neurology* **32**:958–64.

Licht S. (1980) History of electromyography. In: Johson EW, ed. *Practical electromyography*. London: Williams & Wilkins, 403–23.

Livingstone EF, Delisa JA, Halar EM. (1984) Electrodiagnostic values through the thoracic outlet using C8 root needle studies, F-waves, and cervical somatosensory evoked potentials. *Arch Phys Med Rehabil* **65**:726–30.

Logigian EL, Kelly JJ, Adelman LS (1994) Nerve conduction and biopsy correlation in over 100 consecutive patients with suspected polyneuropathy. *Muscle Nerve* **17**:1010–20.

Lussiez B, Courbier R, Toussaint B, Benichou M, Gomis R, Allieu Y. (1993) Paralysie radiale au bras après effort musculaire à propos de 4 cas Etude clinique et physio-pathologique. *Ann Chir Main* **12**:130–5.

Mackinnon SE, Novak CB. (1994) Clinical commentary: pathogenesis of cumulative trauma disorder. *J Hand Surg* **19A**:873–83.

Marie P, Foix C. (1913) Atrophie isolée de l'éminence thénar d'origien névretique. Rôle du ligament annulaire antérieur du carpe dans le pathogénie de la lésion. *Rev Neurol* **21**:647–9.

Matsen FA, Mayo KA, Krugmire RB, Sheridan GW, Kraft GH. (1977) A model compartmental syndrome in man with particular reference to the quantification of nerve function. *J Bone Joint Surg* **59A**:648–53.

Mauguière F, Brunon AM, Echallier JF, Courjon J. (1981) Intérêt des potentiels évoqués somesthésiques précoses dans l'exploraiton des voies de la sensibilité lemniscale: mise au point à propos de 167 observations et revue de la littérature. *Rev Neurol* **137**:1–19.

McDougall AJ, McLeod JG (1996) Autonomic neuropathy, I. Clinical features, investigation, pathophysiology and treatment. *J Neurol Sci* **137**:79–88.

Merlevede K, They P, Van Hees J. (2000) Diagnosis of ulnar neuropathy: a new approach. *Muscle Nerve* **23**: 478–81.

Mittal RL, Gupta BR. (1978) Median and ulnar nerve palsy: an unusual presentation of the supracondyla process. *J Bone Joint Surg* **60A**:557–8.

Narakas A. (1974) Epicondylite et syndrome compressif du nerf radial. *Med et Hygiène* **1129**:2067–8.

Nathan PA, Meadoxs KD, Doyle LS. (1988) Sensory segmental latency values of the median nerve for a population of normal individuals. *Arch Phys Med Rehabil* **69**:499–501.

Netter FH. (1991) Anatomy, physiology, and methabolic disorders, musculoskeletal system. In: *The Ciba collection of medical illustration*. West Caldwell: Ciba-Geigy Corporation.

Nigst H, Dick W. (1979) Syndromes of compression of the median nerve in the proximal forearm pronator teres syndrome; anterior interosseous nerve syndrome. *Arch Orth Traum Surg* **93**:307–12.

Nishida T, Price SJ, Minieka MM. (1993) Medial antebrachial cutaneous nerve conduction in true neurogenic thoracic outlet syndrome. *Electromyogr Clin Neurophysiol* **33**: 285–8.

Parsonage MJ, Turner JWA. (1948) The shoulder girdle syndrome. *Lancet* **i**:973–8.

Pestronk A, Cornblath DR, Ilyas AA, et al. (1988) A treatable multifocal motor neuropathy with antibodies to GM1 ganglioside. *Annals Neurol* **24**:73–8.

Phalen GS. (1966) The carpal tunnel syndrome. Seventeen years' experience in diagnosis and treatment of six hundred and fifty-four hands. *J Bone Joint Surg* **48A**:211–28.

Piadé JP, Pelissier J, Georgescu M, Blotman F, Cadilhac J, Simon L. (1984) Potentiels évoqués somesthésiques de moelle et névralgie cervico-brachiale. *Rev Rhum* **51**:7–13.

Pitres A, Testut L. (1925) *Les nerfs en schémas. Anatomie et physiopathologie. Traité d'anatomie humaine*. Paris: Doin.

Pou-Serradel A, Palazzi-Coll S. (1993) Lésions foiales du nerf radial au cours de la néurolgie amyotrophiante de l'épaule de Parsonage and Turner. In Serratine G, ed. *Système nerveux, muscles et maladies systemiques*. Paris: Expansion Scientifique Française; 222–9.

Preston DC, Logigian EL. (1992) Lumbrical and interossei recording in carpal tunnel syndrome. *Muscle & Nerve* **15**:1253–7.

Rainer WG, Mayer J, Sadler TR. (1973) Effect of graded compression on nerve conduction velocity. *Arch Surg* **107**:719–21.

Reddy MP. (1983) Conduction studies of the medial cutaneous nerve of the forearm. *Arch Phys Med Rehabil* **64**: 209–11.

Ritts GD, Wood MB, Linscheid RL. (1987) Radial tunnel syndrome: a ten year surgical experience. *Clin Osthopea Relat Res* **219**:201–5.

Seror P. (1983) Comparison of the distal motor latency of the first dorsal interosseous with abductor pollicis brevis (report of 200 cases). *Electromyogr Clin Neurophys* **28**:341–5.

Seror P. (1989a) Le test centimétrique: test diagnostic de certitude du syndronme du canal carpien très fruste? *Ann Chir Main* **8**:254–64.

Seror P. (1989b) A la recherche d'une corrélation électro-clinique au cours du syndrome du canal carpien. *Rev Rhum* **54**: 643–8.

Seror P. (1990) Reflexion sur les tests dynamiques en neurophysiologie. In: *EMG 90 7ème Congrès d'EMG de Langue Française Montpellier 3–5 mai 1990*, 153–61.

Seror P. (1991) Carpal tunnel syndrome in the elderly. 'Beware of severe cases'. *Ann Hand Surg*, **10**:217–25.

Seror P. (1992) L'atteinte du nerf cubital au coude: données épidémiologiques, cliniques, électromyographiques (à propos de 312 patients). *Rev Rhum* **59**:813–19.

Seror P. (1993a) Electromyography of the upper limb: technique, application and limits. In: Tubiana et al., eds. *The Hand, Vol IV*. Philadelphia: Saunders.

Seror P. (1993b) Forearm secondary to compression of the medial antebrachial cutaneous nerve at the elbow. *Arch Phys Med Rehabil* **74**:540–2.

Seror P. (1994) Sensitivity of the various tests for diagnosis of carpal tunnel syndrome. *J Hand Surg* **19B**:725–8.

Seror P. (1995a) The value of the special motor and sensory tests for the diagnosis of benign and minor median nerve lesion at the wrist. *Am J Phys Rehabil* **74**:124–9.

Seror P. (1995b) Les potentiels évoqués somesthésiques et les potentiels évoqués moteurs étagés dans l'étude de la conduction nerveuse periphérique proximale. *Ann Chir Main* **14**:182–91.

Seror P. (1996a) Amyotrophie monomélique bénigne et atrophie spinale localisée. *Presse Med* **25**:82.

Seror P. (1996b) Anterior interosseous nerve lesion clinical and electrophysiological features. *J Bone Joint Surg* **78B**:238–41.

Seror P. (1996c) Posterior interosseous nerve conduction a new method of evaluation. *Am J Phys Med Rehabil* **75**:35–9.

Seror P. (1996d) The axonal carpal tunnel syndrome. *Electroencephalogr Clin Neurophysiol.* **101**:197–200.

Seror P. (1996e) Hypertrophie musculaire et neuropathie motrice multifocale. *Presse Med* **25**:1891.

Seror P. (1996f) Les compressions nerveuses tronculaires du membre supérieur au cours de la PR. In: Allieu Y, ed. *La main et le poignet Rhumatoïde*. Paris: Expansion Scientifique.

Seror P. (1997) Le syndrome du canal carpien de la grossesse. *J Gynecol Obstet Biol Reprod* **26**:148–53.

Seror P. (1999a) Electrodiagnostic examination of the anterior interosseous nerve. Normal and pathologic data. *Electromyogr Clin Neurophysics* **39**:183–9.

Seror P. (1999b) Ulnar conduction block at the wrist. *Arch Phys Med Rehabil* **80**:1346–8.

Seror P. (2000) Comparative diagnostic sensitivities of orthodromic and antidromic sensory inching test in mild carpal tunnel syndrome. *Arch Phys Med Rehabil* **81**:442–6.

Seror P. (2001) Brachial plexus neoplastic lesions assessed by conduction study of medial antebrachial cutaneous nerve. *Muscle Nerve* **24**: 1068–70.

Seror P. (forthcoming) Simplified orthodomic inch testing in mild carpal tunnel syndrome. *Muscle Nerve* **25**.

Seror P, Bouche P. (1997) Névralgie amyotrophiante post-opératoire du nerf cubital: 4 cas. *Rev Neurol* **153**:201–4.

Seror P, Alliot F, Cluzan RV, Pascot M. (1999) Resultats d'une consultation neurophysiologique chez des patientes atteintes d'un lymphoêdème secondaire du membre supérieur après cancer du sein et présentant des troubles neurologiques. *J Mal Vasc* **24**:294–9.

Serratrice G. (1963) *Le diagnostic clinique dans les maladies neuro-musculaires*. Paris: Doin.

Serratrice G, Pellissier JF, Pouget J et al. (1987) Les neuropathies allantoïdiennes (tomaculaires): étude de 23 cas. *Sem Hôp* Paris **63**:2353–63.

Serratrice G, Pouget J, Pellissier JF. (1985) Des formes familiales du syndrome de Parsonnage Turner aux hérédopathies tomaculaires du plexus brachial. *Rev Rhum* **52**:625–9.

Seze S, de Dreyfus P. (1964) Acroparesthésies et syndrome du canal carpien problèmes nosologiques (A propos de 110 observations). *Rev Rhum* **3**:560–4.

Shields RW, Jacobs B. (1986) Median palmar digital neuropathy in a cheerleader. *Arch Phys Med Rehabil* **67**:824–5.

Siivola J, Pokela R, Sulg I. (1983) Somatosensory evoked responses as a diagnostic in thoracic outlet syndrome. *Acta Chir Scand* **149**:147–50.

Simpson JA. (1956) Electrical signs in the diagnosis of carpal tunnel and related syndromes. *J Neurol Pyschiatry* **19**:275–80.

Spinner M. (1970) The anterior interosseous nerve syndrome: with special attention to its variations. *JBJS* **52A**:84–94.

Stevens JC, Beard CM, O'Fallon WM, Kurland LT. (1992) Conditions associated with carpel tunnel syndrome. *Mayo Clin Proc* **67**:541–8.

Sunderland S. (1976) The nerve lesion in the carpal tunnel syndrome. *J Neurol Neurosurg Psychiatry* **39**:615–26.

Sunderland SS (1978) *Nerves and nerve injuries.* Edinburgh: Churchill Livingstone.

Swash M, Schwartz MS. (1981) *Neuromuscular diseases.* New York: Springer Verlag.

Testut MF, Bonnevialle P. Mansat M, Guiraud B, Grezes-Rueff Ch, Rascol A. (1984) Apport de l'électromyographie dans le diagnostic de la neuropathie non traumatique du nerf radial au coude. *Lyon Medical* **15 November:** 301–3.

Thompson LL. (1964) *The electromyographer handbook.* Paris: Maloine.

Turner JW, Parsonage MJ. (1957) Neuralgic amyotrophy (paralytic brachial neuritis) with special reference to prognosis. *Lancet* **II**:209–12.

Uncini A, di Muzio A, Awad J, Manente G, Tafuro M, Gambi D. (1993) Sensitivity of three median-to-ulnar comparative tests in diagnosis of mild carpal tunnel syndrome. *Muscle & Nerve* **16**:1366–73.

Weber RJ, Piero DL. (1978) F wave evaluation of thoracic outlet syndrome: a multiple regresson derived F wave latency predicitng technique. *Arch Phys Rehabil* **59**:464–9.

Wu JS, Morris JD, Hogan GR. (1985) Ulnar neuropathy at the wrist: case report and review of literature. *Arch Phys Med Rehabil* **66**:785–8.

Yiannikas C, Walsh JC. (1983) Somatosensory evoked responses in the diagnosis of thoracic outlet syndrome. *J Neurol Neurosurg Psychiatry* **46**:234–40.

Yiannikas C, Shahani BT, Young RR. (1983) The investigation of traumatic lesions of the brachial plexus by electromyography and short latency somatosensory potentials evoked by stimulation of the multiple peripheral nerves. *J Neurol Neurosurg Psychiatry* **46**:1014–22.

3
Patient evaluation of nerve compression in the upper limb

Christine B. Novak

Introduction

The evaluation and management of the patient with nerve compression can be challenging, particularly in the patient with diffuse upper extremity symptoms and multiple level nerve compression. Many tests and measures have been introduced to assess patients with nerve compression, although no one test has been universally accepted as the gold standard (Bell-Krotoski, 1990; Dellon, 1980, 1981; Gelberman et al., 1983; Greenspan and Lamotte, 1993; Grunert et al., 1990; Gunnarsson et al., 1997; Mackinnon and Novak, 1996; Mielke et al., 1996; Moberg, 1991; Novak et al., 1992, 1993a,b,c, 1994; Paley and McMurtry, 1985; Phalen, 1972). Clinical evaluation of the patient with nerve compression requires a systematic approach to identify all levels of nerve compression and associated musculoskeletal disorders.

Histopathology

Understanding the variability of patient signs and symptoms requires an understanding of the histopathology of chronic nerve compression. There are very few reported investigations regarding the histopathology of chronic nerve compression in humans. This limited information is likely related to the limited availability of neural tissue from patients with this disorder. Numerous animal models for chronic nerve compression have been described and much of the available literature on humans has been extrapolated from the animal models (Aguayo et al., 1971; Mackinnon and Dellon, 1986; Mackinnon et al., 1984, 1985, 1986; O'Brien et al., 1987). The histopathology of chronic nerve compression spans a spectrum of changes (Lundborg, 1988; Mackinnon and Dellon, 1988; Mackinnon et al., 1984, 1985; O'Brien et al., 1987). Early changes begin with edema in the perineurial blood–nerve barrier, followed by thickening of the connective tissue in the epineurium. With increased duration of compression, the myelinated fibers will undergo segmental demyelination and then more diffuse demyelination will occur. The unmyelinated fibers will undergo a process of degeneration followed by regeneration. With additional compression, there will be axonal degeneration of the myelinated fibers. These changes occur slowly, dependent on the duration of compression and amount of compressive force. The changes in the nerve, however, may not occur uniformly across the nerve. Those fascicles that are located on the periphery and closer to the compressive forces may undergo changes earlier and more rapidly than the fascicles located in the interior of the nerve (Lundborg, 1988; Lundborg and Dahlin, 1994). These interior fascicles may be more protected by the surrounding fascicles and connective tissue and therefore chronic changes due to compression may be delayed.

Patient symptoms will parallel the histopathologic changes that occur in the nerve, and therefore the clinical manifestation will not be uniform but vary through a range of clinical signs and symptoms (Figure 3.1). The changes that occur with compression of a motor nerve are well

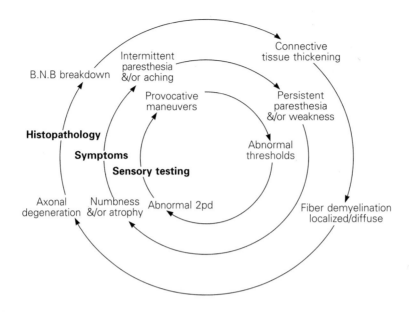

Figure 3.1

The histopathology of chronic nerve compression will begin with edema in the perineurium and progress to axonal degeneration. Similarly, patient symptoms will span a range of patient complaints and the sensitivity of clinical tests will vary through the progression of neural changes.

described; aching, followed by weakness and finally muscle atrophy. Similarly, compression of a sensory nerve will produce sensory complaints that vary, beginning with intermittent paresthesia, progressing to constant paresthesia and finally to constant numbness. The frequency and characteristics of the complaints will depend on the severity of the nerve compression. Patients in the early stages of chronic nerve compression may only have symptoms of intermittent paresthesia with prolonged positioning, i.e. wrist flexion at night may result in compression of the median nerve at the carpal canal, producing paresthesia to the median nerve distribution. As the degree of nerve compression progresses, patients will report more frequent paresthesia and perhaps occasional numbness and/or weakness with severe compression, complaints will progress to constant numbness in the sensory distribution of the entrapped nerve and to muscle atrophy.

Double crush hypothesis

The double crush hypothesis was introduced by Upton and McComas describing an association

between distal nerve entrapments (carpal tunnel syndrome and ulnar neuropathy) and cervical root lesions (Upton and McComas, 1973). They hypothesized that a proximal level of nerve compression will cause the more distal sites to be less tolerant to compression. The clinical association between proximal level nerve compression (cervical root lesions and/or thoracic outlet syndrome) and distal levels of nerve compression has also been supported by others (Hurst et al., 1983; Mackinnon, 1992; Novak et al., 1993b; Omurtag et al., 1996; Upton and McComas, 1973; Wood et al., 1988). Hurst et al. reported a higher incidence of carpal tunnel syndrome in patients with mild proximal impingement resulting from cervical arthritis (Hurst et al., 1985). Wood et al. reported on 165 cases of thoracic outlet syndrome and in 73 cases there was a site of distal nerve compression as confirmed by electrodiagnostic studies (Wood and Biondi, 1990). In our review of 50 patients with thoracic outlet syndrome, we found 64% of patients with positive provocative tests at the carpal tunnel and cubital tunnel (Novak et al., 1993b). The double crush concept was further expanded by Lundborg to include the reverse double crush, where a distal site of entrapment can affect the more proximal sites (Lundborg, 1988). It is the summation of forces along the entire nerve that produces a sensory disturbance in the associated neural distribution. Evaluation at a single compression site may reproduce symptoms, but it would not reveal other sites that are also causing additional compression. For example, the median nerve may be compressed at the carpal tunnel, at the forearm and at the brachial plexus, producing sensory complaints in the median nerve distribution. Evaluation at only the carpal tunnel may reproduce patient symptoms in the median nerve distribution of the hand, but it would not identify more proximal compression sites. If treatment is directed only at the level of the carpal tunnel, it would fail to totally alleviate all symptoms in the patient with undetected proximal sites of compression and thus be classified as a 'treatment failure'. The concept of the double crush on nerve compression would suggest that all sites of potential compression in the upper extremity should be evaluated in order to identify all levels of compression and to formulate a treatment plan to address all sites of compression (Lundborg, 1988; Mackinnon, 1992; Mackinnon and Dellon, 1988; Upton and McComas, 1973).

Evaluation of sites of nerve compression

Many clinical tests and measures have been described to detect and evaluate nerve compression, but none has been accepted as the gold standard (Bell-Krotoski, 1990; Dellon, 1980, 1981; Gelberman et al., 1983; Greenspan and Lamotte, 1993; Grunert et al., 1990; Gunnarsson et al., 1997; Mackinnon and Novak, 1996; Mielke et al., 1996; Novak et al., 1992, 1993a,b,c, 1994; Paley and McMurtry, 1985; Phalen 1972). Because the histopathology of nerve compression and patient symptoms vary through a spectrum of changes, it is unlikely that one test will adequately detect nerve compression through the full spectrum of mild to severe chronic nerve compression (see Figure 3.1). In the early stages of nerve compression, maneuvers of provocation will be most sensitive in eliciting symptoms and thus in detecting sites of nerve compression (deKrom et al., 1990; Dellon, 1980; Gonzalez Del Pino, 1997;

MacDermid, 1991; Williams et al., 1992). At this early stage, all other tests, including electrophysiological tests and sensory assessment, may be negative. With moderate nerve compression, tests of threshold (vibration and cutaneous pressure) will become abnormal and with more severe compression and axonal degeneration, the two-point discrimination (2pd) will become abnormal (Gelberman et al., 1983; Jetzer, 1991; Lundborg et al., 1986, 1992; MacDermid, 1991; Mackinnon and Dellon, 1988; Novak et al., 1992, 1993b; Szabo and Chidley, 1989; Szabo et al., 1984).

Evaluation of patients with potential nerve compression is best achieved with a thorough clinical examination. This should begin with a history and subjective report of symptoms, including exacerbating and relieving activities, postures and positions. Components of the clinical examination will be determined by the subjective patient report. It is necessary to ask specific questions regarding symptoms in the entire upper extremity, including the cervical and scapular region. Patients should be asked specific questions regarding nocturnal symptoms. Patients will often awaken at night with pain, paresthesia and/or numbness or awaken in the morning with these symptoms in the arm and/or cervical region. Complaints of paresthesia and/or numbness to a specific nerve distribution such as the median, ulnar or radial sensory nerve will lead the examiner to the assessment of the associated sites of entrapment in the upper extremity. However, the entire upper quarter should be examined to identify all problems associated with the neural and/or musculoskeletal systems.

Entrapped nerves demonstrate an increased sensitivity to mechanical pressure or tension and therefore provocative maneuvers that increase pressure or tension on the nerve will reproduce symptoms in the sensory distribution of the compressed nerve. Clinical testing for carpal tunnel syndrome is well described and may be extrapolated to the other nerve entrapment sites in the upper extremity (Table 3.1) (Durkan 1997; Gonzalez Del Pino et al., 1997; Gunnarsson et al., 1997; MacDermid 1991; Mackinnon and Novak, 1996; Novak et al., 1992, 1993b, 1994; Paley and McMurtry, 1985; Phalen, 1972, 1996; Williams et al., 1992). In the early stages of nerve compression, pressure provocative or movement provocative maneuvers may be the only positive finding. The provocative tests include Tinel's sign, movements that place pressure on the nerve by tension or compression and direct digital compression on the nerve.

Tinel's sign

A Tinel's sign or direct nerve percussion is performed by applying 4–6 digital taps on the nerve in the known regions of entrapment. A positive response is determined with an 'electric' type response in the appropriate nerve distribution. At the carpal tunnel, the Tinel's sign has been shown to have a sensitivity of 56–67% in those patients with electrodiagnostically confirmed carpal tunnel syndrome (Durkan, 1997; Williams et al., 1992). Williams et al. reported a positive predictive value of 50% with the Tinel's sign. Phalen (1966) described a group of patients with carpal tunnel syndrome (n=654) and 73% of patients had a positive Tinel's sign. A

Tinel's sign should be applied to the median nerve at the carpal tunnel and also on the median nerve in the proximal third of the forearm in the region of the pronator teres. The radial sensory nerve is assessed by applying digital percussion along the nerve beginning at the musculotendinous region of the brachioradialis and the junction of the extensor carpi radialis longus and progressing distally along the lateral border of the forearm to the wrist. The ulnar nerve at the cubital tunnel is assessed by tapping along the ulnar nerve beginning just proximal to the cubital tunnel and continuing along the course of the ulnar nerve to the flexor carpi ulnaris. We previously found that the Tinel's sign had a 70% sensitivity and 98% specificity in patients with cubital tunnel syndrome confirmed with nerve conduction studies (Novak et al., 1994). For the brachial plexus, a Tinel's sign is applied to the brachial plexus supraclavicularly between the scalene muscles. Many patients may report tenderness with digital percussion in the region of the scalene muscles, but a positive

Table 3.1 Provocative tests for nerve entrapment*

	Entrapment Site	Provocative Test	Management
Median nerve	Carpal tunnel	Pressure proximal to carpal tunnel Phalen's test Reverse Phalen's test (Hyperextension Wrist)	Night splint wrist in neutral

	Proximal forearm	Pressure over proximal forearm
		  in region of pronator teres
		Resisted elbow flexion, pronation
		  and long finger flexion
			Stretch pronator teres
			Rest periods in supination

Ulnar nerve	Guyon's canal	Pressure proximal to Guyon's canal	Night splint wrist in neutral

	Cubital tunnel	Elbow flexion and pressure
		  proximal to cubital tunnel
			Elbow pad
			Education: to decrease direct pressure
			  on nerve and avoid elbow flexion

Radial nerve	Forearm	Pressure over junction of
		Brachioradialis/extensor carpi
		  radialis tendon
		Forearm pronation with
		  wrist ulnar flexion
			Positioning in supination and avoid
			  repetitive pronation and supination
			  activities

Brachial plexus	Supraclavicular
	and infraclavicular
		Arm elevation above head
		Pressure over brachial plexus in
		  interscalene region
			Avoid arm elevated positions
			Postural correction
			Stretch shortened muscles and strengthen
			  weakened scapular stabilizers

*Reproduced with permission from Mackinnon SE, Novak CB. Evaluation of the patient with thoracic outlet syndrome. In: Cox JL, Mackinnon SE (eds) *Seminars in thoracic and cardiovascular surgery*, 1996;**8**(2):190–100.

Tinel's sign is recorded only with an 'electric' type response in the upper extremity.

Provocative pressure tests

Provocative maneuvers for the diagnosis of carpal tunnel syndrome have been extensively evaluated with little consensus on the best clinical test. First introduced by Phalen, the wrist flexion test was reported to be 'usually positive' in his review of 654 cases of carpal tunnel syndrome (Phalen, 1966). In patients with limited wrist motion, there may be insufficient wrist flexion to increase the pressure within the carpal canal. In these cases, a wrist flexion test may yield a false negative in patients with true median nerve compression at the wrist. Paley and McMurtry (1985) introduced the pressure provocative test for the median nerve at the carpal tunnel, thereby avoiding the problem of limited wrist flexion in some patients. This pressure test was evaluated by Williams et al. (1992) who showed it to have good sensitivity (100%), specificity (97%) and positive predictive value (100%) in those patients with carpal tunnel syndrome when applying 150 mmHg pressure at the wrist with a sphygmomanometer. A variation of this test was described by Durkan (1997), where the site of compression was at the level of the carpal canal and also just distal to the carpal canal. Durkan (1997) reported a sensitivity of 87% and specificity of 90–95% using this compression test. Gonzalez et al. (1997) evaluated 200 hands with carpal tunnel syndrome and 200 hands in 100 healthy volunteers using Durkan's test and reported 87% sensitivity and 95% specificity. Therefore it appears that direct digital compression of the median nerve is a sensitive test in detecting carpal tunnel syndrome. However, to isolate the site of compression, it is important to ensure that only one entrapment site is placed in a position of provocation. For example, a provocative test, that places the forearm in full supination, the elbow in extension and wrist in flexion and reproduces symptoms into the median nerve distribution, may be concurrently provoking symptoms from both the carpal tunnel and median nerve in the forearm. It would therefore be difficult to determine if the provocation producing the symptoms was a result of the compression from the carpal tunnel or at the level of the pronator teres.

Cubital tunnel syndrome is described as ulnar nerve compression at the cubital tunnel of the elbow. The ulnar nerve is located posterior to the medial epicondyle and with elbow flexion the ulnar nerve is placed on tension. With elbow flexion, the nerve is also in a more superficial position behind the elbow and therefore it is vulnerable to external compression and trauma. With elbow flexion, not only is the ulnar nerve stretched behind the medial epicondyle but the pressure is increased within the cubital tunnel (Gelberman et al., 1998; Pechan and Julis, 1975). Gelberman et al. (1998) evaluated the cross-sectional areas and intraneural/extraneural pressures of the cubital tunnel and ulnar nerve in 20 cadaver arms. The authors found that the mean cross-sectional areas of the cubital tunnel and ulnar nerve were decreased as the elbow was moved from full extension to 135 degrees of flexion and that the intraneural pressures were significantly greater than the extraneural pressures with elbow flexion (Gelberman et al., 1998). Pechan et al. reported increased pressures within the cubital tunnel with elbow flexion and this pressure was further increased with the addition of wrist extension and arm elevation (Pechan and Julis, 1975). The clinical test for cubital tunnel syndrome using elbow flexion was evaluated by Buehler and Thayer (1998) in 13 patients with cubital tunnel syndrome confirmed with electrodiagnostic tests. Their test position included both elbow flexion and wrist extension and it was found to be a useful provocative test in the diagnosis of cubital tunnel syndrome. However, this type of double compression on the ulnar nerve at the cubital tunnel and Guyon's canal makes it difficult to identify the exact location of positive provocation. Rayan et al. (1992) evaluated the elbow flexion test in a normal population and found it to be positive in 10% of the normal subjects tested. Provocation of the ulnar nerve can be increased with the combination of nerve tension and compression. We described a combination test of elbow flexion and pressure on the ulnar nerve at the cubital tunnel (Novak et al., 1994). This pressure flexion test was evaluated in 32 patients with electrodiagnostically confirmed cubital tunnel syndrome and 33 controls. The sensitivity and specificity using elbow flexion alone or digital pressure on the ulnar nerve alone were lower than the test that combined elbow flexion and ulnar nerve pressure (sensitivity 98%, specificity 95%, positive predictive value 91%).

The diagnosis of thoracic outlet syndrome remains extremely controversial particularly in those patients with subjective neurological complaints rather than vascular complaints. Historically, a number of tests were used for the diagnosis of thoracic outlet syndrome and these tests evaluated the vascular integrity of the arm by monitoring the pulse from the radial artery (Luoma and Nelems, 1991; Sanders and Haug, 1991). Adson's test uses a position with the patient's arm down by their side with the head in slight extension and rotated to the affected side. The patient is then asked to inspire deeply and the radial pulse is monitored. Adson's test is often modified to include head rotation to the unaffected side. The costoclavicular maneuver and Halstead test requires the patient to assume a military posture where the shoulders are held in a backward and downward direction, thus narrowing the costoclavicular space. Halstead also described applying traction to the patient's arm. Both of these tests evaluate vascular integrity by monitoring the radial pulse. Tests that evaluate vascular integrity have been criticized for high numbers of false positive and negative diagnostic conclusions (Sanders and Haug, 1991). In the hyperabduction test, the shoulders are hyperabducted to 180 degrees and the elbows are flexed. For Roos' test, the shoulders are abducted to 90 degrees with external rotation (AER) and the elbows are flexed to 90 degrees; the patient then flexes and extends the digits of both hands for 3 minutes (Roos and Owens, 1966). Both the hyperabduction test and Roos' test are considered positive with reproduction of arm symptoms. Sanders reports that the hand motions described by Roos are not necessary in the majority of patients and that assuming the AER position is sufficient to reproduce arm symptoms (Sanders and Haug, 1991). The described position includes both arm elevation and elbow flexion that may provoke both the brachial plexus at the thoracic outlet and the ulnar nerve at the cubital tunnel. We have modified the arm position to include elbow extension rather than elbow flexion to decrease the possibility of irritating the ulnar nerve at the cubital tunnel (Mackinnon and Novak, 1996;

Novak et al., 1993b). In those patients with complaints relating to brachial plexus nerve compression and no evidence of vascular insufficiency, a test is positive with reproduction of patient arm symptoms.

Clinical testing

The pressure and/or provocative maneuvers should be performed at all potential sites of nerve entrapment in the upper extremity (see Table 3.1). These maneuvers are held for a total of 60 seconds and a positive response is indicated by reproduction of sensory alteration in the appropriate sensory distribution. Because of the associated discomfort in testing of the more proximal nerve compression sites, the physical examination should begin distally and progress to the more proximal entrapment sites. The positional maneuvers for evaluation of nerve compression in the upper extremity include positions that increase pressure and/or tension on the nerve. The described positional test for carpal tunnel syndrome is wrist flexion (Phalen's test). Wrist extension will also increase pressure in the carpal tunnel and increase tension on the median nerve (Gelberman et al., 1981). This provocative position, however, has not been tested for sensitivity and specificity in the diagnosis of carpal tunnel syndrome. Forearm supination and elbow extension will stretch the pronator teres and thus compress the median nerve in the forearm. The pressure provocative test for the median nerve at the carpal tunnel is performed by placing digital pressure on the median nerve, proximal to the volar wrist crease. At the forearm, the median nerve can be compressed by placing digital pressure in the region of the pronator teres. Wrist flexion with ulnar deviation will place tension on the radial sensory nerve. The ulnar nerve at the cubital tunnel will be provoked with elbow flexion by increasing tension on the ulnar nerve and also increasing pressure within the cubital tunnel (Gelberman et al., 1998; Pechan and Julis, 1975). Pressure provocation can also be performed by placing pressure on the ulnar nerve just proximal to the cubital tunnel. Positional provocation of the brachial plexus is achieved with arm elevation (Novak et al., 1993b). Pressure provocation for the brachial plexus is achieved by placing pressure supraclavicularly between the scalene muscles.

Combining the provocative tests of movement and pressure increases neural pressure by position and direct compression and thus provokes symptoms more quickly. The carpal tunnel is tested by combining a Phalen's test with direct median nerve compression; place the wrist in flexion with the forearm in neutral and place digital pressure on the median nerve at the volar wrist crease. A positive response would be reproduction of sensory alteration in the median nerve distribution; however, wrist flexion may also compress the ulnar nerve at Guyon's canal thus producing a sensory change in the ulnar nerve distribution (little and/or ring finger). Therefore all reported sensory changes in the hand with wrist flexion testing should be noted. The median nerve in the forearm is compressed by placing the forearm in full supination with the elbow in comfortable extension and wrist in neutral (to minimize provoking the carpal tunnel). Digital pressure is then applied to the median nerve in the region of the pronator teres. A positive response is noted with sensory changes in the median nerve distribution of the hand including the palm. The radial sensory nerve is provoked by placing the forearm in pronation and the wrist in flexion and ulnar deviation. A positive response is recorded with a sensory alteration in the dorsum of the first web space. This position will also stress the extensor tendons in the first dorsal extensor compartment (the abductor pollicis longus and extensor pollicis brevis) and therefore de Quervain's tenosynovitis should be considered in differential diagnosis. Patients with de Quervain's tenosynovitis will have pain with this test and they will not complain of a sensory change in the dorsal first web space. Cubital tunnel syndrome is clinically evaluated by placing the elbow in full flexion, forearm supination and wrist in a neutral position; digital pressure is then placed on the ulnar nerve just proximal to the cubital tunnel. Patients with a positive response will report alteration of sensation in the little and/or ring finger. Patients may also report aching in the medial aspect of the forearm. Brachial plexus nerve compression is evaluated by having the patient raise the hands overhead (with elbow extension and wrist neutral position to minimize provocation from the cubital tunnel or carpal tunnel) (Mackinnon and Novak, 1996; Novak et al., 1993b). Further pressure on the brachial plexus can then be applied by placing downward digital pressure supraclavicularly between the scalene muscles. This test is positive for brachial plexus nerve compression with reproduction of patient symptoms into the upper extremity (Novak et al., 1993b). Alterations of the radial pulse or hand color should be noted, but these signs should not be considered pathognomonic of thoracic outlet syndrome. Complaints of cervical or shoulder pain are also not diagnostic of brachial plexus nerve compression but should indicate the need for a more thorough evaluation of the cervical spine and/or shoulder.

Subjective history should include specific questions regarding discomfort in the cervicoscapular and shoulder region. Patients with brachial plexus nerve compression will often present with concomitant muscle imbalance in the cervicoscapular region. Postural assessment in both standing and sitting is required. In the ideal standing posture, a plumb line that is located slightly anterior to the lateral malleolus will descend through the ear lobe, the cervical vertebral bodies, the shoulder joint, the trunk, the greater trochanter of the femur and slightly anterior to the knee midline (Kendall et al., 1993). The postural faults to the upper body usually include the head anterior to the thorax, scapulae abduction and shoulder internal rotation. This posture will result in alteration of the length and strength of the muscles in the cervicoscapular region, thus altering the cervical and scapular movement patterns. Cervical spine range of motion can be evaluated actively by asking the patient to perform each movement. Evaluation of the cervical active range of motion will reveal movement pattern abnormalities and/or cervical restriction; however, individual muscles should also be assessed for tightness, weakness and tenderness. Spurling's test can be used to screen for foraminal encroachment of the cervical spine. The Spurling's test is performed by placing the patient's head in slight lateral flexion and extension. Downward compression is then placed on the patient's head and a positive response is recorded with a 'spray' of symptoms into the arm. The test is repeated with lateral flexion to the opposite side.

A complete shoulder evaluation is necessary for those patients who complain of pain to the lateral humeral region, or who complain of shoulder discomfort when testing for brachial plexus nerve compression. A shoulder evaluation is performed to rule out pathology specific to the shoulder complex, including rotator cuff tendinitis/impingement. Shoulder range of motion should include both active and passive movements and particular attention should be directed to the associated scapular movements. While performing both shoulder flexion and abduction, the patient should be observed posteriorly for abnormal scapular motion or scapular winging. During the return of the movement from full range, the scapula should be observed for these abnormal motions. Scapular muscle weakness in many cases may only be observed during the eccentric or lengthening contraction which will occur during the return movement from full shoulder flexion or abduction. Patients with suspected rotator cuff tendinitis require a full shoulder assessment beginning with active shoulder range of motion. Patients with a painful arc of motion and/or difficulty performing internal rotation, particularly reaching the hand behind the back, may be impinging the insertion of the rotator cuff on the acromion. Resisted isometric contractions of the muscles of the rotator cuff, in addition to palpation of the insertion of the rotator cuff on the humerus, are used to confirm the diagnosis of rotator cuff tendinitis.

Pain evaluation

Many patients with pain have difficulty in describing and localizing their symptoms and therefore the evaluation of patients with diffuse pain, paresthesia and numbness in the upper extremity can be very confusing. To assess these patients, we use a pain evaluation questionnaire. Our questionnaire is a further modification of the McGill pain questionnaire and Hendler's back pain questionnaire (Chen et al., 1998; Hendler et al., 1985a,b; Mackinnon and Dellon, 1988; Melzack, 1975). This questionnaire will provide more information regarding the quality and location of pain and the impact of the pain on the patient's life. Our pain questionnaire consists of pain descriptors, a body diagram, 10-cm visual analog scales for pain, stress and coping, and questions regarding several areas including pain,

work, home and medications. Each component is scored and categorized as positive if: more than three descriptors are selected; the body diagram does not follow a known anatomic pattern; or the questionnaire score exceeds 20. Those patients who score positive in more than two components are referred for psychological evaluation.

Sensory receptors and sensory testing

To understand the concept of clinical sensory evaluation of the patient with nerve compression, one requires an understanding of the sensory receptor system. The A-beta peripheral nerve fibers convey sensory information from the distal sensory receptors to the somatosensory cortex of the central nervous system. Two types of sensory receptors are present in the glabrous skin of the hand: free nerve endings and specialized encapsulated receptors. It is these encapsulated receptors that permit the perception of the various sensory stimuli in the hand. The response patterns of these afferent mechanoreceptors to different types of stimuli have been predominantly investigated in the animal models and these results have been extrapolated to humans. Mountcastle et al. reported two different types of peripheral touch fiber systems: the quickly and slowly adapting receptor systems (Mountcastle et al., 1967, 1969). In the quickly adapting receptor system, the Pacinian corpuscles were found to be most sensitive to the higher vibration frequencies, while the Meissner corpuscles were more sensitive to the lower frequencies. The Merkel cell neurite complexes are the slowly adapting receptors that respond to touch and encode for cutaneous pressure including indentation or elevation. Talbot et al. (1968) evaluated the mechanoreceptive afferent response patterns in both the primate and human and concluded that similar response patterns exist in both models. These vibratory patterns have been confirmed by others in both the human and primate (Lamotte and Mountcastle, 1979; Vallbo and Hagbarth, 1968).

There have been four types of mechanoreceptors identified in the glabrous skin of the hand and these receptors are classified by the receptor field size and adaptive properties (Dellon, 1981).

The RAI (Pacinian corpuscles) and RAII (Meissner corpuscles) are the rapidly adapting receptors, while the slowly adapting receptors are the SAI (Merkel cell neurite complexes) and the SAII (Ruffini end organs). The rapidly adapting receptors (Meissner and Pacinian corpuscles) respond to movement and vibration. The Meissner corpuscles are located within the dermal papilla and are sensitive to the lower frequencies up to approximately 30Hz. The Pacinian corpuscles are located in the deep dermis and they are more sensitive to the higher vibration frequencies. In the slowly adapting receptor system, the Merkel cell neurite complexes are located in the basal layer of the epidermis and respond to constant touch. In the human glabrous skin, the Ruffini end organs have been recorded electrophysiologically but they have not been identified histologically.

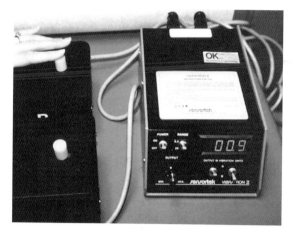

Figure 3.2

The threshold of the quickly adapting receptors can be evaluated with the Vibratron II.

Sensory evaluation

Many tests, measures and assessment tools have been described in the literature with little consensus on a 'gold standard' (Bell-Krotoski, 1990; Dellon, 1980, 1981; Gelberman et al., 1983; Greenspan and Lemotte, 1993; Mackinnon and Novak, 1996; Mielke et al., 1996; Moberg, 1991; Novak et al., 1992, 1993a,b,c, 1994; Paley and McMurtry, 1985; Phalen, 1972). Evaluation of threshold and tactile discrimination are important components in the total evaluation of hand sensibility. In choosing an assessment measure, it is necessary to ascertain the measurement tool that will most accurately evaluate the specific parameter or nerve disorder (compression versus traumatic injury) that is to be evaluated.

Threshold is defined as the minimum stimulus required to elicit a response. Vibration sensation is used to evaluate the threshold of the quickly adapting receptors, while cutaneous pressure thresholds are used to evaluate the threshold of the slowly adapting receptors. Evaluation of tactile discrimination more accurately reflects the innervated receptor field density and this is measured with moving and static two-point discrimination (2pd).

The threshold of the quickly adapting receptors can be measured with vibration using either qualitative or quantitative methods. A tuning fork can be used to evaluate the qualitative response of the patient. The tuning fork is used to apply the vibration stimulus to the digit pulp and the patient is asked to grade the sensation relative to the unaffected side. A low frequency tuning fork (30 cps) will be most useful in the early stages of nerve regeneration following nerve injury. The earliest regenerative sign of the large A-Beta fibers is the perception of low frequency vibration and this sensation will appear prior to light touch (Dellon, 1981). However, with nerve compression, assessment of vibration perception using the higher frequencies (256 cps) will be more sensitive, particularly in the early stages of nerve compression. The tuning fork is applied to the digit pulp by the examiner and the patient is asked if the stimulus feels the same, increased or decreased as compared to the same digit on the contralateral limb. The limitations of using a tuning fork include examiner technique with stimulus application (difficulty of applying the same force each time), patient subjective response and stimuli comparison in patients with bilateral upper extremity nerve compression. Quantitative vibration assessment can be done using either a fixed frequency or multiple frequency vibrometer. The Vibratron II (SensorTek, Clifton, New Jersey) is a fixed frequency (120 cps) variable amplitude vibrometer (Figure 3.2). This vibratron has been shown to have good inter-tester reliability (Gerr and Letz,

1988; Novak et al., 1993c). The patient places the digit to be tested on the stimulus probe and the examiner increases the amplitude until the patient perceives a stimulus. A combined method of limits and forced choice protocol is then used to identify the minimum stimulus that is perceived by the patient (Novak et al., 1993c). This value is recorded in microns of motion on a scale from 0 to 20. In the early stages of nerve compression, the higher frequencies are postulated to exhibit abnormalities before the lower frequencies. Therefore, evaluation at a single frequency of 120 cps with the Vibratron II may not be adequate to detect the early changes associated with nerve compression, particularly if the patient is asymptomatic at rest. In these cases, when only a single frequency vibrometer is available, abnormalities may only be detected with measurement after provocation to a symptomatic state (Novak et al., 1993b). A multiple frequency variable amplitude vibrometer, Bruel and Kjaёr (DK-2850 Naerum, Denmark), permits the evaluation of vibration thresholds at seven frequencies ranging from 8 to 500 Hz (Grunert et al., 1990; Lundborg et al., 1986, 1987, 1992). With the arm supported, the patient places the digit to be examined on the probe. The amplitude of the stimulus is increased until the patient indicates that a stimulus is felt and then the amplitude is decreased until the stimulus is not perceived. This oscillation of stimuli is repeated for 20 seconds and the mean value is recorded as the vibration threshold in decibels. This procedure is then repeated for the remaining six frequencies. The typical pattern for patients with early changes associated with nerve compression is an increased vibration threshold associated with the higher frequencies. Jetzer described an index that evaluates the area beneath the curve formed by the mean vibration threshold at each frequency (Jetzer, 1991). The Jetzer score reflects a composite score formed by the pattern of the actual vibration thresholds. If, however, there are some values above the normal score defined by the B & K vibrometer and other values below the normal score, the differences may be nullified. Therefore, consideration of the original threshold values may more accurately detect subtle changes in the early stages of vibration thresholds.

Cutaneous pressure thresholds are used to evaluate the threshold of the slowly adapting

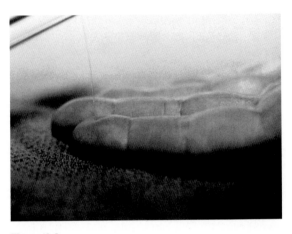

Figure 3.3

Semmes–Weinstein monofilaments can be used to evaluate the threshold of the slowly adapting receptors.

receptors. Evaluation was initially described by Von Frey using various types of hair and they have now been replaced with nylon monofilaments developed by Semmes and Weinstein (Semmes et al., 1960). These nylon filaments vary in diameter thus changing the applied pressure (Figure 3.3). The full set of monofilaments range from 1.65 to 6.65 representing the $\log_{10}$ force in 0.1 milligrams. The monofilament is applied (to the point of filament bowing with the smaller diameter filaments or indentation of the digit pulp with the larger diameter filaments) for a total of 3 seconds to the digit pulp. The patient indicates when a stimulus is perceived and the smallest diameter filament discerned is recorded as the cutaneous pressure threshold. To achieve good reliability in repeated testing, it is important for the examiner to maintain consistent testing technique and filament integrity (Bell-Krotoski, 1990, 1995; Novak et al., 1993c). Another system to measure cutaneous pressure thresholds is the pressure-specified sensory device (N-K Systems, Minneapolis, Minnesota (Dellon, 1997; Dellon et al., 1992, 1997). This system consists of a standard probe, thus only varying the force of application rather than the diameter of the applied stimulus. The 1 mm probe is applied to the digit pulp and the patient responds by pressing a button on the opposite hand when a stimulus is felt. Reports of this instrument have indicated abnormalities in patients with nerve compression (Dellon, 1997; Dellon et al., 1997).

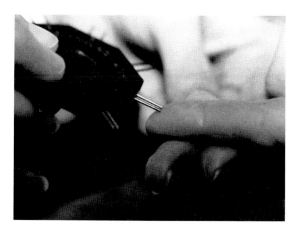

Figure 3.4

The Disk-Criminator can be used to measure moving and static two-point discrimination (2pd).

Moving and static 2pd can be used to evaluate tactile discrimination (Dellon, 1981). Static 2pd was first introduced by Weber. The use of static 2pd was advanced by Moberg and it was functionally integrated in the assessment following nerve injury (Moberg, 1991). Moving 2pd was described by Dellon to reflect assessment of the innervated quickly adapting receptors more accurately (Dellon, 1981). Originally, a bent paper clip was the instrument used to measure 2pd. However, using a paper clip as the measurement tool lacked standardization of the distance between the points and of the blunt end shape. The Disk-Criminator (Neuroregen, Baltimore, Maryland) provides standardized blunt end prongs and interval distances of 1 mm between 2 mm and 15 mm (Figure 3.4). Moving 2pd is evaluated by placing the prongs on the distal digit pulp and moving the disk longitudinally from proximal to distal with sufficient pressure to elicit a response. The patient is then asked if one or two stimuli are felt and the smallest interval that the patient can correctly identify two out of three trials is recorded in millimeters. Static 2pd is evaluated with a similar technique, although the probes are held stationary for 5 seconds. The smallest interval that is correctly identified is determined to be the static 2pd.

Evaluation of hand sensibility should include assessment of each nerve distribution delineated in the patient's subjective symptoms. The little finger is used to evaluate sensation of the ulnar nerve and the index finger is used to evaluate median nerve sensation. The autonomous zone for the sensory distribution of the radial nerve is the dorsal first web space. However, in patients who present with sensory alterations to the thumb, both the median and radial nerves should be evaluated, because of the potential for sensory overlap of the radial sensory nerve and the median nerve.

Motor evaluation

Alterations in the motor system with nerve compression may not become evident until the more severe stages of nerve compression are present. Initially, patients may have some aching in the muscle but this may be associated with muscle strain or overuse rather than nerve compression. Therefore, examination of the muscle should include tests to eliminate muscle strains in the differential diagnosis. As nerve compression becomes more severe, weakness may be present, followed by muscle atrophy. In the upper extremity, the various muscles can be evaluated with manual muscle testing, although

Table 3.2 Test sites for motor evaluation

	Extrinsic muscles	Intrinsic muscles	Sensation
Median nerve	Flexor digitorum profundus of index finger	Thumb abduction	Tip of index finger
Ulnar nerve	Flexor digitorum profundus of little finger	First dorsal interosseus	Tip of little finger
Radial nerve	Wrist extension Finger extension	No muscles intrinsic to hand	Dorsum first web

this is an extremely subjective assessment. Muscle strength can also be assessed and quantified with various commercially available manometers. In the forearm and hand, muscle assessment can be divided in those muscles that are intrinsic or extrinsic to the hand (Table 3.2). Grip and pinch dynamometers can be used to quantify muscle strength and function but these measures may not give the examiner specific information regarding a specific muscle. Lateral key pinch, however, will give good information regarding intrinsic ulnar nerve motor function, as this movement requires maximal effort from the adductor pollicis brevis and the first dorsal interosseus which are innervated by the ulnar nerve. Changes in muscle strength due to nerve compression will occur slowly and predominantly in the later stages of nerve compression and therefore muscle strength assessment is not sensitive to subtle changes in nerve function.

Evaluation of the patient with nerve compression requires a systematic assessment of the motor and sensory components in the upper extremity. Tests of provocation will permit the sites of nerve compression to be identified.

References

Aguayo A, Nair CP, Midgeley R. (1971) Experimental progressive compression neuropathy in the rabbit. Histologic and electrophysiologic studies. *Arch Neurol* **24**:358–64.

Bell-Krotoski JA. (1990) Light touch-deep pressure testing using Semmes-Weinstein monofilaments. In: Hunter JM, Schneider LH, Mackin EJ, Callahan AD, eds. *Rehabilitation of the hand: surgery and therapy.* St Louis, Mo: CV Mosby Company.

Bell-Krotoski JA. (1995) Sensibility testing: current concepts. In: Hunter JM, Mackin EJ, Callahan AD, eds. *Rehabilitation of the hand: surgery and therapy.* St. Louis, Mo: CV Mosby Company, 109–28.

Buehler MJ, Thayer DT. (1988) The elbow flexion test. A clinical test for the cubital tunnel syndrome. *Clin Orthop Rel Res* **233**:213–16.

Chen DL, Novak CB, Mackinnon SE, Weisenborn SA. (1998) Pain responses in patients with upper extremity disorders. *J Hand Surg* **23A**:70–5.

deKrom MCTFM, Knipschild PG, Kester ADM, Spaans F. (1990) Efficacy of provocative tests for diagnosis of carpal tunnel syndrome. *Lancet* **335**:393–5.

Dellon AL. (1980) Clinical use of vibratory stimuli to evaluate peripheral nerve injury and compression neuropathy. *Plast Reconstruct Surg* **65**:466–76.

Dellon AL. (1981) *Evaluation of sensibility and re-education of sensation in the hand.* Baltimore, MD: Williams & Wilkins Company.

Dellon AL. (1997) Computer-assisted quantitative sensorimotor testing in patients with carpal and cubital tunnel syndromes. *Ann Plast Surg* **38**:493–502.

Dellon ES, Keller KM, Moratz V, Dellon AL. (1997) Validation of cutaneous pressure threshold measurements for the evaluation of hand function. *Ann Plast Surg* **38**:485–92.

Dellon ES, Mourey R, Dellon AL. (1992) Human pressure perception values for constant and moving one and two-point discrimination. *Plast Reconstruct Surg* **90**:112–18.

Durkan J. (1997) A new diagnostic test for carpal tunnel syndrome. *J Bone Joint Surg* **73A**:535–8.

Gelberman RH, Hergenroeder PT, Hargens AR, Lundborg G, Akeson WH. (1981) The carpal tunnel syndrome: a study of carpal tunnel pressures. *J Bone Joint Surg* **63A**:380–3.

Gelderman RH, Szabo RM, Williamson RV, Dimick MP. (1983) Sensibility testing in peripheral-nerve compression syndromes. *J Bone Joint Surg* **65A**:632–8.

Gelberman RH, Yamuguchi K, Hollstien SB, et al. (1998) Changes in interstitial pressure and cross-sectional area of the cubital tunnel and of the ulnar nerve with flexion of the elbow. *J Bone Joint Surg* **80A**:492–501.

Gerr FE, Letz R. (1988) Reliability of a widely used test of peripheral cutaneous vibration sensitivity and a comparison of two testing protocols. *Br J Indust Med* **45**:635–9.

Gonzalez Del Pino J, Delgado-Martinez AD, Gonzalez I, Lovic A. (1997) Value of the carpal compression test in the diagnosis of carpal tunnel syndrome. *J Hand Surg* **22B**:38–41.

Greenspan JD, Lamotte RH. (1993) Cutaneous mechanoreceptors of the hand: experimental studies and their implications for clinical testing of tactile sensation. *J Hand Therapy* **6**:75–82.

Grunert BK, Wertsch JJ, Matloub HS, McCallum-Burke S. (1990) Reliability of sensory threshold measurement using a digital vibrogram. *J Occup Med* **32**:100–2.

Gunnarsson LG, Amilon A, Hellstrand P. Leissner P, Philpson L. (1997) The diagnosis of carpal tunnel syndrome. Sensitivity and specificity of some clinical and electrophysiological tests. *J Hand Surg* **22B**:34–7.

Hendler N, Mollett A, Viernstein M, Schroeder D, Rybock J, Campbell J. (1985a) Comparison between the MMPI and the Mensana clinic back pain test for validating the complaint of chronic back pain in women. *Pain* **23**:243–51.

Hendler N, Mollett A, Viernstein M, Schroeder D, Rybock J, Campbell J. (1985b) Comparison between the MMPI and the Hendler back pain test for validating the complaint of chronic back pain in men. *J Neurol Orthop Med Surg* **6**:333–7.

Hurst LC, Weissberg D, Carroll RE. (1985) The relationship of the double crush to carpal tunnel syndrome. *J Hand Surg* **10B**:202–4.

Jetzer T. (1991) Use of vibration testing in the early evaluation of workers with carpal tunnel syndrome. *J Occup Med* **33**:117–20.

Kendall FP, McCreary EK, Provance PG. (1993) *Muscles: testing and function*. Baltimore: Williams & Wilkins.

Lamotte RH, Mountcastle VB. Capacities of humans and monkeys to discriminate between vibratory stimuli of different frequency and amplitude: A correlation between neural events and psychophysical measurements. *J Neurophysiol* **38**:539–59.

Lundborg G. (1988) *Nerve injury and repair*. New York: Churchill Livingstone.

Lundborg G, Dahlin LB. (1994) Pathophysiology of nerve compression. In: Gordon SL, Blair SJ, Fine LJ, eds. *Repetitive motion disorders of the upper extremity*. Rosemont: American Academy of Orthopaedic Surgeons: 381–97.

Lundborg G, Dahlin LB, Lundstrom R, Necking L, Stromberg T. (1992) Vibrotactile function of the hand in compression and vibration-induced neuropathy. *Scand J Plast Reconstruct Hand Surg* **25**:1–5.

Lundborg G, Lie-Stenstrom A, Stromberg T, Pyykko I. (1986) Digital vibrogram: a new diagnostic tool for sensory testing in compression neuropathy. *J Hand Surg* **11A**:693–9.

Lundborg G, Sollerman C, Stromberg T, Pyykko I, Rosen B. (1987) A new principle for assessing vibrotactile sense in vibration-induced neuropathy. *Scand J Work Environ Health* **13**:375–9.

Luoma A, Nelems B. (1991) Thoracic outlet surgery, thoracic surgery perspective. *Neurosurg Clin North Am* **2**:187–226.

MacDermid J. (1991) Accuracy of clinical tests used in the detection of carpal tunnel syndrome: a literature review. *J Hand Therapy* **4**:169–76.

Mackinnon SE. (1992) Double and multiple crush syndromes. *Hand Clin* **8**:369–80.

Mackinnon SE, Dellon AL. (1986) Experimental study of chronic nerve compression. Clinical implications. *Hand Clin* **2**:639–50.

Mackinnon SE, Dellon AL. (1988) *Surgery of the peripheral nerve*. New York: Thieme Medical Publishers.

Mackinnon SE, Dellon AL, Hudson AR, Hunter DA. (1984) Chronic nerve compression: an experimental model in the rat. *Ann Plastic Surg* **13**:112–20.

Mackinnon SE, Dellon AL, Hudson AR, Hunter DA. (1985) A primate model for chronic nerve compression. *J Reconstruct Microsurg* **1**:185–94.

Mackinnon SE, Dellon AL, Hudson AR, Hunter DA. (1986) Chronic human nerve compression – a histological assessment. *Neuropathol Appl Neurobiol* **12**:547–65.

Mackinnon SE, Novak CB. (1996) Evaluation of the patient with thoracic outlet syndrome. *Sem Thoracic Cardiovasc Surg* **8**:190–200.

Melzack R. (1975) The McGill pain questionnaire: Major properties and scoring methods. *Pain* **1**:277–99.

Mielke K, Novak CB, Mackinnon SE, Feely CA. (1996) Hand sensibility measures used by therapists. *Ann Plast Surg* **36**:292–6.

Moberg E. (1991) The unsolved problem – how to test the functional value of hand sensibility. *J Hand Therapy* **4**:105–10.

Mountcastle VB, Talbot WH, Darian-Smith I, Kornhuber HH. (1967) Neural basis of the sense of flutter-vibration. *Science* **155**:597–600.

Mountcastle VB, Talbot WH, Sakata H, Hyvarien J. (1969) Cortical neuronal mechanisms in flutter-vibration studied in unanesthetized monkeys. Neuronal periodicity and frequency discrimination. *J Neurophysiol* **32**:452–84.

Novak CB, Lee GW. Mackinnon SE, Lay L. (1994) Provocative testing for cubital tunnel syndrome. *J Hand Surg* **19A**:817–20.

Novak CB, Mackinnon SE, Brownlee R, Kelly L. (1992) Provocative sensory testing in carpal tunnel syndrome. *J Hand Surg* **17B**:204–8.

Novak CB, Mackinnon SE, Kelly L. (1993a) Correlation of two-point discrimination and hand function following median nerve injury. *Ann Plast Surg* **31**:495–8.

Novak CB, Mackinnon SE, Patterson GA. (1993b) Evaluation of patients with thoracic outlet syndrome. *J Hand Surg* **18A**:292–9.

Novak CB, Mackinnon SE, Williams JI, Kelly L. (1993c) Establishment of reliability in the evaluation of hand sensibility. *Plast Reconstruct Surg* **92**:311–22.

O'Brien JP, Mackinnon SE, MacLean AR, Hudson AR, Dellon AL, Hunter DA. (1987) A model of chronic nerve compression in the rat. *Ann Plast Surg* **19**:430–35.

Omurtag M, Novak CB, Mackinnon SE. (1986) Multiple level nerve compression is frequently unrecognized. *Can J Plast Surg* **4**:165–7.

Paley D, McMurtry RY. (1985) Median nerve compression test in carpal tunnel syndrome diagnosis. Reproduces signs and symptoms in affected wrist. *Orthop Rev* **14**:41–5.

Pechan J, Julis I. (1975) The pressure measurement in the ulnar nerve. A contribution to the pathophysiology of the cubital tunnel syndrome. *J Biomechanics* **8**:75–9.

Phalen GS. (1996) The carpal tunnel syndrome: seventeen years experience in diagnosis and treatment of six hundred and fifty-four hands. *J Bone Joint Surg* **48A**:211–28.

Phalen GS. (1972) The carpal tunnel syndrome. Clinical evaluation of 598 hands. *Clin Orthop* **83**:29–40.

Rayan GM, Jenson C, Duke J. (1992) Elbow flexion test in the normal population. *J Hand Surg* **17A**:86–9.

Roos DB, Owens JC. (1966) Thoracic outlet syndrome. *Arch Surg* **93**:71–4.

Sanders RJ, Haug CE. (1991) *Thoracic outlet syndrome. A common sequela of neck injuries*. Philadelphia: J.B. Lippincott Company.

Semmes J, Weinstein S, Ghent I, Teuber H. (1960) *Somatosensory changes after penetrating brain wounds in man*. Cambridge: Harvard University Press.

Szabo RM, Chidley LK. (1989) Stress carpal tunnel pressures in patients with carpal tunnel syndrome and normal patients. *J Hand Surg* **14A**:624–7.

Szabo RM, Gelberman RH, Dimick MP. (1984) Sensibility testing in patients with carpal tunnel syndrome. *J Bone Joint Surg* **66A**:60–4.

Talbot WH, Darian-Smith I, Kornhuber HH, Mountcastle VB. (1968) The sense of flutter-vibration: comparison of the human capacity with response pattern of mechanoreceptive afferents for the monkey hand. *J Neurophysiol* **31**:301–34.

Upton ARM, McComas AJ. (1973) The double crush in nerve-entrapment syndromes. *Lancet* **2**:359–62.

Vallbo AB, Hagbarth KE. (1968) Activity from skin mechanoreceptors recorded percutaneously in awake human subjects. *Exp Neurol* **21**:270–89.

Williams TM, Mackinnon SE, Novak CB, McCabe S, Kelly L. (1992) Verification of the pressure provocative test in carpal tunnel syndrome. *Ann Plast Surg* **29**:8–11.

Wood VE, Biondi J. (1990) Double-crush nerve compression in thoracic outlet syndrome. *J Bone Joint Surg* **72A**:85–7.

Wood VE, Twito R, Verska JM. (1988) Thoracic outlet syndrome. The results of first rib resection in 100 patients. *Orthop Clin North Am* **19**:131–46.

4

Thoracic outlet syndrome

Christine B. Novak and Susan E. Mackinnon

Introduction

Thoracic outlet syndrome (TOS) is a term commonly used to describe patients with a clinical presentation attributed to compression of the subclavian artery, subclavian vein and/or brachial plexus in the region of the thoracic outlet (Sanders and Haug, 1991). Four types of TOS have been described: arterial, venous, neurogenic with intrinsic atrophy, and neurogenic with no intrinsic atrophy (Roos, 1979; Sanders and Haug, 1991). Compression of the brachial plexus is seen more often than compression of the subclavian vein/artery. Neurogenic TOS associated with intrinsic weakness is rare and compression of the brachial plexus producing paresthesia and numbness in the upper extremity is relatively common. However, this 'less severe' compression of the brachial plexus is most controversial. (Cherington and Happer, 1986; Wilbourn, 1990, 1991). This is likely because the diagnosis is based on clinical presentation and physical examination with the lack of objective findings and a diagnostic quantifiable 'test'.

Anatomy

Several restrictive anatomic structures have been identified in the region commonly referred to as the thoracic outlet (Sanders and Haug, 1991). There is a great deal of confusion regarding the terminology in this region (Ranney, 1996). Anatomists have described the thoracic outlet as the inferior thoracic aperture, the opening into the abdominal area delineated by the lower costal segments. Anatomically, the region between the scalene muscles and the first rib is defined as the thoracic inlet. Clinically, the thoracic outlet has been described in the region of the scalene muscles and the first rib. The clinical syndrome of TOS has three anatomic regions that have been described as contributing to the compression on the neurovascular structures: the scalene triangle, the costoclavicular space, and the pectoralis minor space. The scalene triangle is the area bordered by the anterior scalene muscle, the middle scalene muscle and the first rib. The brachial plexus and the subclavian artery go through the scalene triangle (between the scalene muscles and over the first rib). The subclavian vein passes over the first rib but it is external to the scalene muscles. The costoclavicular space is below the clavicle and above the first rib, bordered anteriorly by the costoclavicular ligament and posteriorly by the middle scalene muscle. The contents of this space include the subclavian vein and artery, the brachial plexus and the subclavius muscle. The subcorocoid space is beneath the corocoid process and the pectoralis minor muscle and it is bordered posteriorly by the ribs. The brachial plexus goes through this space and the nerves can be compressed beneath the pectoralis muscle and around the corocoid process and then further stretched with arm elevation and/or abduction.

Anomalous cervical ribs have been described as a contributing factor to compression of the neurovascular structures, including the brachial plexus, the subclavian artery and/or vein.

Cervical ribs are reported to exist in 0.17 to 0.74% of the population with a higher incidence in women, and rudimentary first ribs are cited in 0.29 to 0.76% of the population (Sanders and Haug, 1991). Of those individuals with cervical ribs, Sanders reported that only 10% develop TOS symptoms and that the onset is usually associated with trauma. Compression of the subclavian artery is most often seen in patients with cervical or rudimentary ribs. Congenital bands and ligaments have been described as contributing to the neurovascular compression in the region of the thoracic outlet (Roos, 1976). The majority of these bands extend from the C-7 transverse process or the tip of the cervical rib to the first rib and lie on the anterior surface of the middle scalene muscle (Roos, 1976). The brachial plexus by its close proximity to the middle scalene muscle may be compressed against the taut ligamentous bands.

There are multiple regions within the thoracic outlet region that may contribute to compression of the brachial plexus, subclavian vein and/or subclavian artery. It is likely that the multiple sites of compression along the brachial plexus produce patient symptoms rather than simply one site of compression producing the symptoms.

Hypothesis for the patient with 'neurovascular compression'

Symptoms resulting from nerve compression will be described by the patient as tingling or numbness in the sensory distribution of the compressed nerve. Patients with TOS usually present with symptoms beyond these, including discomfort and/or pain to the cervicoscapular region. This discomfort does not result from simple nerve compression but more likely from muscle and joint discomfort in the cervicoscapular region. In the majority of patients, the onset of symptoms is described as insidious and likely the result of years of 'bad posture' causing muscle imbalance in the cervicoscapular region. Certain postures and positions of the upper quadrant will have three main effects on the neural and musculoskeletal structures (Figure 4.1) (Mackinnon and Novak, 1994): (1) Increase compression or tension on nerves and vascular structures. (2) Place muscles in lengthened or shortened positions. These muscles will reset at these new lengths over time. If these shortened muscles lie over a nerve or blood vessel, they may then place more pressure on the neural and vascular structures. (3) Result in an imbalance of use of certain muscles such that some muscles are overused and others are underused. Muscles that act in less than ideal lengths will be placed at a mechanical disadvantage. Weak muscle actions will require other muscles to assist with the movement and therefore may cause overuse of the compensatory muscles, creating muscle imbalance. Continued use of these muscles will perpetuate the cycle of muscle imbalance.

Certain positions in the arm that increase nerve tension and/or nerve compression have been well described (Gelberman et al., 1981, 1998; Pechan and Julis, 1975). Wrist flexion increases pressure in the carpal canal which will increase pressure on the median nerve. Wrist extension will also increase pressure in the carpal canal and this position will also increase tension on the median nerve, thus further compromising the median nerve. Elbow flexion will increase the tension on the ulnar nerve and increase the pressure within the cubital tunnel (Gelberman et al., 1998; Pechan and Julis, 1975). This position will increase both the intraneural and extraneural pressure on the ulnar nerve (Gelberman et al., 1998). Arm elevated positions are postulated to increase tension and thus pressure on the brachial plexus. Head forward positions will decrease the length of the scalenes and over time these muscles will reset to this shortened range. Assuming a more upright posture will place a stretch on the scalenes, thus compressing the brachial plexus and subclavian artery between the middle scalene muscle, the anterior scalene muscle and the first rib.

In typical postures with thoracic flexion, with the head anterior to the thorax and the scapulae abducted, the middle and lower trapezius will be elongated and thus weakened. Weakness of the lower scapular stabilizers will result in increased work of the scapular elevators, including the upper trapezius and the levator scapulae muscles. Therefore arm positions, such as shoulder abduction, will have decreased scapular rotation and substitution of scapular elevation. These patients will display hypertrophy and tenderness of the suprascapular region.

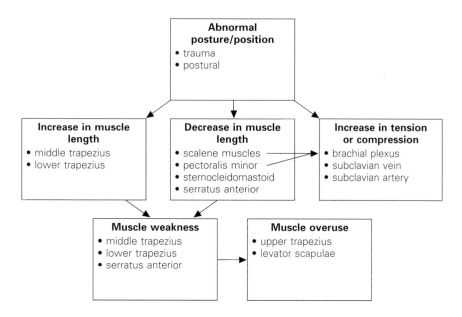

Figure 4.1

Symptoms presenting as 'thoracic outlet syndrome', may be caused by compression of the brachial plexus and by muscle imbalance in the cervicoscapular region. The brachial plexus may be compressed between the scalene muscles and the first rib and/or beneath the pectoralis minor and the corocoid process. Head forward scapular abducted postures will produce lower scapular muscle weakness and overuse of the scapular elevators, thus contributing to the muscle imbalance in the cervicoscapular region. (Reproduced with permission from Novak CB. (1999) Conservative management of thoracic outlet syndrome. *Chest Surg Clin North Am* **9**: 747–60.)

Prolonged abnormal or bad posture will have consequences both in the upper quadrant and arm that may affect the neural and musculoskeletal structures.

Chronic nerve compression and double crush mechanism

It is important to understand the histopathology of chronic nerve compression in order to understand brachial plexus nerve compression. The majority of studies have been performed using an animal model and the findings have been extrapolated to the human. The histopathology of the chronic nerve compression spans a range of changes which will progress dependent on the amount and duration of the compressive forces (Mackinnon and Dellon, 1986). The early changes begin with edema in the perineurium, followed by connective tissue thickening. With increased duration of compression, there will be segmental demyelination localized to the area of the fascicle experiencing the most compression. This is followed by more diffuse demyelination and then finally axonal degeneration. These changes may not occur consistently across the nerve but will vary with the distribution of compressive forces on the nerve. Therefore those fascicles closer to the periphery of the nerve may be affected sooner than the fascicles located in the center of the nerve. With brachial plexus nerve compression, the brachial plexus is hypothesized to be compressed when arm elevated positions are assumed. These positions, however, will also produce discomfort in the arm and/or cervicoscapular region. Patients will therefore attempt to minimize the time in these postures and positions and therefore the duration of nerve compression will be decreased. Since the progression of chronic nerve compression depends upon the duration of compression, brachial plexus nerve compression in the majority of patients does not usually progress to the more severe stages of nerve compression. Patients, with congenital ligamentous bands, however, are more prone to isolated nerve compression presenting with intrinsic muscle atrophy.

The concept of the double crush mechanism suggests that a proximal site of compression will render the more distal entrapment sites less tolerant to compressive forces (Upton and McComas, 1973). Lundborg expanded the double crush mechanism to include the reverse double crush (Lundborg, 1988). Distal nerve impingement will impact the more proximal entrapment sites and these proximal sites will be less tolerant to compression. There are multiple sites in the region of the thoracic outlet that may compress the brachial plexus, and cumulatively these forces will produce symptoms in the upper extremity. In addition, brachial plexus nerve compression may affect the more distal entrapment sites or the distal sites may affect the more proximal compression, making the nerves at these sites less tolerant to compressive forces.

Evaluation and diagnosis

The diagnosis of TOS remains controversial because of the lack of true objective measures and criteria. A large number of radiographical, electrophysiological and clinical tests have been described but none has been universally accepted as the 'gold standard'. The diagnosis of TOS remains a clinical diagnosis, with the exclusion of other pathologies that may cause a similar patient presentation. The most important component of this diagnosis is the patient's subjective complaints and the physical examination. A systematic subjective and physical examination will simplify the complex history, numerous subjective complaints and physical findings in this population of patients.

Review of the history should begin with the mechanism of injury, pain (location, duration, quality, radiation), course of symptoms and treatment outcome to date since onset. Patients often report an onset that is determined to be insidious in nature or a relatively minor trauma with a slowly progressive increase in symptoms. Patients should be furthered questioned regarding a change in their activities at home or at work that may have contributed or exacerbated the presenting symptoms. Patients with a long duration of symptoms will likely describe increased frequency of pain, paresthesia and numbness, in addition to radiation and increased intensity of symptoms.

Pain evaluation

A significant component of TOS patient symptoms is pain, and it is often difficult to ascertain the impact of this pain on the patient. The pain evaluation questionnaire that we use has been modified from the McGill pain questionnaire and Hendler's questionnaire for back pain (Chen et al., 1998; Hendler et al., 1985a,b; Mackinnon and Dellon, 1988; Melzack, 1975; Novak and Mackinnon, 1999). The main components of our pain evaluation are the body diagram, the pain adjectives and the questionnaire. If the patient scores above the expected values in at least two of these components, they are sent for psychological or psychiatric evaluation. We have also included 10-cm visual analog scales to assess average level of pain, emotional stress and coping (at home and at work). These visual analog scales do not have an impact on the scoring of the questionnaire. However, visual analog scales are more sensitive to either positive or negative changes that may occur with treatment.

Clinical findings

Patients usually describe discomfort to the suprascapular, interscapular, subscapular, thoracic and cervical region and radiation of symptoms to the arms. The upper extremity may be described as tired, heavy and weak. Paresthesia and/or numbness to the upper extremity may be limited to a sensory distribution (usually the ulnar nerve). The ulnar nerve is an extension of the brachial plexus lower trunk, which is situated closest to the first rib and therefore may be more likely to be compressed. This nerve compression will produce symptoms to the medial border of the forearm, the ring finger and little finger. Isolated compression of the upper trunk producing symptoms in the median nerve distribution is less common. But in patients with longstanding symptoms, the tingling/numbness may extend to the entire hand and arm. Prolonged positions that compress the brachial plexus (i.e. arm elevation, during sleep) may result in complaints of tingling/numbness to the entire upper extremity. These positions may occur at night or with prolonged arm elevation. Headaches (orbital and/or occipital) are often described and they are likely related to pathology from the cervical spine rather than compression of the brachial plexus. Complaints of facial pain and anterior chest pain are less common. Symptoms to the arm, neck and scapular region are exacerbated by upper extremity activity, particularly head forward postures, overhead arm positions and/or downward loading of the arms. Wasting of the intrinsic muscles of the hand is less commonly seen in patients diagnosed with TOS. Compression at the brachial plexus level rarely produces muscle atrophy except in those patients with an anomalous rib or ligamentous bands. Patients with muscle atrophy should be evaluated for a more distal site of nerve compression at the cubital tunnel and Guyon's canal. Patients with vascular compression of either the subclavian vein or artery will be relatively easy to identify by the clinical presentation of hand swelling, cyanosis, coldness, color changes or digital lesions.

The clinical tests that were originally described in the evaluation and diagnosis of TOS monitored the radial pulse and thus evaluated vascular compression (Figure 4.2). Adson's test, with the patient's arm down by the side, head in slight extension and rotated to the affected side, requires the patient to inspire deeply. The radial pulse is monitored and the test is considered positive with obliteration of the pulse. Adson's test is often modified to include head rotation to the unaffected side. For the costoclavicular maneuver, the patient assumes a 'military type' posture with scapular retraction and the radial pulse is monitored. Halstead modified this maneuver to include downward traction of the patient's arms. Both of these tests are considered positive with obliteration of the radial pulse. Many authors have reported high numbers of both false negative and false positive diagnoses with the use of provocative maneuvers that monitor the radial pulse (Sanders and Haug, 1991). The majority of TOS patients present with symptoms due to compression of the brachial plexus rather than from compression of the vascular structures, and monitoring the radial

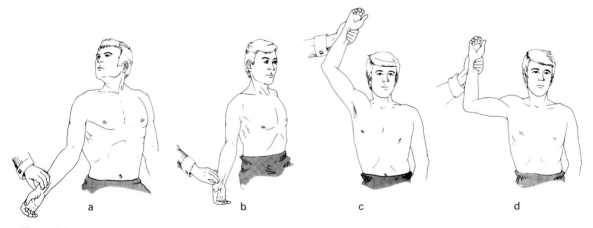

Figure 4.2

Provocative maneuvers for thoracic outlet syndrome. (a) Adson's test positions the patient's arm by the side with the head rotated to the affected side and the patient takes a deep inspiration. The radial pulse is monitored. (b) In the costoclavicular maneuver and Halstead's test the patient assumes a 'military' posture with the shoulders in a retracted and downward direction. The radial pulse is monitored. (c) The hyperabduction test has the patient's arm in 180 degrees hyperabduction with elbow flexion. (d) Roos' test has the patient's arm in 90 degrees of abduction with external rotation and 90 degrees of elbow flexion. (Reproduced with permission from Luoma A, Nelems B. (1991) Thoracic outlet syndrome, thoracic surgery perspective. *Neurosurg Clin North Am* **2**:187.)

artery is not very sensitive to changes in the brachial plexus. Reproduction of patient symptoms should be used as the criterion for a positive test for TOS. The 90-degree shoulder abduction and external rotation test has been found to be a reliable TOS provocative test (Sanders and Haug, 1991). Roos advocated this test with the addition of the patient opening and closing their hands for a total of 3 minutes and considered the test positive with reproduction of patient arm symptoms. Sanders noted that the hand motions are unnecessary and that reproduction of arm symptoms in the majority of TOS patients can be achieved by assuming the abduction with external rotation (AER) position. To avoid provocation at the cubital tunnel and the carpal tunnel, we have modified this test by asking the patient to extend the elbows and maintain the wrist in a neutral position (Mackinnon and Novak, 1996; Novak et al., 1993).

Clinical testing using provocative maneuvers is essential in the assessment of patients with suspected neurogenic TOS and also to identify concurrent distal sites of nerve compression that may be contributing to the symptomatology (see Chapter 3). Provocative testing for other sites of nerve compression including carpal tunnel and cubital tunnel may be extrapolated to the clinical testing for TOS. There have been reports of concurrent carpal tunnel and cubital tunnel syndrome in patients with thoracic outlet syndrome and therefore all potential sites of nerve entrapment in the upper extremity should be evaluated (Novak et al., 1993; Wood and Biondi, 1990).

A Tinel's sign is performed by applying 4–6 digital taps between the scalene muscles in the supraclavicular region. Many patients may report discomfort in this region but a positive Tinel's sign is recorded with complaint of an 'electric shock' sensation. The scalene muscles should also be palpated specifically to evaluate the muscles for tenderness. The provocative maneuver described for TOS requires the patient to raise the arms overhead for 1 minute. The elbows should be in extension, the forearms in neutral and the wrists in neutral to avoid provocation at the cubital tunnel, the median nerve in the forearm and carpal tunnel, respectively. A positive response is recorded with reproduction of patient symptoms in the upper extremity. Pain that is reported in the cervical and/or shoulder region indicates the need for a more in-depth assessment of the cervical spine and/or shoulder.

Evaluation of the cervicoscapular region should begin with postural evaluation. This should include a generalized overview of the entire body in both sitting and standing because posture of the cervical, thoracic and lumbar spine will affect the position of the head and arms. Beginning with standing posture, comparisons are made to the ideal posture (Kendall et al., 1993). When viewed from the side, a plumb line that is dropped anterior to the lateral malleolus will fall anterior to the midline of the knee, through the greater trochanter of the femur and midway through the trunk, glenohumeral joint, cervical spine and ear. The palms of the hands should face the lateral aspect of the thigh and the olecranons should face posteriorly. Patients with TOS often present with a posture that includes the head anterior to the thorax, loss of cervical lordosis, thoracic kyphosis, scapulae abduction and shoulder internal rotation. Postural abnormalities may also be present in the lumbar spine and lower extremities, which will need to be addressed for complete resolution of the problem.

Cervical range of motion can be evaluated for limitation in movement. Head forward postures may result in a loss of cervical lordosis, upper cervical hyperextension and decreased mobility of the cervical spine (McKenzie, 1990). McKenzie's approach to spinal problems may be applied to the TOS patient (McKenzie, 1990). He describes three factors that do occur in the TOS patient; loss of cervical lordosis, bad sitting posture and increased duration in flexion. Following postural assessment and active cervical range of motion, repetitive test movements of the cervical spine are performed. As each movement is performed the range of motion is noted and also the movement's relationship to pain (increases, decreases, centralizes, radiates, no effect). The cervical motions to be tested include protraction, retraction, retraction with extension, flexion, side flexion and rotation. Testing of the motions should be determined by the irritability of the patient's symptoms and all motions need not be evaluated at the first visit.

A Spurling's test is used to evaluate neural encroachment of the cervical vertebral foramina. The patient's head is placed in lateral flexion and slight extension. Compression is then placed downward on the head and a positive response is recorded with a 'spray' of symptoms into the arm. The test is repeated with lateral cervical flexion to the opposite side. The patient may report local cervical pain and this pain may be from other cervical spine pathology (i.e. osteoarthritis, degenerative disc disease) rather than nerve root impingement.

Shoulder evaluation should include both the glenohumeral joint and associated scapular motions. Abnormal scapular mobility may impact the glenohumeral joint particularly the insertion of the rotator cuff leading to rotator cuff tendinitis and/or impingement (Sahrmann, 2002). Assessment should begin with relaxed standing to assess the resting position of the humerus and scapula. The most common postural fault seen with TOS patients is a head forward posture with scapular abduction and internal rotation of the humerus. Head forward postures with scapulae abduction will place the middle and lower trapezius in a lengthened position and the serratus anterior in a shortened position, placing these muscles at a mechanical disadvantage. Movement of the humerus and scapula should be viewed both during the movement and the returning motion from the end point of the range. The patient is asked to raise the arms into forward shoulder flexion and to slowly return the arms to the side, noting the total humeral range of motion, discomfort and associated scapular motion. Similarly, this assessment should also be done through full shoulder abduction. With respect to the scapular motion and humeral movements, shoulder flexion will best evaluate the activity of the serratus anterior muscle and shoulder abduction will bias the middle/lower trapezius muscle. Weakness of the lower scapular stabilizers will result in overuse of the scapular elevators and therefore scapular elevation will be seen as a substitution motion for the scapular rotation required for shoulder abduction and flexion.

Sensory evaluation

A number of tests and measures have been described to evaluate hand sensibility. Many of these tests evaluate different parameters (threshold and tactile discrimination) of the quickly and slowly adapting sensory receptors located in the glabrous skin of the hand (Dellon, 1981). Threshold

is the minimal stimulus that is perceived by the individual and tactile discrimination is an assessment of the sensory receptor innervation density. Measures of threshold (cutaneous pressure or vibration) are postulated to be more sensitive than tactile discrimination (two-point discrimination) measures to assess the early changes that occur with chronic nerve compression.

Threshold of the slowly adapting receptors is assessed with cutaneous pressure thresholds. Semmes Weinstein monofilaments are commonly used to measure pressure thresholds (Semmes et al., 1960). These nylon filaments range in diameter and therefore in the force required to bow the filament when applied to the digit pulp. The monofilament is applied to the finger tip pulp and the smallest filament to elicit a response is recorded as the cutaneous pressure threshold. Computerized pressure devices to measure pressure thresholds have also been introduced (Dellon et al., 1992, 1997). These devices have probes that are applied to the finger tip and the patient indicates with a switch held in the other hand when the sensation is felt.

Vibration thresholds are used to assess the threshold of the quickly adapting receptors. Qualitative assessment can be performed using a tuning fork (Dellon, 1981). The higher frequency tuning forks will be most sensitive in assessing early alterations in sensibility related to nerve compression. The tuning fork is placed on the finger tip pulp and the patient is asked to compare the sensation to the same finger on the contralateral limb. The test is of limited use in patients with bilateral disease and it also depends upon good examiner technique to apply the same amplitude of stimulus each time. Quantification of vibration thresholds can be done with a single frequency vibrometer or a multiple frequency vibrometer. The single frequency vibrometer (Vibratron II, Physitemp, Clifton, New Jersey) is at 120 Hz with variable amplitude and it allows quantification of the minimum vibration stimulus that the patient can perceive. This vibrometer may not be sensitive in patients with early changes due to nerve compression. It is hypothesized that with nerve compression the higher frequencies are first affected and therefore a single frequency at 120 Hz may not detect abnormalities that may be detected at the higher frequencies. In the patient who is asymptomatic at rest with normal baseline vibration thresholds, abnormalities in vibration thresholds may be detected by provocation prior to testing. Novak et al. (1993) evaluated 50 patients with a clinical diagnosis of TOS using the Vibratron II and there was no difference in baseline vibration thresholds. However, vibration thresholds were significantly increased in the little finger following provocation (arm elevation with downward pressure on the brachial plexus). Multiple frequency vibrometers, such as the Bruel & Kjaer vibrometer (Type 9627, Naerum, Denmark) permit the measurement of vibration thresholds at seven frequencies ranging from 8 to 500 Hz. By testing multiple vibration frequencies it is possible to detect abnormalities that might otherwise be unnoticed were only a single vibration frequency to be assessed.

Tactile discrimination is evaluated using moving and static two-point discrimination (2pd) (Dellon, 1981; Mackinnon and Dellon, 1988). Both moving and static may be assessed with a Disk-Criminator (Neuroregen, Bel Air, Maryland). Abnormalities in 2pd will not be evident until the patient has reached the more severe stages of nerve compression and 2pd will not be sensitive to the subtle changes in the early stages of nerve compression. As brachial plexus nerve compression does not usually progress to the more severe stages of nerve compression, 2pd will not yield useful information in the TOS patient.

Because the changes in neural function with brachial plexus nerve compression will be relatively mild and subtle, sensory testing will be normal in the majority of TOS patients. Provocative testing is useful to identify the sites of nerve compression. However, in the majority of patients with isolated brachial plexus nerve compression, there will be normal findings with sensory tests of threshold and tactile discrimination.

Radiographic evaluation

Radiographs of the cervical spine and chest are beneficial in locating cervical ribs, abnormal first ribs and long C-7 transverse processes that may contribute to symptoms in the TOS patients. These standard X-rays may also assist in recognizing other pathologies including cervical spine arthritis, a degenerative disc disease which may be contributing to the patient's symptoms. Computerized axial tomography (CT scans) and magnetic resonance imaging (MRI) are non-invasive studies that may be helpful in identifying other pathology but they have not been shown to be sensitive in confirming the diagnosis of TOS. Bilbey et al. reported abnormalities on CT scans in 60% of their patients and in total 85% of patients had abnormalities identified by X-ray or CT scans (Bilbey et al., 1989). Gebarski et al. evaluated 10 patients with brachial plexopathy and 50 people with non-neurogenic diseases (Gebarski et al., 1982). They reported that CT scans were useful in diagnosing TOS but that the scans were inconclusive in excluding TOS. In our evaluation of 50 TOS patients, CT scans identified compressive abnormalities in 32 patients (Novak et al., 1993). We have found radiographic evaluation to be most useful in identifying other pathology that may produce patient symptomatology. Therefore these tests will be most useful in excluding the diagnosis of TOS but not useful in supporting the diagnosis of TOS.

Electrodiagnostic evaluation

Electrodiagnostic testing to confirm the diagnosis of TOS remains controversial. Jebson introduced the concept of using ulnar nerve motor conduction velocities for the diagnosis of TOS and this practice has been popularized by Urschel et al. (1971). These studies have not been rigorously tested for sensitivity and specificity and remain limited in acceptance for confirming the diagnosis of TOS. Somatosensory evoked potentials (SSEP) have been characterized as a more sensitive test for the TOS diagnosis. Machleder et al. (1987) found that 74% of their patients with TOS had an abnormal SSEP. Yiannikas and Walsh (1983) confirmed the usefulness of SSEP in the diagnosis of TOS in their patients. Using positional stress tests in addition to the SSEP was advocated by both Machleder et al. (1987) and Borg et al. (1988). However, in our investigation using provoked and baseline SSEP for both the median and ulnar nerve, we did not find SSEP helpful in the diagnosis of TOS (Komanetsky et al., 1996). In general, electrodiagnostic tests are best used to identify distal sites of compression, such as carpal and cubital tunnel syndromes.

Vascular testing

The majority of TOS patients present with symptoms resulting from compression of the brachial plexus and only a small percentage of patients will present because of compression to the subclavian vein and/or artery (Sanders and Haug, 1991). Patients who present with extremity temperature changes, edema, cyanosis, intermittent claudication or lesions to the digits should have more in-depth vascular investigations (i.e. Doppler studies, venograms, arteriograms). In the patients with brachial plexus nerve compression, these vascular studies offer very little additional information. Despite the advancement of radiographic and electrodiagnostic studies, the diagnosis of TOS remains a clinical diagnosis. It should be based on subjective complaints, physical examination and the exclusion of other pathologies.

Management

Conservative treatment

Conservative treatment should be directed towards the restoration of cervical range of motion and neural mobility and correction of cervicoscapular muscle imbalance (Novak, 1996; Novak et al., 1995). Conservative management should begin by identifying postures and positions that may be exacerbating and/or perpetuating symptoms (Table 4.1). Patient education is critical to the patient's understanding of these postures and the impact of positioning

on their symptoms. Modification of activities to minimize positions that provoke symptoms is important in controlling symptoms and therefore postural awareness must begin early in the rehabilitation program.

The patient may not be able to modify postures in some activities because of structural constraints. However, changing postures and modifying positions, in those activities that can be changed, may have a great impact on symptoms. Approximately 6 to 8 hours per day are spent sleeping and abnormal postures that are assumed during sleep may irritate the nerves. Irritation of the nerves overnight may result in increased symptoms during the day. Patients should be asked specific questions regarding symptoms at night that awaken the patients and/or if they awaken in the morning with pain, paresthesia or numbness to the arm or cervicoscapular region. Supporting the cervical spine at night may assist in minimizing provocation from the cervicoscapular region and allow the patient to have a more restful night of sleep. The use of prefabricated cervical collars will not be tolerated by the majority of patients due to the excessive cervical extension positioning. We prefer to use cervical rolls that we construct using non-sterile composite padding inserted into 2-inch (5-cm) stockinette. Patients are given two rolls to fully support the cervical spine, although some patients especially those with a short neck will begin with one roll. Some patients may require an accommodation period (up to 2 weeks) to get used to wearing the cervical rolls and they may have to adjust their pillow for comfort. However, the majority of patients report improvement in their sleep, decreased

Table 4.1 Exacerbating and relieving positions in nerve compression

Nerve	Site of entrapment	Exacerbating position	Relieving position
Brachial plexus	Supra/Infraclavicular	Arm elevation	Arms by side Postural correction
Radial nerve	Distal forearm	Forearm pronation with wrist ulnar deviation	Forearm supination and wrist neutral
Ulnar nerve	Cubital tunnel	Elbow flexion Pressure on ulnar nerve at cubital tunnel region	Elbow extension Avoid leaning on ulnar nerve at elbow
	Guyon's canal	Pressure at Guyon's canal	Wrist neutral position
Median nerve	Proximal forearm	Forearm supination with tight pronator teres	Stretch pronator teres muscle
	Carpal tunnel	Wrist flexion and/or extension	Wrist neutral position

night symptoms and less discomfort upon awakening. With improvement in patient symptoms and decreased complaints at night, the patient is progressed to commercially available pillow supports (i.e. cervical rolls inserted into the pillow case).

The degree of postural correction must be initially determined by patient tolerance. Postural overcorrection may increase symptoms to the cervicoscapular region and/or arms. Initially, many patients will not tolerate correction to the 'ideal' posture owing to excessive tension placed on the tight neural and musculoskeletal structures. With an appropriate stretching and strengthening exercise program, 'comfortable' postural correction can be achieved.

Improving cervical and head postures affected by cervical spine restriction are best accomplished following the protocols as outlined by McKenzie (1990). To minimize the probability of irritating the condition, patients should begin in supine, lying with a pillow and towel roll supporting the head and cervical spine. Repetitions of cervical retraction are used to mobilize the cervical spine and thus stretch those structures that are restricting the movement. With repetition of cervical retraction, a decrease and/or centralization of discomfort should be reported. By removing the pillow cervical flexion is decreased and the exercise is progressed until the patient is able to complete full retraction in a flat supine position. If an increase of discomfort is reported or if the symptoms radiate, then the cervical flexion is increased with another pillow and the exercise progression continues until the patient is able to perform cervical retraction with decreasing discomfort. With full cervical retraction, the patient is progressed through the full cervical range of motion as outlined by McKenzie (1990).

Further evaluation of the cervicoscapular muscles usually reveals muscle discrepancies in length. Janda has described a pattern of muscle abnormality and imbalance that is typically seen in patients with 'neurovascular compression' (Janda, 1995; Roos, 1976, 1979; Sanders and Haug, 1991). He describes tightness occurring in the sternocleidomastoid, pectorals, levator scapulae and upper trapezius (Janda, 1995). He also notes weakness in the deep neck flexors and lower scapulae stabilizers. In Janda's description, the role of the scalene muscles remains to be established although others have identified the scalenes as a major component of brachial plexus compression (Roos, 1976, 1979; Sanders and Haug, 1991). We have found in our patients with TOS, that typical postural faults results in tightness of the pectoralis minor, upper trapezius, levator scapulae, sternocleidomastoid, the suboccipitals and the scalenes muscles and in weakness of the middle trapezius, lower trapezius and serratus anterior. Our treatment has been most successful by first stretching the tight muscles followed by strengthening of the weakened lower scapular stabilizers.

Restoration of normal muscle length can be achieved with specific exercises. Patients who report increasing pain, paresthesia and/or discomfort with the exercises are likely being stretched too aggressively. These exercises should be done slowly and taken to the point of tolerance. A number of techniques have been described to assist in restoring muscle length and to decrease trigger point activity. Travell and Simons (1983) describe a 'spray and stretch' technique using a vapocoolant spray. It is important to incorporate an active range of motion and stretching program to complement the spray and stretch. This can be useful in restoring muscle length but the therapist must be aware of the irritability of the condition to avoid increased muscle spasm following treatment. As the irritability decreases, the patient may begin more aggressive stretching.

Stretching exercises are usually designed to elongate tight muscular, ligamentous and capsular structures but one should also be aware of the neural tissue that may be placed on tension. Patients are often instructed in the 'corner stretch' to stretch the pectoralis major. In this position, the shoulder is placed in abduction and external rotation with elbow flexion and the stretch is further stressed by having the patient lean into the corner. This position will not only place the shoulder structures on tension but it will also place the brachial plexus and ulnar nerve on a stretch. Overstretching of the neural structures in this position will quickly exacerbate pain, paresthesia and numbness in the entire upper extremity. In order to 'lean' into the corner, the patient must have good scapular mobility and if the patient has limited scapular retraction, the scapulae will elevate rather than retract. If appropriate scapular retraction takes place, then increased tension is placed on the brachial plexus. Knowledge of neural tension testing and positions is necessary to minimize exacerbation of symptoms with excessive stretching of the neural tissues and to assess neural mobility (Butler, 1991). Care should be given in assessing neural mobility since symptoms can be needlessly exacerbated with overstretching. Segmental stretching with movements of the cervical spine, scapulae and arm will increase the mobility in both the musculoskeletal and neural systems and decrease the risk of exacerbating symptoms (Totten and Hunter, 1991). These stretches can then be progressed to more complex neural stretches over multiple joints.

Physical therapy modalities (i.e. heat, ultrasound, ice, transcutaneous electrical nerve stimulation, iontophoresis) may be used in some patients but are not necessary in the majority of patients. The primary goal of correcting muscle imbalance, postural abnormalities and decreased neural mobility can be addressed with an exercise program. In a select group of patients who require temporary pain relief in order to comply with the exercises, physical therapy modalities may be helpful. However, successful conservative treatment in the majority of patients can be achieved with an exercise program (Novak et al. 1995).

With restoration of cervical and scapular mobility and relative pain control, treatment should be directed towards the return of muscle balance in the cervicoscapular region. The problem in the majority of TOS patients is not simply muscle weakness but muscle imbalance. Therefore strengthening exercises that load the upper extremity muscles and that emphasize power will not correct the problem of muscle imbalance and will likely intensify pain and exacerbate symptoms (Sahrmann, 2002). In most TOS patients, there will be weakness in the middle trapezius, lower trapezius and serratus anterior and this weakness will result in overuse of the muscles that elevate the scapulae. Loading the upper extremity with progressive resisted exercises will increase the use of the scapular elevators and it will not ensure correct recruitment of the lower scapular stabilizers (Novak et al., 1995). These strengthening exercises should begin in gravity assisted positions with an emphasis on the recruitment of the middle trapezius, lower trapezius and serratus anterior. With some patients, these exercises must begin

in gravity eliminated positions. Motor re-education is important to reinforce the recruitment of the correct muscles rather than continue with substitution of the stronger muscles. As the strength of the weaker muscles increases, the exercises can be progressed to be done against gravity and then to resisted exercises, provided that the target muscles can be correctly recruited.

Personal factors including poor aerobic conditioning, obesity and breast hypertrophy may also contribute to TOS symptoms. Orthotic supports are often advocated to assist in maintaining a more erect posture. Many of these supports have straps that cross anteriorly over the pectoral region and then go posteriorly in a figure-of-eight pattern at the back. In many patients, these supports are uncomfortable by placing excess pressure on the brachial plexus beneath the pectoralis minor and/or by placing the patients in positions that are too upright. Postural correction is best attained through an appropriate exercise program rather than an external support. Women with breast hypertrophy may find some relief using a bra that crosses at the back and gently encourages a more upright posture. These types of wider bra straps may also help to decrease the forces caused by the weight of the breast on the supraclavicular region. In some women, a reduction mammoplasty may be recommended to decrease symptoms and to improve posture. A consequence of poor aerobic conditioning is a decreased efficiency of the cardiorespiratory system. Respiratory function will be further compromised with kyphotic postures. A compromise in the respiratory system capacity will result in increased use of the secondary respiratory muscles, including the sternocleidomastoid, the trapezius and the scalene muscles. With increased use of the scalene muscles, there will be resultant hypertrophy and physiological muscle changes. Concurrent adaptive shortening of the scalene muscles will further compress the brachial plexus between the scalene muscles and the first rib. Improvement in posture and trunk position will allow greater chest expansion during the inspiratory phase of respiration. Exercises that encourage lateral costal excursion and diaphragmatic breathing patterns will assist in more efficient inspiration and thus decrease the use of the secondary respiratory muscles. Aerobic exercise should be encouraged and both lateral costal and diaphragmatic breathing patterns should be incorporated in these exercises. In the majority of patients, aerobic exercise must begin with a walking program and be progressed as tolerated. Other aerobic exercises should be evaluated to avoid excessive cervical extension, head forward postures or excessive loading of the upper extremities before the patient is able to tolerate the weight. The problems associated with obesity cannot be overlooked with respect to the effects directly on the nerve and to the effects of increased weight on the upper quarter. For complete relief of symptoms in the obese patients, weight loss is essential, however improvement in symptoms is possible with compliance to postural correction, behavioral modification and to the exercises previously outlined (Novak et al., 1995). The goal of weight loss is often very daunting in the obese patient and therefore these patients should be directed to a nutritionist who can implement a realistic weight loss program.

Surgical management

When all facets of conservative management and behavioral modification have been exhausted and there has been insufficient improvement of symptoms, surgical decompression is often recommended. Informed consent emphasizes the possibility of major or minor nerve injury and failure to relieve symptoms. The patient is encouraged to seriously balance the risks and benefits of this surgery prior to considering surgical intervention. Several operative procedures have been described for thoracic outlet decompression including anterior/middle scalenectomy, anterior scalenotomy, first rib resection and a combination scalenectomy with a first rib resection. These procedures are usually done through a number of surgical approaches (transaxillary, supraclavicular, infraclavicular, transthoracic) depending upon surgeon preference.

Using a supraclavicular approach, the compressive structures in the interscalene region of the brachial plexus and the first rib can be safely released (Mackinnon and Patterson, 1999). Throughout the procedure, loupe magnification, bipolar cautery and a nerve stimulator are used. The incision is made approximately 2 cm above

the clavicle in the supraclavicular fossa. The supraclavicular nerves are identified beneath the platysma and retracted with a vessel loop. The omohyoid muscle is divided and the supraclavicular fat pad is elevated. At this point, both the scalene muscles and the brachial plexus are visualized. The lateral segment of the clavicular head of the sternocleidomastoid muscle is divided and it will be repaired at the end of the operative procedure. The phrenic nerve (on the anterior surface of the anterior scalene muscle) and the long thoracic nerve (on the posterior surface of the middle scalene muscle) must be identified and protected. The anterior scalene muscle is then resected from the first rib. The subclavian artery will be visible beneath the anterior scalene muscle. The brachial plexus is carefully mobilized and the middle scalene muscle is separated from the first rib. At this time, any congenital bands and/or thickening in Sibson's fascia are also divided. Using bone cutting instruments, the first rib is removed back to the articular facets of the costovertebral and costotransverse joints. If cervical ribs or long transverse processes are present, they are removed using a similar bone cutting technique. An opening in the superior dome of the lung pleura is made to assist in blood drainage into the chest cavity away from the operative site. This technique will minimize the chances of a hematoma forming in the region of the brachial plexus. The wound is then closed and a suction drain is sealed after wound closure and maximum lung inflation.

Range of motion of the shoulder and cervical spine are begun on the first postoperative day and full range of motion is anticipated within 3 to 4 weeks following surgery. Soft cervical rolls may be used at night to support the neck and to provide more comfort during sleep. Patients are permitted activity as they can tolerate within their discomfort, although heavy lifting is restricted. Massage and desensitization to the incision region will assist in decreasing any postoperative hypersensitivity and these exercises are begun in the first week following surgery. Progressive resisted strengthening exercises are started 4 to 6 weeks post-operatively. Surgical decompression of the brachial plexus will not address the problem of muscle imbalance in the cervicoscapular region and therefore patients following surgery will need strengthening exercises to address the decreased strength of the lower scapular stabilizers.

The results of patients following surgical decompression of the thoracic outlet have been reviewed (Sanders and Haug, 1991). In that review, Dr Sanders concludes that there is very little difference in results between scalenotomy, transaxillary first rib resection and supraclavicular first rib resection; a good result is reported initially in 90% of patients and this good result is maintained in 65% of patients after 15 years (Figure 4.3) (Sanders and Haug, 1991).

Conclusion

A non-operative approach to TOS is the first method of treatment. Successful conservative management however depends on a thorough assessment and a treatment plan relative to the condition of the patient. Symptom exacerbation with conservative treatment is likely the result of an exercise that is too aggressive for the patient's condition. A treatment plan, that includes patient education, an exercise program addressing muscle imbalance in the cervicoscapular region and decreased neural mobility and behavioral modification at home, work and sleep, will relieve symptoms in the majority of patients with TOS.

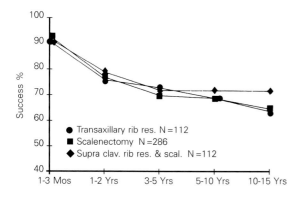

Figure 4.3

As summarized by Sanders, the results from three operations to decompress the interscalene region are presented. These data show similar results from the three operations. (Reproduced with permission from Sanders RJ, Haug CE. (1991) *Thoracic outlet syndrome. A common sequela of neck injuries.* Philadelphia, PA: J.B. Lippincott Company.)

References

Bilbey JH, Muller NL, Connell DG, Luoma AA, Nelems B. (1989) Thoracic outlet syndrome: evaluation with CT. *Radiology* **171**:381–4.

Borg K, Persson HE, Lindblom U. (1988) Thoracic outlet syndrome: diagnostic value of sensibility testing, vibratory thresholds and somatosensory evoked potentials at rest and during perturbation with abduction and external rotation of the arm. *Proceedings on World Congress on Pain.* Amsterdam: Elsevier; 144–50.

Butler DS. (1991) *Mobilisation of the nervous system.* Melbourne: Churchill Livingstone.

Chen DL, Novak CB, Mackinnon SE, Weisenborn SA. (1998) Pain responses in patients with upper extremity disorders. *J Hand Surg* **23A**:70–5.

Cherington M, Happer I. (1986) Surgery for thoracic outlet syndrome may be hazardous to your health. *Muscle Nerve* **9**:632–4.

Dellon AL (1981) *Evaluation of sensibility and reeducation of sensation in the hand.* Baltimore: Williams & Wilkins.

Dellon ES, Keller KM, Moratz V, Dellon AL. (1997) Validation of cutaneous pressure threshold measurements for the evaluation of hand function. *Ann Plastic Surg* **38**:485–92.

Dellon ES, Mourey R, Dellon AL. (1992) Human pressure perception values for constant and moving one and two-point discrimination. *Plast Reconstruc Surg* **90**:112–18.

Gebarski KS, Glazer GM, Gebarski SS. (1982) Brachial plexus: anatomic, radiologic and pathologic correlation using computed tomography. *J Comput Assist Tomog* **6**:1058–63.

Gelberman RH, Hergenroeder PT, Hargens AR, Lundborg G, Akeson WH. (1981) The carpal tunnel syndrome: a study of carpal tunnel pressures. *J Bone Joint Surg* **63A**: 380–3.

Gelberman RH, Yamaguchi K, Hollstien SB, et al. (1998). Changes in interstitial pressure and cross-sectional area of the cubital tunnel and of the ulnar nerve with flexion of the elbow. *J Bone Joint Surg* **80A**:492–501.

Hendler N, Mollett A, Viernstein M, et al. (1985a) Comparison between the MMPI and the Mensana clinic back pain test for validating the complaint of chronic back pain in women. *Pain* 23:243–51.

Hendler N, Mollett A, Viernstein M, et al. (1985b). A comparison between the MMPI and the Hendler back pain test for validating the complaint of chronic back pain in men. *J Neurol Orthop Med Surg* 6:333–7.

Janda V. (1995) Muscles and motor control in cervico-genic disorders: assessment and management. In: Gheit R, ed. *Clinics in Physical Therapy.* New York: Churchill Livingstone; 153–66.

Kendall FP, McCreary EK, Provance PG. (1993) *Muscles: testing and function.* Baltimore: Williams & Wilkins.

Komanetsky RM, Novak CB, Mackinnon SE, Russo M, Padberg A. (1996) Somatosensory evoked potentials fail to diagnose thoracic outlet syndrome. *J Hand Surg* 21A:662–6.

Lundborg G. (1988) *Nerve injury and repair.* New York: Churchill Livingstone.

Machleder HI, Moll F, Nuwer M, Jordan S. (1987) Somatosensory evoked potentials in the assessment of thoracic outlet syndrome. *J Vasc Surg* 6:177–84.

Mackinnon SE, Dellon AL. (1986) Experimental study of chronic nerve compression. Clinical implications. *Hand Clin* 2:639–50.

Mackinnon SE, Dellon AL. (1988) *Surgery of the peripheral nerve.* New York: Thieme Medical Publishers.

Mackinnon SE, Novak CB. (1994) Clinical commentary: pathogenesis of cumulative trauma disorder. *J Hand Surg* 19A:873–83.

Mackinnon SE, Novak CB. (1996) Evaluation of the patient with thoracic outlet syndrome. *Sem Thoracic Cardiovasc Surg* 8:190–200.

Mackinnon SE, Patterson GA. (1999) Supraclavicular first rib resection. *Chest Surg Clin N Am* 9:761–70.

McKenzie RA. (1990) *The cervical and thoracic spine.* Waikanae, New Zealand: Spinal Publications.

Melzack R. (1975) The McGill pain questionnaire: major properties and scoring methods. *Pain* 1:277–99.

Novak CB. (1996) Conservative management of thoracic outlet syndrome. *Sem Thoracic Cardiovasc Surg* 8:201–7.

Novak CB, Mackinnon SE. (1999) Evaluation of the patient with thoracic outlet syndrome. *Chest Surg Clin North Am* 9:725–46.

Novak CB, Collins ED, Mackinnon SE. (1995) Outcome following conservative management of thoracic outlet syndrome. *J Hand Surg* 20A:542–8.

Novak CB, Mackinnon SE, Patterson GA. (1993) Evaluation of patients with thoracic outlet syndrome. *J Hand Surg* 18A:292–9.

Pechan J, Julis I. (1975) The pressure measurement in the ulnar nerve. A contribution to the pathophysiology of the cubital tunnel syndrome. *J Biomechanics* 8:75–9.

Ranney D. (1996) Thoracic outlet: an anatomical redefinition that makes clinical sense. *Clin Anat* 9:50–2.

Roos DB. (1976) Congenital anomalies associated with thoracic outlet syndrome. *Am J Surg* 132:771–8.

Roos DB. (1979) New concepts of thoracic outlet syndrome that explain etiology, symptoms, diagnosis and treatment. *Vasc Surg* 13:313–21.

Sahrmann SA. (2002) *Diagnosis and treatment of movement impairment syndromes.* St Louis: Mosby.

Sanders RJ, Haug CE. (1991) *Thoracic outlet syndrome. A common sequela of neck injuries.* Philadelphia, PA: J.B. Lippincott Company.

Semmes J, Weinstein S, Gheit I, Teuber H. (1960) *Somatosensory changes after penetrating back wounds in man.* Cambridge: Harvard University Press.

Totten PA, Hunter JM. (1991) Therapeutic techniques to enhance nerve gliding in thoracic outlet syndrome and carpal tunnel syndrome. *Hand Clin* 7:505–20.

Travell JG, Simons DG. (1983) *Myofascial pain and dysfunction. The trigger point manual.* Baltimore, MD: Williams & Wilkins.

Upton ARM, McComas AJ. (1973) The double crush syndrome in nerve-entrapment syndromes. *Lancet* ii:359–62.

Urschel HC, Razzuk MA, Wood RE, Parekh M, Paulson DL. (1971) Objective diagnosis (ulnar nerve conduction velocity) and current therapy of the thoracic outlet syndrome. *Ann Thoracic Surg* 12:608–20.

Wilbourn AJ. (1990) The thoracic outlet syndrome is over-diagnosed. *Arch Neurol* 47:228–30.

Wilbourn AJ. (1991) Thoracic outlet syndromes – plea for conservatism. *Neurosurg Clin North Am* 2:235–45.

Wood VE, Biondi J. (1990) Double-crush nerve compression in thoracic outlet syndrome. *J Bone Joint Surg* 72A:85–7.

Yiannikas C, Walsh JC. (1983) Somatosensory evoked responses in the diagnosis of thoracic outlet syndrome. *J Neurol Neurosurg Psychiatry* 46:234–40.

5
Median nerve compression in the forearm

Rahul K. Nath

Introduction

Median nerve injury about the elbow is an overlooked cause of morbidity and must be considered in cases of median nerve dysfunction where pathology in the carpal tunnel is not present. Equally important, compression in the forearm must always be evaluated even in the presence of diagnosed carpal tunnel syndrome. Median nerve anatomic relations in the forearm are complex, and a thorough knowledge of their interactions is important to understanding management of injury (Dawson et al., 1983; Kaplan and Spinner, 1980; Mackinnon and Dellon, 1988; Omer, 1988; Spinner, 1978b; Sunderland, 1978). Appropriate management of acute and chronic injuries must also take into account the concept of multiple crush syndrome, and its emphasis on sequential anatomic sites of nerve compression along the course of the median nerve (Mackinnon and Dellon, 1988).

Inherent in the theory of multiple crush syndrome is the need for surgical release of anatomic compression points in the forearm. These areas are comprised of various muscle and fibrous arch anomalies along the course of the median nerve, and diagnosis is based on physical examination and electrical studies localizing the specific site of compression. Management generally consists of surgical release of all compression points distal to and including the site of a given injury. Knowledge of nerve anomalies such as the Martin–Gruber anastomosis is important in diagnosing the level of injury and management (Mannerfelt, 1966).

Injury to the median nerve can occur at any level from the axilla to the hand. In the forearm, injury tends to be caused by compression at anatomic squeeze points, not by acute penetrating trauma. The onset can be acute, as in blunt injury, or chronic as in repetitive work injury.

The two entrapment neuropathies that involve the median nerve in the forearm are the pronator teres syndrome and anterior interosseous nerve compression. An understanding of the anatomic relationships of the median nerve in the forearm will allow an appreciation of the pathophysiologic mechanisms responsible for the clinical features of compression.

Surgical anatomy

Compression of the median nerve in the forearm is a function of the interaction between median nerve structure and the anatomic sites it traverses on its path through the forearm (Figure 5.1). Variations in nerve and musculoskeletal anatomy can result in abnormal extrinsic pressures being applied to the nerve, with clinical consequences. Therefore, systematic analysis of the possible sites of compression will require a thorough knowledge of median nerve anatomic variations and anomalies, as well as of their surrounding structures.

Median nerve anatomic considerations

The median nerve arises from roots C-5 through T-1 in the brachial plexus. Many proximal variants are possible (Kerr, 1918). Distally, beneath the

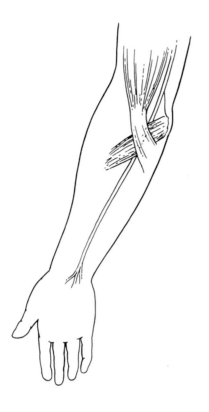

Figure 5.1

Right median nerve course through the forearm. Lacertus fibrosus and pronator teres shown superficial to nerve.

interosseous nerve (Winkelman and Spinner, 1973). This branch is susceptible to injury in isolation from the median nerve as a consequence of its extended course through the forearm. Symptoms of injury include paresthesia or pain in the third web space distribution of the hand.

The median nerve can be acted upon by adjacent structures to suffer compressive injury. These structures can be classified as ligamentous, vascular and anomalous anatomic causes. The common factor is direct physical compression of the median nerve resulting in symptoms of nerve injury. Acute and chronic or repetitive trauma can result in conduction block and symptoms of median nerve functional impairment (Dawson et al., 1983; Omer, 1988; Stewart, 1987).

Provocative tests to diagnose these sites of compression are designed to stretch the various locations of entrapment, thereby mimicking the impingement on the adjacent nerve and causing a conduction block.

This compression is initially equivalent to a first degree Sunderland injury or neurapraxic injury, but can progress with time to an axonal injury (Mackinnon and Dellon, 1988; Sunderland, 1978). It is possible to reverse anatomic signs of compression by relieving the compression. There is compelling histomorphometric data that axonal drop-out is reversed and presumably function is improved as a result (Mackinnon and Dellon, 1988).

Ligamentous causes of compression

Median nerve compression in the forearm is classically associated with entrapment by the tendon of the pronator teres muscle (Bell and Goldner, 1956; Gessini et al., 1983; Hartz et al., 1981; Kelly and Jackson, 1976; Kojima et al., 1968; Kopell and Thompson, 1958; Morris and Perers, 1976; Omer, 1988; Spinner, 1978b). However, the original entity probably describes many different compression points related to neighboring anatomic structures. These are not truly anomalous anatomic structures, but simply variants of normal that may nevertheless predispose to impingement. From proximal to distal, the median nerve travels between the brachialis muscle and the lacertus fibrosus, then beneath the pronator teres, the leading edge of the flexor

elbow two major variations are important. One is the presence of a Martin–Gruber anastomosis, which describes an anatomic connection between the median and ulnar nerves in the forearm. The connection carries median motor fibers to all the intrinsic muscles of the hand, and must be kept in mind when analyzing a particular clinical situation in relation to nerve injury in the forearm. For example, in the presence of a Martin–Gruber anastomosis, a high complete injury to the ulnar nerve might present with sensory findings alone. Conversely, a high injury of the median nerve will result in complete loss of hand intrinsic function in this situation. The Martin–Gruber anastomosis is present in 10–25% of the population (Mannerfelt, 1966).

The third web space sensory branch of the median nerve has been reported to arise several centimetres distal to the take-off of the anterior superficialis arch and the flexor pollicis longus (Mackinnon and Dellon, 1988).

Hypertrophy of the brachialis is known to cause compression of the nerve as it travels beneath the lacertus fibrosus and bicipital aponeurosis (Martinelli et al., 1982). Multiple anatomic configurations of the pronator teres and the flexor superficialis can similarly result in clinically significant compression.

The primary anatomic consideration with the pronator and superficialis muscles is the presence of fascial arches of one or both muscles. Entrapment can occur beneath fascial arches in any anatomic location, owing to the presence of cutting edges along the arch. These cause impingement upon the nerve during contraction of the arch muscle and also by generalized swelling of surrounding soft tissues after repetitive motion.

Dellon and Mackinnon designed an anatomic study to define the specific patterns of fascial development of the pronator and superficialis muscles (Figure 5.2). Based on 31 cadaver dissections, three basic patterns were identified: the presence of no arches, one arch, or two arches. The superficial head of the pronator teres was found to be present in all specimens and

continuous with the forearm fascia through the lacertus fibrosus. The median nerve traveled beneath the superficial head of the pronator in all instances. In 6% of the specimens, the deep head of the pronator was missing and in these instances no arches were present. In the remaining arms, a deep head was present and in this case formed one of the arches described. The association of the superficialis origin to its arch formation is complex, and in about one-third of specimens dissected, a fascial arch was present. A superficialis arch did not exist in the absence of a pronator arch (Dellon and Mackinnon, 1987).

The importance of these arches arises in the context of heavy work requiring flexion of the fingers and forearm pronation. Hypertrophy of the muscles in response to workload can significantly increase the chances of median nerve compression. The anterior interosseous nerve is also at risk if it arises on the radial side of the median nerve instead of a posterior origin (Mackinnon and Dellon, 1988). Furthermore, acknowledging the presence of two arches is critical in surgical management of median nerve impingement. The surgeon must always look for a second arch to provide a complete release.

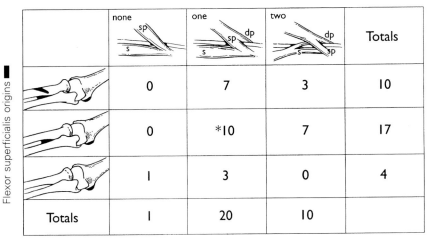

Number of arches

Flexor superficialis origins		none	one	two	Totals
		0	7	3	10
		0	*10	7	17
		1	3	0	4
	Totals	1	20	10	

* one with no PT deep head
sp superficial head of pronator
dp deep head of pronator
s superficialis
median nerve

Figure 5.2

Forearm musculotendinous arches affecting median nerve. (Redrawn with permission from Mackinnon SE, Dellon AL. (1988) Median nerve entrapment in the proximal forearm and brachium. In: Mackinnon SE, Dellon AL, eds. *Surgery of the peripheral nerve*. New York: Thieme.)

Abnormal musculoskeletal structures

The flexor pollicis longus muscle takes origin from the proximal radius and the interosseous membrane (Mangini, 1960; Nebot-Cegarra et al., 1991). An important anomaly of the flexor pollicis longus was initially described by Gantzer and bears his name (Kaplan, 1960; Mangini, 1960). Gantzer's muscle is an extension of the flexor pollicis longus and was found by Mackinnon and Dellon in 45% of their forearm dissections (Dellon and Mackinnon, 1987). It is joined to the flexor pollicis longus by a tendinous band which may be 3 cm long. This can cause a compression of the anterior interosseous nerve and must be searched for in any decompressive surgery of the median nerve. Spinner and Hill have suggested that the most common cause for anterior interosseous nerve compression is an abnormal fibrous band from the pronator teres (Hill et al., 1985; Spinner, 1970). More rarely, compression is caused by abnormal origins of the palmaris profundus and flexor carpi radialis brevis (Spinner, 1978a; Reimann et al., 1944).

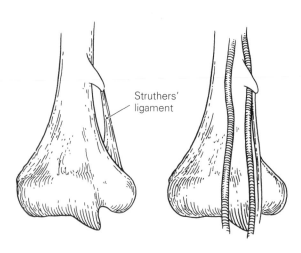

Figure 5.3

Struthers' ligament, right elbow. Median nerve and ulnar artery travel beneath ligament. (Redrawn with permission from Mackinnon SE, Dellon AL. (1988) Median nerve entrapment in the proximal forearm and brachium. In: Mackinnon SE, Dellon AL, eds. *Surgery of the peripheral nerve*. New York: Thieme.)

Compression of the median nerve by a supracondylar process and ligament of Struthers 3–6 cm proximal to the elbow has been reported (Barnard and McCoy, 1946; Dellon, 1986; Struthers, 1848, 1854). Struthers' ligament is quite rare, found in only 0.7% of the population (Figure 5.3) (North and Kaul, 1996).

Vascular causes

Unnamed crossing vessel leashes can occur anywhere in the forearm along the course of the median nerve, and can be causes of impingement. Penetration of the nerve by a large median artery has been reported (Gainor and Jeffries, 1987; Jones and Ming, 1988; Proudman and Menz, 1988). Thrombosis of an ulnar collateral artery and abnormal radial arteries have caused compression at various points along the nerve (Feldmeier et al., 1977; Hartz et al., 1981).

Traumatic etiology

Acute penetrating trauma to the deep structures of the forearm can injure the median nerve at any point (Danielsson, 1980; Molner and Paul, 1972; Omer, 1974). Closed injuries are less common (Spinner, 1978a), but one crucial clinical situation must be recognized: complete supracondylar humeral fracture with displacement of the fragments often entraps the median nerve within the fracture and causes a complete injury of the median nerve (Henrikson, 1966; Lipscomb and Burleson, 1955; Rana et al., 1974; Spinner and Schreiber, 1969). This situation is a neurological emergency and early diagnosis with open visualization of the fracture site must be undertaken within hours of the injury. Normalization of median nerve position and reduction of the fracture are required, along with management of attendant brachial artery injuries.

Subacute and chronic trauma relates to repetitive elbow motion in the workplace or through such activities as tennis, rowing and hammering nails (Hartz et al., 1981; Kopell and Thompson, 1958; Lorei and Hershman, 1993). The presence of cubital bursitis is also associated with median nerve irritation (Karanjia and Stiles, 1988).

Diagnosis

The diagnosis of median nerve injury is primarily based on physical examination in the context of a thorough understanding of median nerve functional anatomy. Direct penetrating trauma localizes the site of injury in a straightforward manner. Motor losses may involve thumb abduction and opposition, flexion of the distal thumb phalanx, profundus flexion of the index and long fingers, forearm pronation, and radial wrist flexion. Sensory loss will affect the pulps of the thumb, index and long fingers, along with the radial half of the ring finger. The various combinations of sensory and motor deficits will generally suggest the level of injury.

It is important to understand that carpal tunnel syndrome frequently exists in the same clinical context as forearm compression of the median nerve. Although carpal tunnel syndrome is much more common than forearm compression, both must be looked for in any case of median nerve deficit. Electrophysiological studies are invaluable in confirming carpal tunnel syndrome, but are generally of less help in forearm compression. It has been suggested that electromyography is more specific than nerve conduction velocity in forearm compression (Aiken and Moritz, 1987; Bell and Goldner, 1956; Buchthal et al., 1974; Morris and Perers, 1976). Classically, the pronator teres is spared, although needle evidence of injury to all the other median-innervated muscles of the forearm and hand is present. In the presence of a Martin–Gruber anastomosis, forearm compression may look like a combined ulnar and median nerve deficit. Meticulous physical examination and provocative testing are the mainstays for ruling out forearm compression.

Physical examination will typically include elicitation of Tinel's sign over the median nerve in the proximal forearm as well as at the wrist. Provocative testing will be useful in isolating the site of compression. Specific maneuvers will be described below.

Pronator teres syndrome

The pronator teres is the major pronator of the forearm, and as such will tend to become hyper-trophic or inflamed by constant repetitive pronation movements (Adelman and Elsner, 1982). Activities such as tennis, wringing of clothes, and industrial jobs requiring heavy pronation and supination will precipitate symptoms of median nerve compression if the particular arch system present in the individual predisposes to anatomic compression as outlined previously.

Symptoms of pronator syndrome generally consist of muscle aches in the forearm following exertion in pronation. Coexistent symptoms might include weakness of median innervated muscles and paresthesia in the median nerve sensory territory (Hartz et al., 1981; Kopell and Thompson, 1958; Mackinnon and Dellon, 1988; Martinelli et al., 1982; Morris and Perers, 1976; Spinner and Schreiber, 1969).

The first physical examination maneuver should be deep percussion of the median nerve beneath the proximal volar forearm muscles. The presence of a Tinel's sign will suggest impingement neuropathy. Direct deep compression of the

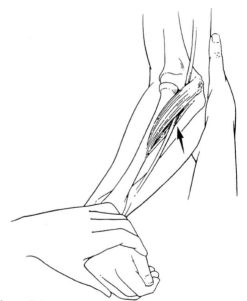

Figure 5.4

Discomfort on resisted pronation implies entrapment beneath pronator teres muscle or arch. Arrow denotes point of median nerve compression beneath pronator teres muscle. (Redrawn with permission from Mackinnon SE, Dellon AL. (1988) Median nerve entrapment in the proximal forearm and brachium. In: Mackinnon SE, Dellon AL, eds. *Surgery of the peripheral nerve.* New York: Thieme.)

median nerve often produces a dull ache, again suggestive of entrapment beneath an anatomic structure at that location. Elicitation of symptoms through provocative testing is useful. Production of symptoms on resisted pronation implies entrapment beneath a component structure of the pronator teres (Figure 5.4). Resisted forearm flexion and supination suggest impingement beneath the lacertus fibrosus (Figure 5.5), and resisted superficialis flexion of the long finger indicates the presence of an arch of the superficialis origin with entrapment beneath (Figure 5.6). Weakness of individual muscle testing may be found on occasion (Mackinnon and Dellon, 1988).

Mackinnon and Dellon (1988) have described a provocative test for pronator syndrome, consisting of provocation of symptoms of paresthesia in the median nerve distribution of the hand with the wrist and the elbow in extension, the forearm in supination, and pressure over the median nerve at the leading edge of the pronator muscle. They also emphasized that the sensory findings in patients with just carpal tunnel syndrome will exclude the distribution of the palmar cutaneous branch of the median nerve. By contrast, there will be sensory complaints in the palmar cutaneous branch in patients with pronator syndrome.

Anterior interosseous nerve syndrome

The anterior interosseous branch of the median nerve is primarily motor to the flexor pollicis longus muscle (Cragg, 1974), the profundus supply of the index finger and the long finger; additionally, the pronator quadratus muscle is supplied. It also innervates the volar wrist capsule, but has no cutaneous distribution (Farber and Bryan, 1968; Fearn and Goodfellow, 1965; Gardner-Thorpe, 1974; Schmidt and Eiken, 1971; Spinner, 1970). A complete injury to the nerve therefore presents with inability to flex the distal phalanges of the thumb and index finger, and a

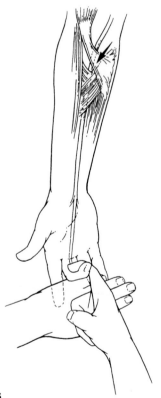

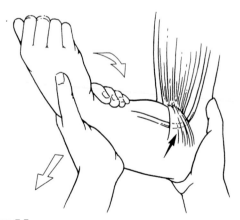

Figure 5.5

Discomfort on resisted supination and elbow flexion implies compression by lacertus fibrosus. Closed arrow denotes point of median nerve compression beneath lacertus fibrosus. Open arrows show direction of examiner's manipulation, with patient in resistance. (Redrawn with permission from Mackinnon SE, Dellon AL. (1988) Median nerve entrapment in the proximal forearm and brachium. In: Mackinnon SE, Dellon AL, eds. *Surgery of the peripheral nerve*. New York: Thieme.)

Figure 5.6

Discomfort on resisted middle finger superficialis implies presence of tight superficialis arch. Arrow denotes point of median nerve compression beneath superficialis arch. (Redrawn with permission from Mackinnon SE, Dellon AL. (1988) Median nerve entrapment in the proximal forearm and brachium. In: Mackinnon SE, Dellon AL, eds. *Surgery of the peripheral nerve*. New York: Thieme.)

variable paralysis of the distal interphalangeal joints of the long finger (Figure 5.7). Pronator quadratus testing can be performed by placing the elbow in flexion and testing pronation.

Electromyography can confirm the pattern of injury, and in some instances rule out a tendinous injury mimicking anterior interosseous palsy. Tendon ruptures can occur in the context of rheumatoid arthritis, synovitis, or bony spurs in the carpal canal, and often result in similar inability to form an 'O' with the thumb and index finger pulp tips (Mannerfelt and Norman, 1969; Nalebuff and Potter, 1968). Electromyography will show normal pronator quadratus function in the tendon ruptures and abnormal signal in anterior interosseous palsy.

Operative techniques for decompression

The patient, having been diagnosed with entrapment neuropathy of the median nerve in the forearm, is brought to the operating room and placed in the supine position. A tourniquet is placed and an incision made after exsanguination of the arm. An 'S'-shaped incision is designed along the radial border of the pronator muscle. The incision must extend from proximal to the antecubital crease to the proximal third of the forearm, with the transverse component of the 'S' being along the antecubital crease. Dissection proceeds through the subcutaneous tissues, using only bipolar electrocautery. Great care should be taken to avoid injury to branches of the lateral antebrachial cutaneous and medial antebrachial cutaneous nerves (Figure 5.8).

The upper arm fascia is entered and the lacertus fibrosus excised along the median border of the biceps tendon. Palpation for a supracondylar spur and Struthers' ligament should be performed, and these structures resected if present. Dissection proceeds distally, beneath the superficial head of the pronator teres. A high origin of the superficial head must be resected, taking care to preserve branches to the muscle that arise off the medial aspect of the median nerve. The median nerve is traced distally, removing any crossing vessels and fibrous bands. The first arch is now approached, formed by the deep and superficial heads of the pronator. The arch is excised and dissection

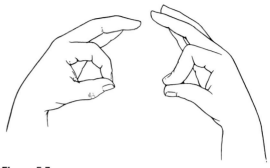

Figure 5.7

Inability to flex right distal interphalangeal joints of thumb and index finger is suggestive of anterior interosseous nerve palsy. This must be differentiated from tendon attrition and rupture.

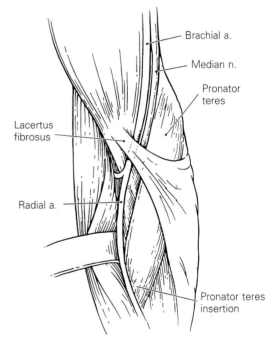

Figure 5.8

Initial exposure of right median nerve and overlying structures.

continues along the course of the median nerve (Figure 5.9). The second or superficialis arch is searched for by palpation along with Gantzer's muscle, and both resected if present (Figure 5.10) (Mackinnon and Dellon, 1988).

Once all potentially compressive structures have been released, attention is turned to the nerve itself. Careful examination under magnification

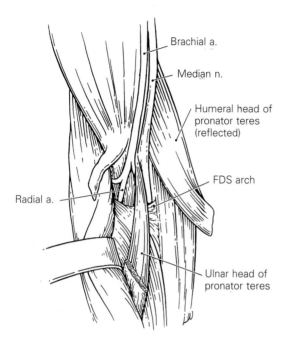

Figure 5.9

Release of lacertus fibrosus and superficial head of pronator teres reveals underlying second fibrous superficialis arch if present.

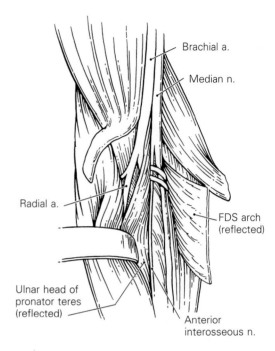

Figure 5.10

Superficialis arch must be resected if present. Crossing vessels should also be excised and neuroplasty of median nerve performed.

will detect the presence of narrowing or thickening at sites of compression. Pseudoneuromas may be present with chronic and severe compression. Meticulous external and internal neuroplasty is now performed at apparent sites of compression using microsurgical technique under high magnification. At the conclusion of surgery, the tourniquet is released and hemostasis is obtained. Unipolar electrocautery is not recommended, for fear of injuring peripheral nerves by transmitted current. A drain should be used to evacuate minor bleeding overnight. A light dressing is placed and immediate postoperative movement is established to prevent scar tethering of the median nerve within the operative field.

Exploration of anterior interosseous nerve for decompression essentially follows the same procedures as in the pronator syndrome. The added maneuvers relate to following the nerve beneath the superficial head of the pronator through its course to the deep volar compartment underneath a possible superficialis arch. As

with the main median nerve the anterior interosseous nerve is examined for the presence of crossing vessels and random fascial bands which are excised.

An important consideration in planning median nerve decompression in the forearm is to rule out preoperatively the presence of coexistent ulnar nerve compression in the cubital tunnel. If significant impingement is present in that location, then ulnar anterior submuscular transposition can be performed at the same sitting.

Results of median nerve decompression in the forearm

Outcomes from these procedures are generally good, with success rates quoted between 77 and 92% in some series (Hartz et al., 1981; Olehnik et al., 1994). Complete relief of symptoms, however, has been said to be much less frequent, about 25% (North and Kaul, 1996).

Summary

The median nerve is susceptible to compression at several points along its anatomic course. In the forearm, fascial and vascular structures may impinge upon the nerve, and are postulated to become significant clinically upon repetitive pronation/supination activities. Diagnosis of entrapment neuropathies of the median nerve in the forearm depends primarily on history and physical examination, although electrophysiological testing may add useful data in some instances. Management of confirmed entrapment neuropathy is usually best undertaken by operative release of impinging structures. A defined proximal-to-distal dissection will identify the specific anatomic sites of compression which are then released. A thorough microsurgical neuroplasty of obvious constriction zones along the nerve follows. Early postoperative mobilization of the nerve will promote gliding within the wound bed so as not to allow tethering and compression by surgical scar. Results of surgical intervention are good when patients are properly selected.

Mackinnon has suggested that pronator syndrome can often be treated conservatively with stretching exercises of pronator teres; she also emphasizes that anterior interosseous palsy is often related to a neuritis (Kihol and Nevin 1952).

References

Adelman S, Elsner K. (1982) Arm pain in a dentist: pronator syndrome. *J Am Dent Assoc* **105**:61–2.

Aiken BM, Moritz MJ. (1987) Atypical electromyographic findings in pronator teres syndrome. *Arch Phys Med Rehabil* **68**:173–5.

Barnard LB, McCoy SM. (1946) The supercondyloid process of the humems. *J Bone Joint Surg* **28**:845–50.

Bell GE Jr, Goldner JL. (1956) Compression neuropathy of the median nerve. *South Med J* **49**:966–72.

Buchthal F, Rosenthalk A, Trojaborg W. (1974) Electrophysiological findings in entrapment of the median nerve at the wrist and elbow. *J Neurol Neurosurg Psychiatry* **37**:340–60.

Cragg C. (1974) Isolated paralysis of the flexor pollicis muscle. An unusual variation of the anterior interosseous nerve syndrome. Case report. *Scand J Plast Reconstr Surg* **8**:250– 2.

Danielsson LG. (1980) Iatrogenic pronator syndrome: case report. *Scand J Plast Reconstr Surg* **14**:201–3.

Dawson DM, Hallett M, Millender LH. (1987) *Entrapment neuropathies*. Boston, MA: Little, Brown.

Dellon AL, Mackinnon SE. (1987) Musculoaponeurotic variations along the course of the median nerve in the proximal forearm. *J Hand Surg* **12B**:359–63.

Dellon AL. (1986) Musculotendinous variations about the medial humeral epicondyle. *J Hand Surg* **11B**:175–8l.

Farber JS, Bryan RS. (1968) The anterior interosseous nerve syndrome. *J Bone Joint Surg* **58**:521–3.

Fearn CB, D'a Goodfellow JW. (1965) Anterior interosseous nerve palsy. *J Bone Joint Surg* **47B**:91–5.

Feldmeier C, Hauer G, Wilhelm K. (1977) Vascular causes of median and ulnar nerve compression syndromes. *Handchiurgerie* **9**:189–91.

Gainor BJ, Jeffries JT. (1987) Pronator syndrome associated with a persistent median artery. A case report *J Bone Joint Surg* **69A**:303–4.

Gardner-Thorpe C. (1974) Anterior interosseous nerve palsy: spontaneous recovery in two patients. *J Neurol Neurosurg Psychiatry* **37**:1146–50.

Gessini L, Jandolo B, Pietrangeli A. (1983) Entrapment neuropathies of the median nerve at and above the elbow. *J Surg Neurol* **19**:112–16.

Hartz CR, Linscheid RL, Gramser RR, et al. (1981) The pronator teres syndrome. Compressive neuropathy of the median nerve. *J Bone Joint Surg* **63A**:885–90.

Henrikson B. (1966) Supracondylar fractures of the humerus in children. *Acta Chir Scand (Suppl)* **369**:l.

Hill NA, Howard FM, Huffer BR. (1985) The incomplete anterior interosseous nerve syndrome. *J Hand Surg* **10A**:4–16.

Jones NF, Ming NL. (1998) Persistent median artery as a cause of pronator syndrome. *J Hand Surg* **13A**:728–30.

Kaplan EB, Spinner M. (1980) Normal and anomalous innervation patterns in the upper extremity. In: Omer G, Spinner M, eds. *Management of peripheral nerve problems*. Philadelphia: WB Saunders.

Kaplan EB. (1960) Correction of a disabling flexion contraction of the thumb. *Bull Hosp Joint Surg* **42A**:467–70.

Karanjia ND and Stiles PJ. (1988) Cubital bursitis. *J Bone Joint Surg* **70B**: 832–3.

Kelly MJ, Jackson BT. (1976) Compression of median nerve at the elbow. *BMJ* **2**:283–6.

Kerr AT. (1918) The brachial plexus of nerves in man, variations in its formation and branches. *Am J Anat* **23**:285–395.

Kihol LG, Nevin S. (1952) Isolated neuritis of the anterior interosseous nerve. *BMJ* **i**:850–1.

Kojima T, Harase M, Ietsune T. (1968). Pronator syndrome: report of six cases. *Orthop Surg (Jpn)* **19**:1147–8.

Kopell HP, Thompson WAL. (1958) Pronator syndrome. *N Engl J Med* **259**:713–15.

Lipscomb PR, Burleson RJ. (1955) Vascular and neural complications in supercondylar fractures of the humerus in children. *J Bone Joint Surg* **37A**:487–92.

Lorei MP, Hershman EB. (1993) Peripheral nerve injuries in athletes. Treatment and prevention. *Sports Med* **16**:130–47.

Mackinnon SE, Dellon AL (1988) Median nerve entrapment in the proximal forearm and brachium. In: Mackinnon SE, Dellon AL, eds. *Surgery of the peripheral nerve*. New York: Thieme.

Mangini U. (1960) Flexor pollicis longus muscle. Its morphology and clinical significance. *J Bone Joint Surg* **42A**:467–47.

Mannerfelt L, Norman O. (1969) Attrition ruptures of flexor tendons in rheumatoid arthritis caused by bony spurs in the carpal tunnel. *J Bone Joint Surg* **51B**:270–7.

Mannerfelt L. (1966) Studies on the hand in ulnar nerve paralysis. *Acta Orthop Scand (Suppl.)* **87**:1–5.

Martinelli P, Gabollini AS, Poppi N, et al. (1982) Pronator syndrome due to thickened bicipital aponeurosis. *J Neurol Neurosurg Psychiatry* **45**:181–2.

Molner W, Paul DJ. (1972) Complications of axillary arteriotomies. *Radiology* **104**:269–76.

Morris HH, Perers BH. (1976) Pronator syndrome: clinical and electrophysiologic features in seven cases. *J Neurol Neurosurg Psychiatry* **39**:461–4.

Nalebuff EA, Potter TA. (1968) Rheumatoid involvement of tendon and tendon sheaths in the hand. *Clin Orthop* **59**:147–59.

Nebot-Cegarra J, Perez-Berruezo J, Reina de la Torre F. (1991) Variations of the pronator teres muscle: predispositional role to median nerve entrapment. *Arch Anat Histol Embryol.* **74**:35–45.

North ER, Kaul MP. (1996) Compression neuropathy: Median. In: Peimer CA, ed. *Surgery of the hand and upper extremity*. New York: McGraw-Hill.

Olehnik WK, Manske PR, Szerzinski J. Median nerve compression in the proximal forearm. *J Hand Surg* **19A**:121–6.

Omer GE Jr. (1974) Injuries to nerves of the upper extremity *J Bone Joint Surg* **56A**:1615–24.

Omer GE, Spinner M. (1988) *Management of peripheral nerve problems*. Philadelphia, PA: WB Saunders.

Proudman TW, Menz PJ. (1988) An anomaly of the median artery associated with the anterior relation to the pronator teres. *Acta Neurochir (Wien)* **91**:144–6.

Rana NA, Kenwright J, Taylor RG, Rushworth G. (1974) Complete lesion of the median nerve associated with dislocation of the elbow joint. *Acta Orthop Scand* **45**:365–9.

Reimann AF, Daseler EH, Anson BJ, Beaton LE. (1944) The palmaris longus muscle and tendon. The study of 1600 extremities. *Anat Rec* **89**:495–505.

Schmidt H, Eiken O. (1971) The anterior interosseous nerve syndrome. *Scand J Plast Reconstr Surg* **5**:53–6.

Spinner M, Schrieber SN. (1969) The anterior interosseous nerve paralysis as a complication of supercondylar fractures in children. *J Bone Joint Surg* **51A**:1584–90.

Spinner, M. (1970) The anterior interosseous nerve syndrome with special attention to its variations. *J Bone Joint Surg* **52A**:84–94.

Spinner M. (1978a) *Injuries to the major branches of peripheral nerves in the forearm,* 2nd edn. Philadelphia, PA: WB Saunders.

Spinner M. (1978b) The median nerve. In: Spinner M, ed. *Injuries to the major branches of peripheral nerves in the forearm*, 2nd edn. Philadelphia, PA: WB Saunders: 208–11.

Stewart JD. (1987) *Focal peripheral neuropathies*. New York: Elsevier.

Struthers J. (1854) On some points in the abnormal anatomy of the arm. *Br For Med Chir Rev* **14**:170–9.

Struthers J. (1848) On a peculiarity of the humerus and humeral artery. *Monthly J Med Sci* **28**:264–7.

Sunderland S. (1978) Median nerve lesions. In: Sunderland S, ed. *Nerve and Nerve Injuries*. Edinburgh: Churchill Livingstone.

Winkelman NZ, Spinner M. (1973) A variant high sensory branch of the median nerve to the third web space. *Bull Hosp Joint Dis* **54**:161–3.

6
Distal ulnar nerve compression

Carolyn M. Lévis

Introduction

Distal ulnar nerve compression primarily results from entrapment of this nerve at the wrist. Compression of the nerve at the elbow and through the forearm is discussed elsewhere in this book (Chapter 7). Several etiologies and compressive structures have been identified at the level of the wrist and proximal hand. The unique relationship of the ulnar nerve to these structures and the prevalence of wrist trauma pose potential sites of entrapment. Anatomic variations of the ulnar nerve in this area and the proximity to the median nerve make the diagnosis challenging.

Anatomic history

Early descriptions of distal ulnar nerve compression center about the work of Jean Casimir Felix Guyon, a French anatomist who was interested in the 'Ollier Phenomenon' of small areas of skin distention over the volar–ulnar palm when pressure is applied to the base of the hypothenar eminence. Early in his career, he described the relationship of the ulnar nerve as it traveled from the forearm to the hand through a three-sided space in the hypothenar region of the palm and presented this work in 1861 at the Anatomical Society of Paris. This region was subsequently referred to as the 'loge de Guyon' (*loge*, fr. canal). His anatomic work described the course of the nerve through this region and the other contents of this space: the ulnar artery and venae comitantes (Guyon, 1861).

Other authors have described this anatomic region as a 'tunnel' between the pisiform and hamate, in which the ulnar nerve could be compressed. McFarlane et al. (1976) were among the first to report that the 'pisohamate tunnel' represents a site of potential impingement of the motor branch of the ulnar nerve by the fibrous origin of the hypothenar muscles. Further reports have expanded the terminology used to describe this area. Denman (1978) referred to the region as the 'space of Guyon' and purposed to 'define the space of Guyon with precision'. This anatomic study described the components of the space as: the *hiatus*; space bounded by the pisiform ulnarly, the proximal edge of the flexor retinaculum on the deep aspect and the distal edge of the volar carpal ligament superficially, the *floor*; flexor retinaculum fibers radially, pisohamate ligament ulnarly, the *roof*; fibrous tissue and the hypothenar fatpad (Denman, 1978). To distinguish this space from the *pisohamate tunnel*, Denman recommended that this term be reserved for the description of that part of the space that extends dorsally carrying the motor branch of the ulnar nerve. He subsequently referred to the remainder of the space as the *pisoretinacular space*.

This relatively small region has intrigued surgeons to such an extent that further anatomic descriptions and terminology have been presented to further define it. Jay Ramsey Hunt is credited with the first report of distal ulnar nerve compression suggesting various sites of potential entrapment (Hunt, 1908). Gross and Gelberman have referred to this region as the *distal ulnar tunnel* and detailed the anatomy extensively into three distinct zones (Gross and

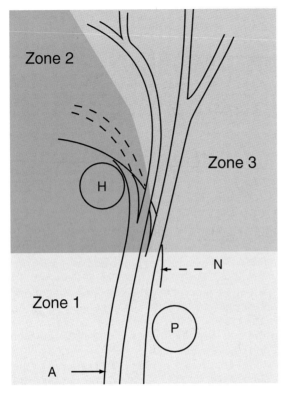

Figure 6.1

Zones of Guyon's canal. H, hamate; P, platform, A, ulnar artery; n, ulnar nerve. (Redrawn with permission from Gross ME, Gelberman RH (1985) Anatomy of the distal ulnar tunnel. *Clin Orthop* **196**: 238–47.)

Gelberman, 1985; Figure 6.1). The zones that they have described are based on the internal topography of the ulnar nerve. The authors have reviewed the reported cases of distal ulnar nerve compression, differentiating the clinical features as they pertain to the pathology located in each zone of the tunnel. Among the cases of nerve compression with both motor and sensory deficits, 83% involved ganglions or fractures in zone I. 72% of the cases with pure motor deficits involved ganglions or fractures in zone II.

Thrombosis or anomalous muscles were found in Zone III in cases of isolated sensory deficits (Figure 6.2).

Although many authors have suggested these anatomically based terms for distal ulnar nerve compression, we will use what is arguably the most familiar term for this region, viz. Guyon's canal.

Cobb et al. (1996) redefined the boundaries of Guyon's canal based upon anatomic dissection and histologic study. They reported that the roof of the Guyon's canal 'does not directly connect to the hamate bone ... the roof of this space extends radially to the hook of the hamate and attaches to the flexor retinaculum (transverse carpal ligament)'. Their description emphasizes that the ulnar artery, venae comitantes and the sensory branch of the ulnar nerve pass radial to the hook of the hamate and lie on the transverse carpal ligament. The significance of this point should be noted during carpal tunnel decompression (Cobb et al., 1996; Figure 6.3).

Causes of ulnar nerve compression

Vascular anomalies: The early literature has several reports of ulnar nerve impingement from traumatic aneurysms or thrombosis of the ulnar artery (Axe and McClain, 1986; Costigan et al., 1959; Jackson, 1954; Kleinert and Boliantis, 1965; Middleton, 1933;

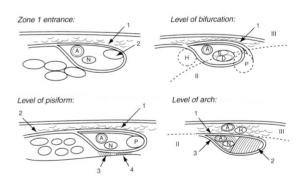

Figure 6.2

Cross section of the distal ulnar tunnel. *Entrance to Zone 1:* A, artery; N, nerve; 1, palmar carpal ligament; 2, tendon of flexor carpi ulnaris. Level of pisiform: P, pisiform; 1, palmaris brevis; 2, transverse carpal ligament; 3, pisohamate ligament; 4, pisometacarpal ligament. *Level of bifurcation of nerve:* H, hamate; S, D, superficial and deep branches of ulnar nerve; 1, palmaris brevis; II, Zone 2; III, Zone 3. *Level of the hypothenar arch:* 1, fibrous arch of muscles; 2, abductor digiti minimi; 3, flexor digiti minimi. (Redrawn with permission from Gross ME, Gelberman RH (1985) Anatomy of the distal ulnar tunnel. *Clin Orthop* **196**: 238–47.)

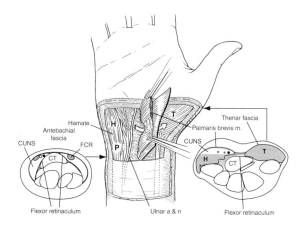

Figure 6.3

Anatomy of Guyon's canal. CT, carpal tunnel; CUNS, carpal ulnar neurovascular space; FCR, flexor carpi radialis; H, hamate; P, pisiform; T, thenar muscle. (Redrawn with permission from Cobb TK, Carmichael SW, Cooney WP. (1996) Guyon's canal revisited: an anatomic study of the carpal ulnar neurovascular space. *J Hand Surg* **21A**: 861–9.)

Smith, 1962). Since then, numerous case reports of ulnar nerve compression from a vascular source have been reported (Grossman and Becket, 1996; Kalisman et al., 1982; Kay et al., 1988; Koch et al., 1998; Segal et al., 1992; Vandertop and van't Verlaat, 1985; Yoshi et al., 1999).

Soft tissue masses: Ganglions in the region of Guyon's canal have been described by many authors as a source of impingement of both the sensory and motor branches of the ulnar nerve (Kuschner et al., 1988; Mallet and Zikha 1955; Moneim, 1992; Puig et al., 1999; Richmond, 1963; Seddon, 1952; Seror et al., 2000). Other soft tissue masses causing distal ulnar nerve impingement include lipomas (Galeano et al., 2001; White and Hauna, 1962; Zahawi, 1984), giant cell tumors (Hages et al., 1961; Milberg and Kleinert, 1980; Rengachary and Arjunan, 1981), intraneural cyst (Bowers and Doppelt, 1979) and uremic tumoral calcinosis (Garcia et al., 2000). Compression of the dorsal sensory branch of the ulnar nerve by a ganglion or proliferative synovium on the ulnar border of the hand has also been described (Lucas, 1984), as well as compression from a wristwatch (Stopford, 1922).

Anomalous muscles, either in location or size, or accessory muscles are a frequent source of distal ulnar nerve compression. Abnormalities of the palmaris longus (Regan et al., 1981; Thomas, 1958), flexor carpi ulnaris (Kang et al., 1997; Papierski, 1996; Pribyl and Moneim, 1994; Zook et al., 1988), and flexor digiti minimi (Spinner et al., 1996) have been described. Accessory muscles that have been found to cause distal ulnar nerve compression include: accessory flexor digiti minimi (Salzebach, 1977; Weeks and Young, 1982); accessory abductor digiti minimi (Al-Qattan, 1993; James et al., 1987; Luethke and Dellon, 1992; Netscher and Cohen, 1997; Vanderpool et al., 1968); and accessory palmaris longus (Santoro et al., 2000).

Fractures and/or dislocations of the carpal bones and of the distal radius and ulna have been described as sources of impingement of the ulnar nerve (Bishop and Beckenbaugh, 1988; Dunn, 1972; Foucher et al., 1985; Murphy and Parkhill, 1990; Nisenfield and Neviaser, 1974; Vance and Gelberman,1978; Yamada et al., 1995; Zoega, 1966). The nerve may be directly injured by the fractured bone such as with a hamate fracture or by traction, impingement or scarring during healing of fracture fragments.

Other sources: Repetitive trauma in the form of vibration or impact of the ulnar nerve and/or artery against the hook of the hamate is described by some as 'hypothenar hammer syndrome' and may be a source of compression of the ulnar nerve as well as the ulnar artery (Conn et al., 1970).

The literature is replete with reports of sports-related causes of ulnar nerve compression in the wrist and palm that can occur from direct trauma to the nerve from repetitive, vigorous micro-injury leading to swelling and ischemia of the nerve, or possibly from prolonged gripping of bicycle handlebars with wrist extension (Anonymous, 1975; Eckman et al., 1975; Hankey and Gubbay, 1988; Howse, 1994; Hoyt, 1976; Maimaris and Zadek, 1990; Richmond, 1994). Both motor and sensory abnormalities on EMG and nerve conduction studies were noted in four long-distance tour cyclists, associated with persistent paresis over several months (Noth et al., 1980). Andersen and Bovim reported that in a survey of 160 touring cyclists, 19% had weakness in the hand and 30% had numbness in the hand, including half with ulnar-sided parathesias only (Andersen and Bovim, 1997).

Anatomy of the ulnar nerve

The ulnar nerve is one of the terminal components of the medial cord of the brachial plexus with contributions from C-8 and T-1 nerve roots. The fibers run in the lower trunk which form a portion of the medial cord before ultimately becoming the ulnar nerve. It travels distally through the arm, with the medial head of triceps on its medial border, and approaches the forearm through a tunnel bounded by the medial epicondyle superiorly and laterally, the condylar groove of the olecranon on its deep side and superficially by the connective tissue traversing these two bony landmarks. As it enters the forearm, it splits the two heads of the flexor carpi ulnaris muscle and proceeds, along with the ulnar artery and vena comitantes, in a straight line towards the radial aspect of the pisiform. The nerve lies in the interval between the flexor carpi ulnaris and the flexor digitorum profundus muscles. The nerve innervates the flexor carpi ulnaris muscle via a branch at the elbow and the flexor digitorum profundus muscle (the ulnar two muscle bellies) through a branch in the mid forearm.

There are three fascicular groups of the ulnar nerve in the forearm. The ulnar group becomes the dorsal sensory branch of the ulnar nerve which exits the main nerve 7–9 cm proximal to the distal wrist crease and passes dorsally to the ulnar hand, ring and small fingers. The central fascicular group represents the motor fibers to the intrinsic muscles in the hand and once the dorsal sensory fibers exit dorsally, the motor bundle is now the ulnar of the two remaining groups. The radial fibers therefore are the sensory branches to the ulnar half of the ring and little fingers. At the level of the distal volar wrist crease, the motor fibers pass ulnar to the pisiform, deep to the sensory fibers and over the pisohamate ligament and course deep to the fibrous arch of the hypothenar muscles into the hand. The anatomy through this pisohamate distal ulnar tunnel has been well described by Gross and Gelberman (1985).

Diagnosis

As with all nerve evaluations, a review of systems may reveal comorbidities such as diabetes mellitus. Distal ulnar nerve entrapment is suspected in cases of motor weakness in the *hand* and diminished sensation in the palmar aspect of the ring and little fingers and the ulnar palm. Parasthesias that include the dorsal aspect of the ring and little fingers suggest a more proximal level of entrapment of the nerve including the dorsal sensory branch. The history may reveal acute or repetitive hand/palm trauma. A thorough motor examination includes: inspection for muscle atrophy (see Figure 6.4); the evaluation of the flexor digitorum profundus (to determine level of compression) to the ring and little fingers; the hypothenar muscles; the interossei and the adductor pollicis; as well as pinch and grip strength. Tenderness in the palm, particularly point tenderness in the palm at or beyond the pisiform, should suggest possible compression of the ulnar nerve in the hand. Provocative maneuvers of compression of the ulnar nerve in the palm causing parasthesias and vascular assessment for bruits and thrills and perfusion of the hand with Allen's test should all be performed. Sensory evaluation of the ring and little fingers and ulnar palm as well as the dorsal ulnar hand (to determine level of compression), includes moving and static two-point discrimination. Other sensory modalities such as temperature and pain can be used to rule out central nervous system causes for muscle atrophy. Similarly, all muscles in the upper extremity should be evaluated for signs of weakness to localize the point of impingement or lesion in the neck or extremity such as at the root, trunk or cord levels. This evaluation may elicit conflicting diagnoses such as sparing of the ulnar intrinsic muscles in a high ulnar nerve lesion or proximal level of compression that should provoke one to consider the anatomic variant of a Martin–Gruber connection. This variation in anatomy is present in 15–20% of upper extremities when motor fibers traveling in the median or anterior interosseous nerve crossover in the forearm and proceed to the hand by way of the ulnar nerve. Similarly, in a ulnar nerve injury or compression in the forearm, clawing may be present in three or four fingers in the presence of the Riche–Cannieu anomaly, where median nerve motor fibers cross to the ulnar nerve in the hand and forearm (Kaplan and Spinner, 1980). Other variations of the innervation exist in the hand such as ulnar nerve to flexor

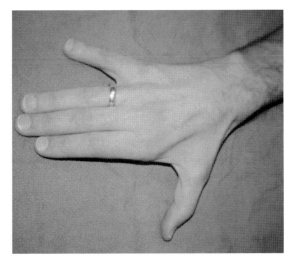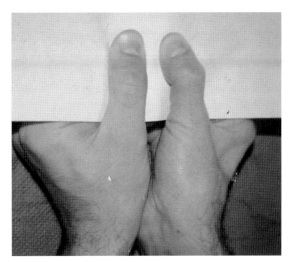

Figure 6.4

(a) Marked intrusion muscle atrophy of a patient with distal ulnar nerve compression. (b) Same patient attempting lateral pinch, with evidence of Fromeits sign and atrophy of the first dorsal inteosseous and abductor pollicis muscles.

pollicis brevis (50%), abductor pollicis brevis in 2.5% and opponens pollicis in 10% of anatomic dissections by Harness and Sekeles (1971).

Although ganglions are the most common cause of distal ulnar nerve compression, they are rarely identified on physical exam. Ultrasound can be used if a cystic mass or vascular cause is suspected (Nakamiohi et al., 2000; Puig et al., 1999). CT scans or MRI can be used to delineate the presence and exact location of masses in the palm. If an associated hook of hamate fracture is suspected, a carpal tunnel view or a CT scan through the carpus may reveal this as a source of distal ulnar nerve compression.

Nerve conduction studies and EMG should be performed to quantitatively assess nerve compression and, in particular, careful inching studies can be used to determine the anatomic area of entrapment. In particular, motor or sensory fibers may be spared which can isolate the compression to a particular pathology within Guyon's canal.

Treatment

In the absence of pathology in the palm, such as ganglia or aneurysms or acute trauma causing compression, non-surgical management of distal ulnar nerve entrapment includes the use of neutral splints to prevent provocative wrist positions such as flexion or extension. Anti-inflammatory agents can be used as well as other disease modifying drugs to treat underlying arthropathies such as rheumatoid arthritis. It is fair to say, however, that the non-surgical treatment for distal ulnar nerve compression is less effective or established than for carpal tunnel syndrome.

In cases where a diagnosis has been made of distal ulnar nerve compression in the presence of a discrete lesion such as a ganglion, anomaly or fracture or symptoms which persist following a trial of non-operative management, decompression of the ulnar nerve through the palm is unwanted. The other clinical scenario worth mentioning, which is frequently encountered by hand surgeons, is a regenerating proximal ulnar nerve following a laceration. A nerve that is regenerating following repair or grafting can be slowed as it traverses through a known site of compression (Mackinnon and Dellon, 1988). Therefore, this region through the pisohamate tunnel should be released either acutely at the time of the nerve repair or as the nerve regeneration proceeds distally to the wrist and hand as determined by the advancing Tinel's sign.

Although the carpal tunnel has been approached with the use of limited incisions and endoscopic techniques, (Agee et al., 1992; Chow, 1989), these minimal access procedures are not appropriate for distal ulnar nerve compression. Open decompression should be considered the gold standard method for releasing the ulnar nerve through the distal ulnar tunnel.

Surgical release of the ulnar nerve through the wrist and palm includes adequate anesthesia using regional (intravenous or brachial plexus block) or less commonly, general anesthesia and the use of a forearm or arm tourniquet. The surgical incision is made at the radial axis of the ring finger which is at the interval between the palmar cutaneous branches of the ulnar and median nerves. The incision also lies between the pisiform ulnarly and proximally and the hamate radially and distally. Proximal exposure may be required depending on the pathology, therefore the incision is extended in a zig-zag fashion across the distal wrist crease to the forearm. The decompression begins proximally in the distal forearm by incising the skin, identifying and retracting the flexor carpi ulnaris tendon ulnarly. Immediately deep to the tendon is the neurovascular bundle of the ulnar nerve and artery with the venae comitantes. As the incision is extended into the palm, the palmaris brevis muscle origin will need to be divided. The volar carpal ligament, which develops from the fibers of the transverse carpal ligament, the palmaris longus and the abductor digiti minimi fascia, is divided. Careful, blunt dissection is required to ensure that small nervelets of the palmar cutaneous branch of the ulnar nerve are not divided in the subcutaneous tissues at the distal end of the volar carpal ligament. Division of any small branches can lead to a painful neuroma or hypersensitive scar postoperatively. At this point in the procedure, a carpal tunnel release can also be performed when indicated by dividing the transverse carpal ligament in a distal-to-proximal direction through this same skin incision. This is performed frequently since median nerve compression through the wrist is very common and the release can easily be accomplished concomitantly to avoid a second procedure through the same region in the future. Silver et al. (1985) reported that 34% of patients with carpal tunnel syndrome have signs and symptoms consistent with distal ulnar nerve compression. As the fibers of the volar carpal ligament are divided proximally, the ulnar artery

and venae comitantes are visualized and are carefully retracted ulnarly, thereby exposing the sensory branch which is also moved towards the pisiform (Figure 6.5). At this point, further decompression of the motor branch of the ulnar nerve can be accomplished. With the ulnar artery, venae comitantes and sensory component of the ulnar nerve retracted ulnarly, the hook of the hamate can be palpated and the origin of the flexor digiti minimi on the hamate visualized as it forms a fibrous arch. At the proximal edge of the arch, the motor branch is identified as it passes between the pisohamate ligament and the flexor digiti minimi (Figure 6.6). A narrow elevator may be placed deep to this arch to protect the motor branch beneath, as the proximal edge of the arch is divided, which can be a restrictive fibrous edge of fascia in many patients.

If necessary, in cases of previous trauma such as fracture, soft tissue injury or secondary surgery when the scar may encroach on the nerve, external neurolysis is performed by incising the epineurium of the motor and sensory branches using loope magnification.

Throughout the dissection, any lesion that has previously been identified will be addressed and

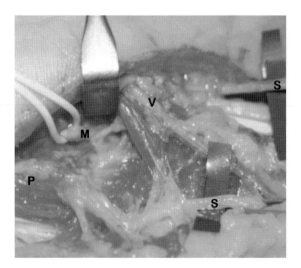

Figure 6.5

Dissection of ulnar nerve through the palm: P, pisiform; V, ulnar artery and venae comitantes retracted radially; M, motor branch of ulnar nerve passing through pisohamate ligament and flexor digiti minimi; S, sensory branch of ulnar nerve.

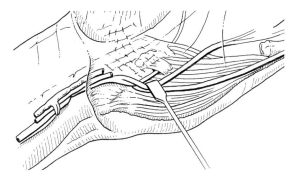

Figure 6.6

Anatomy of deep motor branch traveling deep to the arch of the hypothenar origin. Note the change in position of the motor fascicles from ulnar to radial as the nerve travels distally. (Adapted from Mackinnon SE, Dellon AL (1988) Ulnar nerve entrapment at the wrist. In: *Surgery of the peripheral nerve.* New York: Thieme Medical: 197–216, with permission.)

excised during the decompression. Ultimately, the tourniquet is deflated and hemostasis is confirmed with the bipolar cautery and the skin is closed with 4-0 or 5-0 nylon suture. The incision is dressed and the wrist held in neutral to 20° of wrist extension, often with a carpal tunnel style splint for 48 hours, during which the patient is advised to exercise the digits, but keep the hand elevated while sleeping or sitting. Range of motion and use of the hand for non-repetitive tasks are then encouraged during the day to promote nerve glide while use of a night splint is then recommended for 2 weeks for comfort. The use of a sling is discouraged to avoid unnecessary stiffness of the elbow and shoulder. After the sutures are removed at 2 weeks, the patients are advised to gently massage the incision to promote desensitization and prevent hypertrophy of the scar.

Results

Although there are no reports in the literature that specifically identify the complication rate following distal ulnar nerve decompression, Mackinnon and Dellon (1988) identified hypothenar tenderness and scar hypertrophy or tenderness as the most common adverse outcome.

Similarly, the literature has a paucity of postoperative results of decompression of the nerve at this level. Mackinnon and Dellon (1988) reviewed the results of 43 cases in the literature and found excellent results in 86% and good results in 9%. A subsequent report by Zoch et al. (1990) reviewed the results of ulnar nerve decompression in Guyon's canal in 22 patients, seven of whom had decompression of the ulnar nerve at the elbow simultaneously. All patients had sensory symptoms originally, while 13 had sensory and motor deficiencies. The cause of compression included a ganglion, thrombosed aneurysm of the ulnar artery and fibrotic arch of the hypothenar muscles. In 21 patients, the sensation was improved or normalized. In seven of the 13 patients reported with motor abnormalities, three normalized or improved function while four remained unchanged.

Discussion

Although there are more common compressive neuropathies in the upper extremities, such as the median nerve in the carpal tunnel and the ulnar nerve in the cubital tunnel, distal ulnar nerve compression must be considered in cases of parasthesias and weakness in the hand. Numbness involving the palmar but not the dorsal aspect of the little and ring fingers and weakness of the intrinsic hand muscles should lead one to consider a distal level of ulnar nerve entrapment. A precise history and clinical examination will direct the diagnosis to the correct site of compression. Structural abnormalities are frequently the underlying cause and should be searched for in the evaluation. Surgical decompression is usually necessary when a mass, displaced fracture or dislocation is the source of impingement. Surgery must address both the sensory and motor branches through Guyon's canal to ensure a favorable outcome.

References

Agee JM, McCarroll HR Jr, Tortosa RD, Berry DA, Szabo RM, Peimber CA. (1992) Endoscopic release of the carpal tunnel: A randomized prospective multicenter study. *J Hand Surg* **17A**:987–95.

Al-Qattan NM. (1993) Accessory abductor digiti minimi muscle originating proximal to the wrist causing symptomatic ulnar nerve compression. *Ann Plast Surg* **30**(5):480.

Andersen KV, Bovim G. (1997) Impotence and nerve entrapments in long distance amateur cyclists. *Acta Neurol Scand* **95**(4):233–40.

Anonymous (1975). Handlebar palsy [Letter]. *N Engl J Med* **292**(13):702.

Axe MJ, McClain EJ. (1986) Complete involvement of the ulnar nerve secondary to an ulnar artery aneurysm. A case report. *Am J Sports Med* **14**(2):178–80.

Bishop AT, Beckenbaugh RD. (1988) Fracture of the hamate hook. *J Hand Surg* **13**(1):135–9.

Bowers WH, Doppelt SH. (1979) Compression of the deep branch of the ulnar nerve by an intraneural cyst. Case report. *J Bone Joint Surg* **61A**(4):612–13.

Chow JYC. (1989) Endoscopic release of the carpal ligament: a new technique for carpal tunnel syndrome. *Arthroscopy* **5**:19.

Cobb TK, Carmichael SW, Cooney WP. (1996) Guyon's canal revisited: an anatomic study of the carpal ulnar neurovascular space. *J Hand Surg* **21A**(5):861–9.

Conn J Jr., Bergan JJ, Bell JL. (1970) Hypothenar hammer syndrome: post-traumatic digital ischemia. *Surgery* **68**:1122–28.

Costigan DG, Riley JM, Coy FE. (1959) Thrombofibrosis of the ulnar artery in the palm. *J Bone Joint Surg* **41A**:702–4.

Denman EE. (1978) The anatomy of the space of Guyon. *Hand* **10**:69.

Dunn WA. (1972) Fractures and dislocations of the carpus. *Surg Clin North Am* **52**:1513.

Eckman PB, Pearlstein G, Altorcchi PH. (1975) Ulnar neuropathy in bicycle riders. *Arch Neurol* **2**:130–1.

Foucher G, Schuind F, Merle M, Brunelli F. (1985) Fractures of the hook of the hamate. *J Hand Surg* **10**:205–10.

Galeano M, Colonna M, Risitano G. (2001) Ulnar tunnel syndrome secondary to lipoma of the hypothenar region. *Ann Plast Surg* **46**(1):83–4.

Garcia S, Cofan F, Combalia A, Campistol JM, Oppenheimer F, Ramon R. (2000) Compression of the ulnar nerve in Guyon's canal by uremic tumoral calcinosis. *Arch Orthop Trauma Surg* **120**(3–4):228–30.

Gross MS, Gelberman RH. (1985) Anatomy of the distal ulnar tunnel. *Clin Orthop* **196**:238–47.

Grossman JA, Becker GA. (1996) Ulnar neuropathy caused by a thrombosed ulnar nerve vein. Case report and literature review. *Ann Chir Main Memb Super* **15**(4):244–7.

Guyon F. (1861) Note sur une disposition anatomique propre a la face anterieure de la region du poignet et non encore decrite pa le docteur. *Bull Soc Anat Paris* **6**:184–6.

Hankey GJ, Gubbay SS. (1988) Compressive mononeuropathy of the deep palmar branch of the ulnar nerve in cyclists. *J Neurol Neurosurg Psychiatry* **51**(12):1588–90.

Harness D, Sekeles E. (1971) The double anastomotic innervation of the thenar muscles. *J Anat* **109**:461–66.

Hayes JR, Mulholland RC, O'Connor BT. (1961) Compression of the deep palmar branch of the ulnar nerve. *J Bone Joint Surg* **43A**:469.

Howse C. (1994) Wrist injuries in sport. *Sports Med* **17**(3):163–75.

Hoyt CS. (1976) Ulnar neuropathy in bicycle riders. *Arch Neurol* **33**(5):372.

Hunt JR. (1908) Occupational neuritis of the deep palmar branch of the ulnar nerve. *J Nerve Ment Dis* **35**:676–89.

Jackson JP. (1954) Traumatic thrombosis of the ulnar artery in the palm. *J Bone Joint Surg* **36B**:438.

James MR, Rowley DI, Norris SH. (1987) Ulnar nerve compression by an accessory abductor digiti minimi muscle presenting following injury. *Injury* **18**(1):66–7.

Kalisman M, Laborde K, Wolff TW. (1982) Ulnar nerve compression secondary to ulnar artery false aneurysm at the Guyon's canal. *J Hand Surg* **7**(2):137–9.

Kang HJ, Yoo JH, Kang ES. (1997) Ulnar nerve compression syndrome due to an anomalous arch of the ulnar nerve piercing the flexor carpi ulnaris: a case report. *J Hand Surg* **21A**(2):277–8.

Kaplan EB, Spinner M. (1980) Normal and anomalous innervation patterns in the upper extremity. In: Omer GE, Spinner M, eds. *Management of peripheral nerve problems* Philadelphia PA: WB Saunders: 75–99.

Kay PR, Abraham JS, Davies DR, Bertfield H. (1988) Ulnar artery aneurysms after injury mimicking acute infection in the hand. *Injury* 19(6):402–4.

Kleinert HE, Boliantis GJ. (1965) Thrombosis of the palmar arterial arch and its tributaries: etiology and newer concepts in treatment. *Trauma* 5:447–57.

Koch H, Haas F, Pierer G. (1998) Ulnar nerve compression in Guyon's canal due to a haemangioma of the ulnar artery. *J Hand Surg* 23(2):242–4.

Kuschner SH, Gelberman RH, Jennings C. (1988) Ulnar nerve compression at the wrist. *J Hand Surg* [Am] 13:577–80.

Lucas GL. (1984) Irritative neuritis of the dorsal sensory branch of the ulnar nerve from underlying ganglion. *Clin Orthop*, Jun: 216–19.

Luethke R, Dellon AL. (1982) Accessory abductor digiti minimi muscle originating proximal to the wrist causing symptomatic ulnar nerve compression. *Ann Plast Surg* 28(3):307–8

Mackinnon SE, Dellon AL. (1988) Nerve repair and nerve grafting. In *Surgery of the peripheral nerve.* New York: Thieme Medical: 89–129.

Mackinnon SE, Dellon AL. (1988) Ulnar nerve entrapment at the wrist. In *Surgery of the peripheral nerve.* New York: Thieme Medical: 197–216.

Maimaris C, Zadeh HG. (1990) Ulnar nerve compression in the cyclist's hand: two case reports and review of the literature. *Br J Sports Med* 24(4):245–6.

Mallet BI, Zikha KJ. (1955) Compression of the ulnar nerve at the wrist by the ganglion. *Lancet* 1:890.

McFarlane RM, Mayer JR, Huggil JV. (1976) Further observations on the anatomy of the ulnar nerve at the wrist. *Hand* 8:115.

Middleton DS. (1933) Occupational aneurysms of palmar arteries. *Br J Surg* 21:215–18.

Milberg P, Kleinert HE. (1980) Giant cell tumour compression of the deep branch of the ulnar nerve. *Ann Plast Surg* 4:426.

Moneim MS. (1992) Ulnar nerve compression at the wrist. Ulnar tunnel syndrome. *Hand Clin* May: 337–44.

Murphy TP, Parkhill WS. (1990) Fracture-dislocation of the base of the fifth metacarpal with an ulnar motor nerve lesion: case report. *J Trauma* 30(12):1585–7.

Nakamichi K, Tachibana S, Kitajima I. (2000) Ultrasonography in the diagnosis of ulnar tunnel syndrome caused by an occult ganglion. *J Hand Surg* 25B(5):503–4.

Netscher D, Cohen V. Ulnar nerve compression at the wrist secondary to anomalous muscles: a patient with a variant of abductor digiti minimi. *Ann Plast Surg* 39(6):647–51.

Nisenfield G, Neviaser RJ. (1974) Fracture of the hook of the hamate: a diagnosis easily missed. *J Trauma* 14:612.

Noth J, Dietz V, Mauritz KH. (1980) Cyclist's palsy: neurological and EMG study in 4 cases with distal ulnar lesions. *J Neurol Sci* 47(1):111–16.

Papierski P. Ulnar neuropathy at the wrist associated with a recurrent branch through the flexor carpi ulnaris tendon. *J Hand Surg* 21B(3):347–8.

Pribyl CR, Moneim MS. (1994) Anomalous hand muscle found in the Guyon's canal at exploration for ulnar artery thrombosis. A case report. *Clin Orthop* 306:120–3.

Puig S, Turkof E, Sedivy R, Ciovica R, Lang S, Kainberger FM. (1999). Sonographic diagnosis of recurrent ulnar nerve compression by ganglion cyst. *J Ultrasound Med* 18(6): 433–6.

Regan PJ, Feldberg L, Bailey BN. (1991) Accessory palmaris longus muscle causing ulnar nerve compression at the wrist. *J Hand Surg* 16A(4):736–8.

Rengachary SS, Arjunan K. (1981) Compression of the ulnar nerve at Guyon's canal by soft tissue giant cell tumour. *Neurosurgery* 8:400–5.

Richmond DA. (1963) Carpal ganglion with ulnar nerve compression. *J Bone Joint Surg* 45B:513.

Richmond DR. (1994) Handlebar problems in bicycling. *Clin Sports Med* 13(1):165–73.

Salzebach S. (1977) Ulnar tunnel syndrome caused by anomalous muscles. Case report. *Scand J Plast Reconstr Surg* 11(3):255–8.

Santoro TD, Matloub HS, Gosain AK. (2000) Ulnar nerve compression by an anomalous muscle following carpal tunnel release: a case report. *J Hand Surg* 25A(4):740–4.

Seddon HJ. (1952) Carpal ganglion as a cause of paralysis of the deep branch of the ulnar nerve. *J Bone Joint Surg* 34B:386–90.

Segal R, Machiraju U, Larkins M. (1992) Tortuous peripheral arteries: a cause of focal neuropathy. Case report. *J Neurosurg* **76**(4):701–4.

Seror P, Lestrade M, Vacher H. (2000) Ulnar nerve compression at the wrist by a synovial cyst successfully treated with percutaneous puncture and corticosteroid injection. *Joint Bone Spine* **67**(2):127–8.

Silver MA, Gelberman RH, Gellman H, et al. (1985) Carpal tunnel syndrome: associated abnormalities in ulnar nerve function and the effect of carpal tunnel release on these abnormalities. *J Hand Surg* **10A**:710.

Smith JW. (1962) True aneurysms of traumatic origin in the palm. *Am J Surg* **104**:7–13.

Spinner RJ, Lins RE, Spinner M. (1996) Compression of the medial half of the deep branch of the ulnar nerve by an anomalous origin of the flexor digiti minimi. A case report. *J Bone Joint Surg* **78A**(3):427–30.

Stopford JSB. (1922) Neuritis produced by a wristlet watch. *Lancet* **1**:993–4.

Thomas CG. (1958) Clinical manifestations of an accessory palmaris muscle. *J Bone Joint Surg* **40A**:929.

Vance RM, Gelberman RH. (1978) Acute ulnar neuropathy with fractures at the wrist. *J Bone Joint Surg* **60A**:692–95.

Vanderpool DW, Chalmers J, Whiston TB. (1968) Peripheral compression lesions of the ulnar nerve. *J Bone Joint Surg* **50**:792.

Vandertop WP, van't Verlaat JW. (1985) Neuropathy of the ulnar nerve caused by an aneurysm of the ulnar artery at the wrist. A case report and review of the literature. *Clin Neurol Neurosurg* **87**(2):139–42.

Weeks PM, Young VL. (1982) Ulnar artery thrombosis and ulnar nerve compression associated with an anomalous hypothenar muscle. *Plast Reconstr Surg* **69**(1):130–1.

White WL, Hauna DC. (1962) Troublesome lipomata of the upper extremity. *J Bone Joint Surg* **1A**:247.

Yamada K, Sekiya S, Oka S, Norimatsu H. (1995) Lunate dislocation with ulnar nerve paresis. *J Hand Surg* **20B**(2):206–9.

Yoshii S, Ikeda K, Murakami H. (1999) Ulnar nerve compression secondary to ulnar artery true aneurysm at Guyon's canal. *J Neurosurg Sci* **43**(4):295–7.

Zahrawi F. (1984) Acute compression ulnar neuropathy at Guyon's canal resulting from lipoma. *J Hand Surg* **9A**:238–40.

Zoch G, Meissl G, Millesi H. (1990) Results of decompression of the ulnar nerve in Guyon's canal. (In German). *Handchir Mikrochir Plast Chir* **22**(3):125–9.

Zoega H. (1966) Fracture of the lower end of the radius with ulnar nerve palsy. *J Bone Joint Surg* **48B**:514–16.

Zook EG, Kucan JO, Guy RJ. (1988) Palmar wrist pain caused by ulnar nerve entrapment in the flexor carpi ulnaris tendon. *J Hand Surg* **13A**(5):732–5.

7
Ulnar nerve compression

Greg Watchmaker

Historical introduction

The term 'cubital tunnel syndrome' was coined by Feindel and Stratford (Feindel and Stratford, 1958). The first reports of ulnar compression at the elbow, however, are credited to Panas (Panas, 1878) who emphasized the role of previous local trauma or facture. He described this condition as 'post-traumatic ulnar neuritis'. Adson described his treatment of ulnar nerve compression in which one-third of the patients had not previously suffered a fracture (Adson, 1918). Feindel felt the cause of such 'idiopathic' ulnar neuropathy was from a thick fibrous band running between the two heads of the flexor carpi ulnaris. Geoffrey Osborne received credit a year earlier for this discovery (Osborne, 1957).

The first surgical procedure on the ulnar nerve at the elbow was described by Earle who performed a nerve resection for severe neuralgia (Earle, 1816). Several reports of resection or division of the nerve and repair followed (Calder, 1833; Sherren, 1908). Sheldon recognized the permanent deficit resulting from nerve division and cautioned against it (Sheldon, 1921). The first anterior transposition is reported to have been performed by Roux of Lausanne in 1897 (Platt, 1926; Davidson, 1935). Two years later, Farquhar Curtis presented a patient to the New York Neurological Society in whom he transposed the nerve anteriorly. Earlier attempts to deepen the postcondylar groove were discarded because of fibro-osseous scarring.

Anatomy and sites of compression

The nerve fibers that form the ulnar nerve exit the spinal cord via the C-8 and T-1 nerve roots. The ulnar nerve proper is the terminal branch of the medial cord of the brachial plexus (Figure 7.1a). The nerve crosses the axilla medial to the axillary artery and descends anterior to the triceps (Figure 7.1b). An unusual site of nerve compression occurs high in the arm secondary to the chondroepitrochlearis muscle (Spinner et al., 1991). This uncommon muscle arises from the sixth and seventh ribs and crosses the axilla to insert upon the medial epicondyle. It is readily identified on physical exam by an accessory anterior axillary fold.

In the middle third of the arm, the nerve pierces the intermuscular septum and continues down the arm immediately posterior to the septum (Figure 7.1c). Proximal to the elbow, a potential site of compression has been identified as 'the arcade of Struthers'. Struthers' article in 1848 deals more with median nerve compression and the ligament which bears his name than with an arcade across the ulnar nerve (Struthers, 1848). Several authors have found the ulnar nerve compressed by thin ligamentous bands in the zone where it pierces the intermuscular septum (Ochiai et al., 1992). Mackinnon failed to find an arcade at this level in her series of more than 500 ulnar nerve explorations (Mackinnon and Dellon, 1988). The arcade was felt to be an iatrogenic artifact following incomplete release of the medial intermuscular septum.

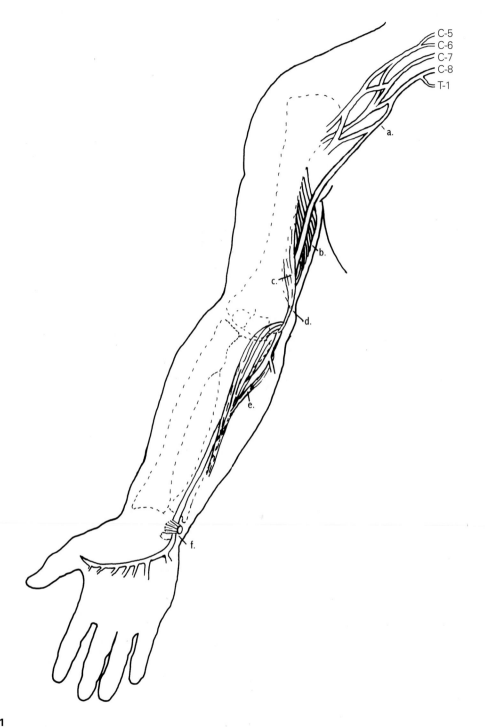

Figure 7.1

The course of the ulnar nerve from brachial plexus to hand: (a) nerve arises from medial cord, (b) descends anterior to triceps, (c) posterior to intermuscular septum, (d) entering fibro-osseous cubital tunnel, (e) entering forearm between heads of flexor carpi ulnaris, and (f) crossing wrist through Guyon's canal.

As the nerve approaches the elbow, it enters a fibro-osseous tunnel (Figure 7.1d). The roof of the tunnel (superficial) is a fascial bridge between the medial epicondyle and olecranon. O'Driscoll has referred to this bridge as the 'cubital tunnel retinaculum' and noted its anatomic variants (O'Driscoll et al., 1991). In individuals with a thickened retinaculum, compression of the nerve occurs with elbow flexion. In 11% of individuals, an anconeous epitrochlearis muscle will be found covering the tunnel (Dellon, 1986). Rarely, this muscle has been found compressing the nerve (Dahners and Wood, 1984). Excessive elbow exercise may cause the epitrochlearis muscle to become hypertrophied and compressive (Hodgkinson et al., 1994). In individuals with an underdeveloped retinaculum, ulnar nerve subluxation is more likely. Recurrent subluxation may contribute to nerve dysfunction (Rayan, 1990).

The floor of the tunnel (deep) is the ulnar groove of the medial epicondyle of the humerus. In 28% of individuals, the medial head of the triceps extends within the floor of the tunnel proximally (Dellon, 1986). In three-quarters of such individuals, the ulnar nerve partially subluxes out of the tunnel. A prominent medial head has clinically been found to compress the nerve (O'Hara and Stone, 1996). The medial head of the triceps may also play a role in patients with cubitus varus deformity. The forward, medial movement of the triceps head may compress the nerve in such individuals (Ogino et al., 1986). Abnormal insertions of the triceps muscle into the medial epicondyle has also been implicated in ulnar neuropathy (Matsuura et al., 1994).

More distally, as the nerve crosses the elbow joint, the floor is composed of the joint capsule and portions of the medial collateral ligament (O'Driscoll et al., 1991). Inflammatory arthritis, including rheumatoid disease and calcium pyrophosphate dihydrate crystal deposition disease, can cause thickening of the joint capsule and ligament (Taniguchi et al., 1996). This protrudes the floor of the tunnel and can compress the nerve leading to neuropathy (Balagtas-Balmaseda et al., 1983).

Fractures about the elbow can also lead to synovial cysts that compress the nerve directly (Laurencin et al., 1994). Hemarthrosis of the elbow joint can secondarily cause compression (Renwick and Moneim, 1993). Recurrent elbow dislocation may injure the nerve through repeated traction (Malkawi, 1981). Swelling from a distal rupture of the biceps tendon is more commonly associated with median nerve symptoms, but may also cause ulnar neuropathy.

Standard radiographs of the elbow for non-traumatic ulnar neuropathy rarely demonstrate pathology. Special views to assess the depth of the groove and adjacent trochlear lip osteophytes may be helpful (St John and Palmaz, 1986). Twenty per cent of patients with neuropathy were found to have osteophytes adjacent to the groove compared with none of the normal individuals.

Magnetic resonance imaging is not commonly used to establish a diagnosis of cubital tunnel compression. Nerve swelling (74%) and nerve signal increase (97%), however, are sensitive and specific markers of this problem (Britz et al., 1996).

Individuals suffering severe burns develop heterotopic calcification, 2% of the time. It most frequently occurs about the elbow and may result in bony encasement of the ulnar nerve with concomitant compression (Vorenkamp and Nelson, 1987). The surgeon caring for burned patients must be aware of this possibility, as numbness is often attributed to the associated finger burns.

In the forearm, the ulnar nerve passes between the two heads of the flexor carpi ulnaris (FCU) where they join. Seventy-three per cent of dissected specimens have a fibrous band (Osborne's band) bridging the two FCU heads (Dellon, 1986). In the proximal forearm, the ulnar nerve is found deep to the FCU. Rarely, the nerve has been found compressed distally where it exits from the FCU muscle (Campbell et al., 1988). In the mid-forearm, compression is possible by fibrovascular bands coursing over the nerve. These bands originate from the ulnar artery and supply the distal belly of the FCU (Holtzman et al., 1984). A subcutaneous lipoma in the distal two-thirds of the forearm can also cause ulnar neuropathy by direct compression. The nerve becomes compressed against the ulna when the forearm is rested on a firm surface. A similar condition of direct compression occurs in drivers' elbow (Abdel-Salam et al., 1991).

Intraneural anatomy and innervation

The ulnar nerve gives no branches proximal to the elbow except for an occasional articular branch. The most proximal motor branch in the forearm arises approximately 1.6 cm distal to the epicondyle and innervates the FCU (Watchmaker et al., 1994). Subsequent branches arise to innervate the FCU and FDP from both radial and ulnar sides of the nerve. The fascicular anatomy within the nerve is highly variable at the elbow. Some dissected specimens have a single large fascicle comprising the entire nerve while others have more than a dozen fascicles.

The blood supply of the ulnar nerve about the elbow is derived from branches of the brachial artery and ulnar artery. Above the elbow, the superior ulnar collateral artery (SUCA) branches from the brachial artery to join the ulnar nerve in the middle or distal third of the arm (Prevel et al., 1993). The posterior ulnar recurrent artery (PURA) arises from the ulnar artery near its origin and supplies the ulnar nerve below the elbow. Both the SUCA and PURA were found in all dissected extremities. The inferior ulnar collateral artery (IUCA) makes only a minor contribution to the nerve and was found in 5 of 18 specimens studied by Prevel.

The effects of dissection and stretching of peripheral nerves has been examined in laboratory models. Longitudinal stretch of nerves more than 15% causes complete arrest of blood flow in the nerve (Ogata et al., 1986). Local extraneural dissection of the nerve from surrounding tissues resulted in a variable reduction up to 80% depending on the region of dissection. At the elbow, Ogata evaluated the effect of medial epicondylectomy versus anterior transposition on blood flow. There was a significant decrease (>50%) in ulnar nerve perfusion immediately after dissection for transposition. By day 3–4, perfusion returned to normal or above normal flows. Medial epicondylectomy was not associated with this transient decrease in perfusion.

To preserve blood supply during transposition, Sugawara has investigated vascularized transposition (Sugawara, 1988). The technique of vascularized transposition has also been demonstrated (Messina and Messina, 1995).

Tunnel physiology and neural pathology

Nerve excursion and tunnel pressures

The arcade bridging the two heads of the FCU is a zone of high pressure in patients with clinical neuropathy (Werner et al., 1985). Tunnel pressure when the elbow was extended and forearm muscles relaxed was 7–10 mmHg. Passive elbow flexion resulted in pressures of 41–86 mmHg while stimulated flexion resulted in pressures of 163–247 mmHg. Cadaveric study of cubital tunnel pressures has also shown increasing values with elbow flexion (Pechan and Julis, 1975). Resting pressures measured 7 mmHg, while the highest pressures (46 mmHg) were recorded in full elbow flexion with the wrist extended. The volume of the cubital tunnel is greatest with the elbow in full extension and 45% less in flexion (Apfelberg and Larson, 1973).

Pressure upon the nerve can be increased by intraneural masses such as synovial cysts or hemangiomas (Ferlic and Ries, 1990; Inhofe and Moneim, 1996; Kline and Moore, 1992). Direct blunt trauma to the nerve may induce swelling and subsequent compression. Rarely in this situation, an X-ray may reveal calcific neuritis in which the outline of the nerve becomes visible (Ametewee, 1986).

Histology/pathology

Similar to other peripheral nerves, the ulnar nerve is composed of a variable number of fascicles held together by interstitial epineurium and wrapped by an outer epineurium. Dellon has demonstrated histologic changes in cadaveric ulnar nerves with known cubital tunnel syndrome, including thinned myelin layers and Renault bodies (Dellon and Mackinnon, 1988). Similar cadaveric examination on individuals without known neuropathy, however, demonstrated intercalated, demyelinated segments, and reduced myelinated fiber density (Neary and Eames, 1975). Some changes within the nerve, therefore, are expected and may be secondary to normal stretch and relaxation as the elbow moves.

Iatrogenic injury

Ulnar neuropathy is a well documented potential complication following general anesthesia (Warner et al., 1994). One-third of nerve injury claims against anesthesiologists in the United States involve ulnar neuropathy at the elbow. Warner found a rate of one patient per 2,729 with persistent neuropathy in this retrospective postoperative review of non-cardiac patients. Risk factors included male gender, duration of hospitalization greater than 2 weeks, and extremes of body habitus. Patients having all three risk factors suffered a 1:200 rate of neuropathy. Neither the anesthetic technique nor patient position increased this risk. Prospective evaluation of 6,538 patients undergoing surgery found a 0.26% risk of developing neuropathy (Alvine and Schurrer, 1987). The prognosis of postoperative neuropathy is poor whether treated surgically or medically (Miller and Camp, 1979).

Cardiac surgery has a much higher incidence of neuropathy (Casscells et al., 1993). Twenty-six per cent of patients, who were prospectively studied, demonstrated ulnar nerve symptoms after cardiac surgery. All of these patients had abnormalities on their presurgical nerve screening. No patients who had normal presurgical nerve studies developed symptoms postoperatively. A careful preoperative assessment, therefore, can potentially identify patients at risk for this complication.

An uncommon but reported cause of iatrogenic ulnar nerve injury includes cutaneous cryotherapy treatment (Finelli, 1975). Application of liquid nitrogen to the skin for an extended period over the cubital tunnel can cause direct axonal damage.

Diagnosis

Differential diagnosis

The diagnosis of cubital tunnel syndrome depends on a complete medical history, detailed examination, and neurodiagnostic testing. Several systemic illnesses including diabetes, hypothryoidism, polyneuropathy, renal failure and vitamin deficiency can impair function of all peripheral nerves including the ulnar nerve and should be noted. Compression of the ulnar nerve at sites other than the elbow is less common including ulnar tunnel compression at the wrist, tethering across a cervical rib, and C-8 or T-1 root compression.

Its lack of elbow symptoms and sparing of more proximal muscle groups and sensory territories differentiate ulnar tunnel compression at the wrist from cubital tunnel syndrome. Compression at the wrist spares the FCU and FDP muscles in the forearm. It also spares the dorsal ulnar sensory branch which provides sole innervation to the dorsum of the little finger. Assessing weakness in flexion of the little finger distal interphalangeal joint is useful in addition to EMG study of each of the muscle groups.

Nerve root compression or plexopathy may easily be confused with cubital tunnel syndrome. The C-8 and T-I nerve roots provide the motor fibers that travel through the ulnar nerve to supply all ulnar innervated muscles. Patients with more proximal compression, however, will often have more proximal symptoms as well. A cervical spine X-ray is necessary to evaluate foraminal narrowing or spurs in these patients. Attention to the presence of anomalous ribs should be made. Forearm sensory testing can also help separate these two diagnoses. The MABC sensory territory (inner forearm) is spared in cubital tunnel compression since this nerve is a direct branch from the plexus. Intrinsic hand muscle testing can also aid in this differential. Although the ulnar nerve supplies most intrinsic hand muscles, it does not innervate the thenar muscles. These muscles are innervated by C-8, T-1 fibers which travel in the median nerve.

Presentation and symptoms

The most common presenting symptoms include: numbness in the ring and little fingers, weakness of grip, hand clumsiness, atrophy of the hand muscles, and elbow discomfort. In most individuals, sensory complaints proceed motor deficits. A history of the patient's job activities, home activities and athletic endeavors should focus on repetitive flexion and extension use of the elbow. Relief during vacations from work or exacerbations during certain activities are also important clues to causation. A medical history should include questions concerning diabetes, alcoholism, inflammatory joint problems, and thyroid function. A history of recent surgery or postsurgical rehabilitation activities should also be discussed. Although ulnar neuropathy following general anesthetic has been discussed, we have also treated a number of patients who first developed ulnar neuropathy after beginning postoperative cardiovascular rehabilitation that included repetitive elbow flexion–extension exercises with weights.

Clinical examination and tests

Examination of the patient with suspected ulnar neuropathy should begin by excluding more proximal compression. The patient with neck pain or limited motion may have radiculopathy in the C-8 nerve root. Cervical spine X-rays should be examined in such patients. Thoracic outlet syndrome may also mimic this neuropathy. Such patients may have paresthesias in the medial arm and forearm that will alert the clinician to more proximal compression. Provocative maneuvers such as Wright's test, Roos' test (hand elevation with clinched fists), and a supraclavicular Tinel's sign also favor proximal compression.

Examination should include elbow range of motion and carrying angle (valgus deformity). Inspection of the elbow should note whether inflammation about the joint or olecranon bursa exists. Palpation over the medial and lateral epicondyles may reveal concomitant epicondylitis. Occasionally, an enlarged or subluxing ulnar nerve can be directly palpated.

Tinel's sign of the ulnar nerve may or may not be useful since many normal individuals have positive tests (Rayan et al., 1992). This test is considered positive only if it produces symptoms in the distribution of the ulnar nerve and not if it causes local discomfort.

The 'elbow flexion–pressure provocative test' combines two maneuvers which directly increase the pressure within the cubital tunnel. The test is performed by placing the elbow in maximal flexion and applying digital pressure on the cubital tunnel (Novak et al., 1994). The sensitivity and specificity of this test was greater than 90% at 30 seconds. The obvious drawback in this

technique is the difficulty in applying a uniform pressure between patients.

The elbow flexion test has also been investigated in combination with full wrist extension (Buehler and Thayer, 1988). All patients with electrophysiologic evidence of cubital tunnel syndrome noted an increase in pain, numbness or tingling in the ulnar nerve distribution during this 3-minute positional test. A similar maneuver performed in normal volunteers revealed a 13% false positive test rate (Rayan et al., 1992).

Clinical examination of the hand should include assessment of sensibility, motor function and muscle atrophy. Sensory testing involves two-point discrimination, Semmes–Weinstein monofilament testing, and vibratory perception. Both filament and vibratory testing have been shown more sensitive than two-point testing (Dellon, 1980).

Motor function may be tested directly or noted by its effects on hand posture and use. Pinch strength is usually affected more than grip as the ulnar nerve innervates both the first dorsal interosseous muscle and the adductor pollicis. These two muscles account for the majority of pinch strength. The patient may compensate for these muscle weaknesses by flexing the thumb interphalangeal joint (Froment's sign) during pinch (Froment, 1918). Wartenberg's sign consists of an abducted little finger with metacarpophalangeal extension (Wartenberg, 1939). This is due to a combination of weakness in the fourth palmar interosseous muscle and the abducting vector of force of the extrinsic extensor tendons to the little finger. Weakness of ring and little finger profundus muscle strength can help localize ulnar nerve compression. Branches to the FDP bellies occur in the forearm and would be spared in more distal compression at the wrist. Independent profundus testing can be unreliable, however, since the profundus bellies are shared to some degree with their median innervated counterparts to the index and long fingers. Clawing of the ring and little fingers with hyperextension of the metacarpophalangeal joints and flexion of the proximal interphalangeal joints is also secondary to intrinsic weakness. The intrinsic muscles are responsible for initiating metacarpophalangeal flexion and performing proximal interphalangeal extension.

The crossed finger test is a simple maneuver which evaluates the action of the first volar and second dorsal interossei (Earle and Vlastou, 1980). The test is easy to explain to patients and is specific to ulnar innervated muscles.

Intrinsic muscle atrophy in the hand may accompany advanced compression. Flattening of the metacarpal arch with hollowing between the metacarpal shafts is due to intrinsic wasting. A deep depression in the first web space is caused by first interosseous wasting, and scalloping on the ulnar border by hypothenar wasting (Figure 7.2).

Electrodiagnostic testing

Nerve conduction velocity and needle EMG examination of ulnar innervated muscles can provide objective information in the patient with clinical ulnar neuropathy. Shortcomings in the ability of surface conduction tests to detect abnormalities should temper complete reliance on these data. Small changes in arm position, temperature and electrode placement can yield false positive or negative results. The specific technique of testing (motor, sensory, ortho-dromic, inching, etc.) also varies significantly in clinical practice and in literature reviews. Fifteen per cent of normal volunteers have been found to have abnormal studies (Odusote and Eisen, 1979).

Needle EMG evaluation of the upper extremity and paraspinal muscles provides valuable infor-mation in diagnosis and exclusion of more proxi-mal or distal compression.

Importance of elbow position

Nerve conduction is useful to assess peripheral nerves secondary to slowing at sites of compres-sion. The ulnar nerve at the elbow, however, is subject to testing errors from a number of sources including stretching of the nerve with elbow motion and segment length mismeasure-ment (Checkles et al., 1971). Mismeasurement errors become significant as the tested segment length is reduced (Kincaid et al., 1986).

When the elbow is flexed, the ulnar nerve elongates. Since impulse propagation primarily occurs through saltatory (jumping) conduction

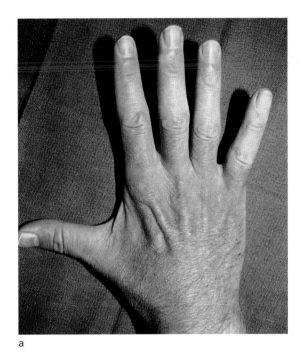

a

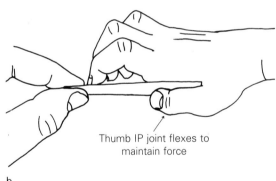

Thumb IP joint flexes to maintain force

b

Figure 7.2

Wasting of the first dorsal interosseous muscle appears as a hollow on the radial side of the index extensor tendon. (b) Froment sign is exhibited when the patient attempts to perform thumb to index finger side pinch. The patient will recruit the flexor pollicis longus to aid pinch which results in interphalangeal joint flexion.

between nodes of Ranvier, the nerve will appear to conduct faster when it is stretched as the internodal distance increases. Kincaid et al. demonstrated this in the ulnar nerves of normal volunteers (Figure 7.3). When the elbow was flexed 135 degrees, the conduction velocity artifact was eliminated. A drop in motor conduction velocity greater than 11.4 m/s was deemed abnormal.

Elbow position and details of electrodiagnostic testing are important when reviewing studies on this topic and one's own results of treatment. An example is a study of the natural history of mild cubital tunnel syndrome where testing was performed with the elbow in an extended position (Eisen and Danon, 1974). The mean drop in conduction velocity across the elbow was only 8 m/s which would fall in the normal range for this elbow position. Following surgery, conduction velocity measurements become more problematic. Dellon et al. have demonstrated that nerve testing in elbow extension is more accurate in the post-transposition patient (Dellon et al., 1987).

Testing technique

Simpson has been credited with the first utilization of electrodiagnostic studies for ulnar neuropathy in 1956 (Raynor et al., 1994; Simpson, 1956). Initial motor studies, however, proved insensitive in patients with mild clinical findings. While 67% of patients with ulnar motor weakness and sensory loss may have positive motor studies, only 9% of patients with paresthesias alone have positive motor studies (Raynor et al., 1994). Several techniques including sensory antidromic, sensory orthodromic, segmental and inching have focussed on improving the sensitivity and specificity of ulnar nerve testing.

Early attempts to obtain sensory potentials yielded amplitudes too low to be reproducibly measured (Gilliatt et al., 1958). Electronic averaging and filtering now allows sensory conduction testing unless the nerve is significantly impaired. Raynor et al. found sensory nerve study abnormalities in 19% of patients with clinical ulnar neuropathy and normal motor studies.

Inching studies measure conduction and latency shifts over one-inch intervals across the elbow. Short segment incremental studies (SSIS) are even more detailed. One-centimeter segments are studied along the course of the nerve at the elbow (Campbell et al., 1992). Theoretically, SSIS have a greater ability to localize the site of pathology by localizing latency changes of more than 4 ms over 1-cm segments. Among 33 patients, 14 pure retroepicondylar compressions were found, 11 humeral ulnar arcade compressions, and 3 distal

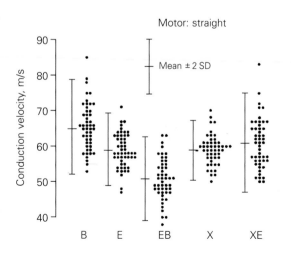

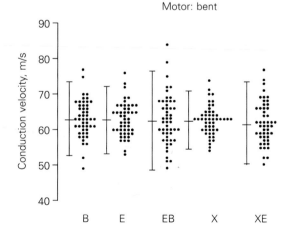

Figure 7.3

Across the elbow conduction velocity as a function of elbow position demonstrates the importance of measuring conduction in a flexed position to prevent a false positive result.

compressions at the FCU exit site. SSIS data correlate closely with intraoperative nerve conduction studies (Campbell et al., 1988). In practice, however, this will probably not influence a surgeon's choice of treatment except for distal findings of compression.

Treatment

Current treatment for cubital tunnel syndrome includes conservative methods aimed at relieving irritation and compression, and surgical methods to decompress the nerve with or without transposition anteriorly.

Conservative treatment

Once a diagnosis of cubital tunnel compression is suspected or has been demonstrated, the patient should be instructed on methods to minimize additional nerve compromise. This includes a trial of anti-inflammatory medication, elbow use modification, and soft splinting.

The physician should discuss avoidance of work or off-work activities that involve tightly flexed elbow positions or repetitive elbow flexion. If the patient works at a keyboard frequently, the keyboard should be lowered to waist height so that the elbows may be at 30 degrees or less flexion. If the job requires prolonged telephone conversations, a headset will prevent holding the elbow flexed. The patient should be instructed to sleep with the elbows extended (usually by placing the palms together and pinning them between the knees). While driving, the elbow should not be rested on the door rest.

Rigid elbow splints may not be well tolerated by the patient; however, a soft padded splint can be helpful. The elbow pad can be slid on like a sock and should have padding to cover the medial/posterior elbow. At night, the elbow pad should be turned 180 degrees so that the padding rests in the antecubitus. Bunching of the padding with elbow flexion will promote the patient to sleep in a more extended position. A firmer style of night-time splint has been studied in France with good success (Seror, 1993). That padded splint allows motion from 15–60 degrees.

We routinely reexamine the patient after 3–6 weeks of conservative treatment. If the symptoms persist, a nerve study is recommended. Elbow radiographs are recommended in older individuals, those with a history of trauma, and individuals with a component of joint pain or swelling.

Cortisone injections are not routinely recommended for cubital tunnel syndrome. The nerve occupies the tunnel with little room to spare, therefore, injections risk being deposited either outside the tunnel or inside the nerve. The only exception may be in the patient with significant medial epicondylitis where a more anterior injection may be carefully attempted. Care must be taken to avoid subcutaneous placement of the cortisone since fat atrophy will leave the nerve even more vulnerable to trauma. Repeated injections have resulted in such atrophy 23% of the time (Pechan and Kredba, 1980).

If the conservatively treated patient has progression of numbness or weakness or has evidence of axonal loss on EMG we begin to discuss surgery at the 6-week follow-up visit. Depending on the individual and severity of symptoms, we will often try several additional months of soft splinting and elbow rest. Failing this treatment, we recommend proceeding with transposition. Our recommended surgery is submuscular transposition with pronator step-cut in all individuals. For completeness, other techniques are also reviewed below.

In-situ decompression/medial epicondylectomy

Simple decompression of the roof of the cubital tunnel with or without medial epicondylectomy was described in the 1950s (King and Morgan, 1950). As described by Kuschner, a 10–15 cm incision just anterior to the epicondyle is incised (Kuschner, 1996). The nerve is unroofed but not dissected from its bed. Next, a subperiosteal dissection of the medial epicondyle is followed by osteotome resection. The periosteal sleeve is closed after bone wax application. The skin is closed without drain, and a long arm splint is applied. Tada emphasizes the importance of a

Figure 7.4

(a) The incision is marked, the elbow is propped on a towel roll. (b) Two branches of the posterior division of the MABC nerve. One courses safely in the reflected flap, the other crosses the incision and will also be preserved (right is proximal for all photographs). (c) A loop around the ulnar nerve proximal to the cubital tunnel and a blue background slipped between the ulnar nerve and the medial intermuscular septum. (d) The ulnar nerve has been released from the cubital tunnel, also note preservation of the MABC nerve. (e). A motor branch arises several centimeters distal to the medial epicondyle and prevents adequate transposition. (f) The motor branch has been neurolysed proximally to allow the nerve adequate transposition. (g) The flexor–pronator muscle step-cut is designed such that the nerve will lay without tension well away from the bony epicondyle. (h) After transposition and repair of the muscle in a lengthened fashion, a finger should pass with little tension along side the ulnar nerve.

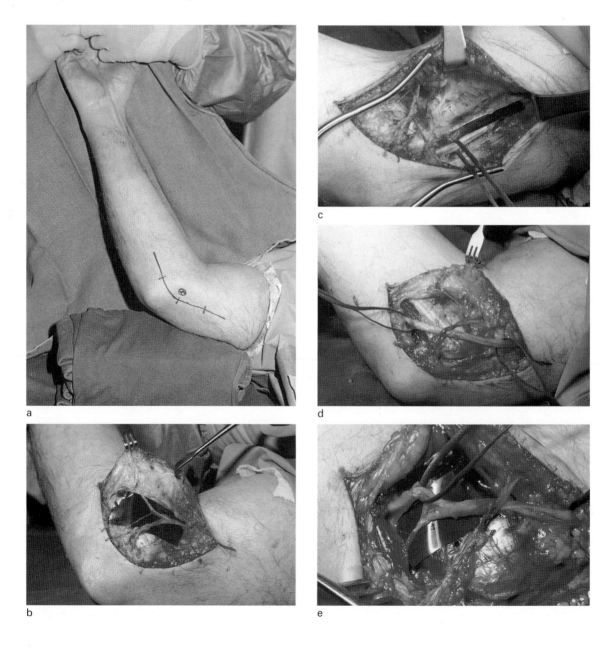

a

b

c

d

e

complete bony resection that prevents continued entrapment of the nerve (Tada et al., 1997).

Endoscopic decompression using a 3 cm incision and glass tube has been described (Tsai et al., 1995). Visualization of potential sites of compression is limited with this technique and follow-up has been short. This technique should still be considered experimental until additional studies are completed.

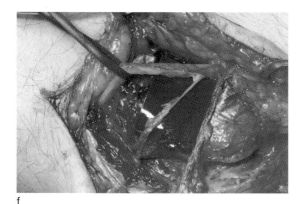

f

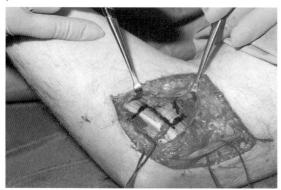

g

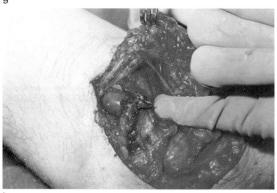

h

Transposition

Current techniques of transposition include anterior subcutaneous, intramuscular, and submuscular placement of the nerve. As described below in the results section, little prospective, randomized data exist to compare these three techniques, therefore the surgeon's training and personal experience often dictate the operation undertaken.

Subcutaneous technique

Subcutaneous transposition has the theoretical appeal of less tissue dissection along with removal of the nerve from the cubital tunnel. Several techniques have been described, which all share complete release of the nerve including resection of the medial intermuscular septum and some means to prevent the nerve from subluxing back into the cubital tunnel. A fasciodermal sling fashioned from the antebrachial fascia is commonly employed (Eaton et al., 1980).

Submuscular transposition technique

The patient is positioned supine with the shoulder at the edge of the operating table and armboard. The entire extremity and shoulder and axilla are prepped and draped. A sterile tourniquet is placed over cast padding high on the arm. After exsanguination and cuff inflation, the elbow is placed on a stack of sterile towels and flexed by the assistant (Figure 7.4). A gently curving incision is incised over the course of the nerve and extending 8 cm proximal and distal to the epicondyle. A useful landmark proximally is the intermuscular septum that can be palpated

Immediate attention should be directed toward identification of the MABC nerve branches. Rapid dissection down to the cubital tunnel will lead to transection or avulsion of these branches. Instead, dissection should begin proximally where the basilic vein runs several centimeters anterior to the septum in the subcutaneous fat. On either side of the basilic vein are the anterior and posterior branches of the MABC nerve. The branch on the lateral side (far side during this dissection) of the vein is the anterior branch which need not be further explored as its branches course lateral to the site of surgery. The branch on the medial side of the vein (near side) should be followed distally where it will give rise to fibers which cross the incision. We mark these branches with a marking pen at this point to better keep them in view during the remainder of the surgery. If a smaller branch is inadvertently avulsed later in the case, the marking aids in its identification and reflection away from the incision line.

The ulnar nerve is easily identified proximal to the cubital tunnel where it courses immediately posterior to the intermuscular septum. Gentle circumferential dissection of the nerve proceeds in a proximal to distal direction so the nerve may be transposed. Branches that arise near the elbow may hinder adequate anterior transposition of the ulnar nerve. The surgeon may safely divide small branches that are occasionally found to arise at or above the medial epicondyle. These branches do not innervate the FCU nor FDP muscles but are thought to provide sensory fibers to the elbow joint. Any branches distal to the medial epicondyle, however, should be preserved. Watchmaker et al. have shown that proximal intraneural dissection may be performed safely as described by Learmonth without disrupting intraneural fibers (Watchmaker et al., 1994; Learmonth, 1942). Most patients will require such neurolysis in order for the nerve to be adequately transposed away from the epicondyle. Leaving the nerve tethered about the epicondyle has been found commonly in failed transpositions. The patient often complains of pain with elbow motion due to adherence of the nerve to the epicondyle and traction neuritis.

A common mistake proximally is inadequate resection of the septum. We place an army-navy retractor on either side of the septum to reflect the biceps and triceps and then bipolarly cauterize any perforating veins. Most individuals have a small plexus just proximal to the epicondyle. The septum is then excised down to periosteum of humerus. A finger passed proximally confirms that no shelf of fascia has been left intact. A common mistake distally is kinking of the nerve where it enters the plane of the FCU muscle. Adequate distal release allows the nerve to take a straight or gently curving course.

Once the nerve has been dissected and inspected, the flexor pronator origin step-cut incision is made (Figure 7.5). Incision through the fascia is followed by division of the muscle with the bipolar cautery. All strands of intermuscular fascia must be excised where the nerve is to lie.

The nerve is then transposed and inspected for any areas of kinking or tethering. The flexor–pronator origin is repaired in a lengthened fashion. A finger passed alongside the nerve will confirm no pressure along its course. The tourniquet is deflated and meticulous hemostasis obtained. If the dissection has proceeded carefully, little bleeding occurs and no drain is necessary. The MABC nerve branches are reexamined after which the skin is closed in a deep dermal and subcuticular layer. A soft bulky dressing which incorporates several layers of fiberglass or plaster keeps the elbow at 45–60 degrees.

Results

McGowan proposed a grading system for ulnar neuropathy (McGowan, 1950). This system was based primarily on motor weakness.

Grade I: no measurable weakness.

Grade II: weakness with no wasting.

Grade III: muscle wasting evident.

Dellon proposed a more comprehensive classification (Dellon, 1989).

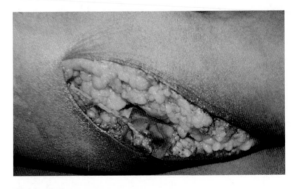

Figure 7.5

An MABC nerve neuroma, which caused pain with elbow motion or minor local trauma. The neuroma should be dissected proximally and buried without tension in the biceps muscle.

Mild –   Sensory: paresthesias come and go, vibration sensation increased.

Motor: subjective weakness, clumsiness or loss of coordination.

Tests: elbow flexion test and/or Tinel's sign may be positive.

Moderate – Sensory: paresthesias come and go, vibration sensation normal or decreased.

Motor: measurable weakness in pinch and/or grip strength.

Tests: elbow flexion and/or Tinel's positive, finger crossing +/- abnormal.

Severe –   Sensory: paresthesias are persistent, vibratory perception decreased. Abnormal two-point discrimination (m2pd >3 mm, static >5).

Motor: measurable weakness in pinch/grip plus muscle atrophy.

Tests: positive elbow flexion and/or positive Tinel's, finger crossing. Usually abnormal.

Regretfully, most study authors choose to develop their own grading systems which hampers comparison of results. Dellon summarized the existing state of affairs regarding surgical intervention for cubital tunnel syndrome (Dellon, 1989). A meta-analysis of 50 published reports comprising more than 2000 patients concluded that there were no statistically significant guidelines for choosing one operation over another. An important finding in this study was the lack of success of conservative treatment for moderate or severe patients.

Conservative results

Several studies have investigated the long-term success of conservative treatment. Eisen and Danon found that most patients with mild symptoms and no motor deficit recovered nerve function within 1 year (Eisen and Danon, 1974). Seventy per cent of the electrodiagnostic studies in this patient group, however, were normal.

Seror demonstrated that night-time splint usage resulted in motor and sensory nerve conduction improvement along with clinical improvement in 16 of 17 patients (Seror, 1993). Payan reported on two patients who were followed conservatively with serial EMG studies (Payan, 1970). The patient with mild neuropathy improved but the patient with wasting remained symptomatic.

The results of cortisone injections at the elbow have been studied in a randomized, prospective study (Hong et al., 1996). Injection was found to offer no benefit.

Dellon et al. have performed a prospective 8-year trial of conservative treatment (Dellon et al., 1993). This included instructing the patient to avoid sleeping with the elbow bent, not holding the telephone with a bent elbow, reading with a book on a stand, and padding or altering the work environment. This treatment was continued for 3–6 months unless persistent paresthesias or muscle wasting occurred. Fifty-eight per cent of patients with intermittent paresthesias (score 1) at entry into the study continued to have symptoms when treated conservatively whereas 80% of patients with abnormal innervation density (score 5–7) continued to have symptoms. Dellon went on to investigate those patients who failed conservative treatment and underwent submuscular transposition and found that 90% improved, mostly by 3 or more score levels.

Epicondylectomy/decompression results

Nathan et al. performed simple decompression in 131 patients with an emphasis on return to work (Nathan et al., 1995). They found 89% good or excellent results and an average time of 20 days off work. Thomsen showed similar good results with simple decompression (Thomsen, 1977). A retrospective comparison of 148 patients with subcutaneous transpositions vs. simple decompressions failed to show a statistical difference in outcome (Davies et al., 1991). A similar comparison by Chan et al. showed 82% improvement in both groups (Chan et al., 1980). Surgery was more successful in patients with symptoms less than 1 year.

The results of simple decompression were compared with submuscular anterior transposition in 79 patients by Bimmler's group. At a mean follow-up of 76 months, they found a 73% objective rate of improvement following transposition and 55% after simple decompression which was not statistically significant (Bimmler and Meyer, 1996). Manske evaluated the success of simple decompression in patients with no atrophy nor weakness and found improvement in 22 of 27 patients (Manske et al., 1992). Steiner et al. also reported good outcome in patients with motor weakness and atrophy (Steiner et al., 1996). Craven and Green reported excellent results with medial epicondylectomy (Craven and Green, 1980). All but two of their 30 patients had almost immediate pain relief, and a return to normal nerve conduction. The results of medial epicondylectomy in 30 patients were retrospectively reviewed by Froimson and Zahawi who found complete return of nerve function in McGowen grade I patients, but less success in grade II and III patients. Robinson et al. similarly showed good improvement in grade I patients (Robinson et al., 1992). Goldberg experienced good results with McGowen grade I patients but prolonged and limited improvement with grade III patients (Goldberg et al., 1989).

Medial epicondylectomy using King's method (King and Morgan, 1959) showed improvement in 93% of patients provided that a sufficient bony resection was performed (Tada et al. 1997). Heithoff et al. demonstrated that the potential pitfalls of this operation including loss of pinch and grip strength were uncommon (Heithoff et al., 1990).

Transposition results

One study comparing in-situ decompression, subcutaneous transposition and submuscular transposition found no statistically significant difference among the three although there were more poor results with in-situ decompression (Adellar et al., 1984). Only 8 of the 37 operations yielded good results that were defined as complete resolution of motor and sensory symptoms. Preoperative intrinsic wasting and fibrillations were correlated with poor postoperative outcome 77% of the time.

Experimentally, Dellon has investigated the difference between submuscular and intramuscu-

lar transposition in the primate (Dellon et al., 1986). Neither significant adherence nor difference in fiber diameter was found between the two transposition beds. Kleinman and Bishop have reported good clinical results with the intramuscular technique (Kleinman and Bishop, 1989).

Intraneural pressure following surgery, however, is very technique dependent. Simple decompression or medial epicondylectomy do not change intraneural pressure much while subcutaneous and submuscular transposition (without step lengthening the flexor origin) increase it significantly (Dellon et al., 1994). Submuscular transposition with flexor–pronator lengthening is the only technique to reduce pressure on the nerve (see pressure graph in Dellon et al., 1994). Review of 33 patients undergoing this technique revealed subjective symptomatic improvement in 94% of patients (Nouhan and Kleinert, 1997).

Advocates of submuscular transposition argue that the nerve is padded in a less vulnerable location. Comparison of subcutaneous to submuscular transposition in 51 patients, however, has shown no increased vulnerability of the nerve (Stuffer et al., 1991). Even patients with severe ulnar neuropathy appear to benefit from surgery (Friedman and Cochran, 1986). Despite abnormal EMG results in 91% and a mean nerve conduction of 32 m/s, improvement was noted an average of 4.4 months postoperatively. Advanced age, duration of symptoms, and diabetes did not correlate with worse results. Harrison, on the other hand, found that muscle wasting was unlikely to improve if present for more than one year preoperatively (Harrison and Nurick, 1970). Manicol and LeRoux et al. similarly found that patients with symptoms greater than 1 year had inferior results (LeRoux et al., 1990; Manicol, 1979).

Reexploration/complications

Poor results in the treatment of cubital tunnel syndrome may be divided into those resulting from improper or insufficient diagnosis, those resulting from conservative or surgical treatment, and those resulting from our current inability to help all such patients despite proper care.

Improper diagnosis includes failure to rule out other possible sites of compression or metabolic causes of neuropathy. As mentioned previously, cervical level or other proximal compression may mimic this neuropathy. A detailed examination and EMG evaluation are necessary to exclude other sites of compression that will not be helped by attention to the elbow.

Conservative complications

Poor results from conservative management are common in advanced neuropathy. The surgeon, however, should not be deterred from offering a prolonged conservative regimen in the mild patient. It would be unacceptable, however, to delay surgery in the face of advancing weakness and wasting. Bednar characterizes conservative mismanagement as: (1) treating patients with moderate or severe disease, (2) prescribing conservative treatment in the non-compliant patient, and (3) failing to follow patients for signs of progression (Bednar et al., 1994).

Surgical complications

Surgical complications can be further divided into those caused by inadequate release or transposition, and those caused by injury to adjacent normal structures.

The most common iatrogenic injury we see is MABC nerve injury. Despite extensive literature describing the preservation of this nerve's branches, many surgeons continue to transect them (Dellon and Mackinnon, 1985; Masear et al., 1989; Race and Saldana, 1991). We believe three factors likely account for this fact. First, identification of the MABC branches is sometimes difficult. This difficulty is readily overcome by identifying them proximally near the basilic vein at the beginning of the case. Second, performing the remainder of the operation beneath these branches can sometimes be tedious. Overaggressive retraction can result in their avulsion. This problem should be properly managed by proximal dissection of the branch and reflection away from the incision. Third, this operation continues to be performed by many surgeons who do not specialize in upper extremity nerve problems and who do not remain abreast of the literature describing long-term pain from MABC nerve mishandling.

Problems following MABC nerve division include anesthesia in the skin posterior or distal to the incision and painful scar neuromas. Scar desensitization therapy can improve patients; however, persistent neuromatous incision line pain should prompt exploration at 4–6 months.

Elbow contractures are a theoretical but uncommon complication in ulnar nerve surgery. Loss of several degrees of elbow extension (9 degrees average) following failed transposition has been reported (Gabel and Amadio, 1990). More commonly we find an intact but painful range of motion which on exploration is associated with scarring of the nerve to the medial epicondyle. This tethering prevents normal nerve excursion with elbow motion that leads to traction neuritis. This is best treated by adequate transposition away from the epicondyle. Several other investigators have documented fibrosis in the region anterior to the medial epicondyle (Amadio, 1986; Rogers et al., 1991). Gabel et al. found such fibrosis in 24 of 30 reexplorations. Similar scarring is problematic after medial epicondylectomy. Rogers et al. found that reexploration was usually successful in relieving pain; however, recovery of sensibility and motor function were unpredictable (Rogers et al., 1991).

Incomplete resection of the medial intermuscular septum is also frequently encountered at reoperation (Broudy et al., 1978).

Reexploration was associated with a poor outcome if prior surgery induced significant scarring or was associated with severe preoperative dysesthesia or pain (Leffert, 1982). Kinking of the nerve at the intermuscular septum was found in 9 of 10 nerves reexplored by Broudy et al. (1978).

References

Abdel-Salam A, Eyres KS, Cleary J. (1991) Drivers' elbow: a cause of ulnar neuropathy. *J Hand Surg* **16B**:436–7.

Adelaar RS, Foster WC, McDowell C. (1984) The treatment of the cubital tunnel syndrome. *J Hand Surg* **9**:90–5.

Adson AL. (1918) The surgical treatment of progressive ulnar paralysis. *Minn Med* **1**:455–60.

Alvine FG, Schurrer ME. (1987) Postoperative ulnar-nerve palsy. Are there predisposing factors? *J Bone Joint Surg* **69**:255–9.

Amadio PC. (1986) Anatomical basis for a technique of ulnar nerve transposition. *Surg Radiol Anat* **8**:155–61.

Ametewee K. (1986) Acute cubital tunnel syndrome from post traumatic calcific neuritis. *J Hand Surg* **11B**:123–4.

Apfelberg DB, Larson SJ. (1973) Dynamic anatomy of the ulnar nerve at the elbow. *Plas Reconstr Surg* **51**:76–81.

Balagtas-Balmaseda OM, Grabois M, Balmaseda PF, Lidsky MD. (1983) Cubital tunnel syndrome in rheumatoid arthritis. *Arch Phys Med Rehabil* **64**:163–71.

Bednar MS, Blair SJ, Light TR. (1994) Complications of the treatment of cubital tunnel syndrome. *Hand Clin* **10**:83–92.

Bimmler D, Meyer VE. (1996) Surgical treatment of the ulnar nerve entrapment neuropathy: submuscular anterior transposition or simple decompression of the ulnar nerve? *Annales de Chir de la main* **15**:148–57.

Britz GW, Haynor DR, Kuntz C, Goodkin R, Gitter A, Maravilla K, Kliot M. (1996). Ulnar nerve entrapment at the elbow: correlation of magnetic resonance imaging, clinical, electrodiagnostic, and introperative findings. *Neurosurgery* **38**:458–65.

Broudy AS, Leffert RD, Smith RJ. (1978) Technical problems with ulnar nerve transposition at the elbow: findings and results of reoperation. *J Hand Surg* **3**:85–9.

Buehler MJ, Thayer DT. (1988) The elbow flexion test. *Clin Orthop Rel Res* **233**:213–16.

Calder FWG. (1833) Effects of a division of the ulnar nerve. *Lancet* **1**:489–90.

Campbell WW, Pridgeon RM, Sahni SK. (1988) Entrapment neuropathy of the ulnar nerve at its point of exit from the flexor carpi ulnaris muscle. *Muscle Nerve* **11**:467–70.

Campbell WW, Pridgeon RM, Sahni KS. (1992) Short segment incremental studies in the evaluation of ulnar neuropathy at the elbow. *Muscle Nerve* **15**:1050–4.

Campbell WW, Sahni SK, Pridgeon RM, Riaz G, Leshner RT. (1988) Intraoperative electroneurography:

management of ulnar neuropathy at the elbow. *Muscle Nerve* **11**:75–81.

Casscells CD, Lindsey RW, Ebersole J, Li B. (1993) Ulnar neuropathy after median sternotomy. *Clin Orthop Rel Res* **291**:259–65.

Chan RC, Paine KWE, Varughese G. (1980) Ulnar neuropathy at the elbow: comparison of simple decompression and anterior transposition. *Neurosurgery* **7**:545–50.

Checkles NS, Russakov AD, Piero DL. (1971) Ulnar nerve conduction velocity: effect of elbow position on the measurement. *Arch Phys Med Rehabil* **52**:362–5.

Craven PR, Green DP. (1980) Cubital tunnel syndrome. Treatment by medial epicondylectomy. *J Bone Joint Surg* **62A**:986–9.

Curtis BF. (1898) Traumatic ulnar neuritis–transplantation of the nerve. *J Nerve Ment Dis* **25**:480–1.

Dahners LE, Wood FM. (1984) Anconeous epitrochlearis, a rare cause of cubital tunnel syndrome: a case report. *J Hand Surg* **9A**:579–80.

Davidson AJ, Horowitz MT. (1935) Late or tardy ulnar paralysis. *J Bone Joint Surg* **17**:8744–56.

Davies MA, Vonau M, Blum PW, Kwok BCT, Matheson JM, Stening WA. (1991) Results of ulnar neuropathy at the elbow treated by decompression or anterior transposition. *Aust NZ J Surg* **61**:929–34.

Dellon AL. (1980) Clinical use of vibratory stimuli to evaluate peripheral nerve injury and compression neuropathy. *Plas Reconstr Surg* **65**:466.

Dellon AL. (1986) Musculotendinous variations about the medial humeral epicondyle. *J Hand Surg* **11B**:175–81.

Dellon AL. (1989) Review of treatment results for ulnar nerve compression at the elbow. *J Hand Surg* **14**:688–700.

Dellon AL, MacKinnon SE. (1985) Injury to the medial antebrachial cutaneous nerve during cubital tunnel surgery. *J Hand Surg* **10B**:33–6.

Dellon AL, Mackinnon SE. (1988) Human ulnar neuropathy at the elbow: clinical, electrical, and morphometric correlations. *J Reconstr Micro* **4**:179–84.

Dellon AL, Hament W, Gittelshon A. (1993) Nonoperative management of cubital tunnel syndrome: an 8-year prospective study. *Neurology* **43**:1673–7.

Dellon AL, Chang E, Coert JH, Campbell KR. (1994) Intraneural ulnar nerve pressure changes related to operative techniques for cubital tunnel decompression. *J Hand Surg* **19**:923–30.

Dellon AL, Mackinnon SE, Hudson AR, Hunter DA. (1986) Effect of submuscular versus intramuscular placement of ulnar nerve: experimental model in the primate. *J Hand Surg* **11B**:117–9.

Dellon AL, Schlegel RW, Mackinnon SE. (1987) Validity of nerve conduction velocity studies after anterior transposition of the ulnar nerve. *J Hand Surg* **12**:700–3.

Earle AS, Vlastou C. (1980) Crossed fingers and other tests of ulnar nerve motor function. *J Hand Surg* **5**:560–5.

Earle H. (1816) Cases and observations illustrating the influence of the nervous system in regulating animal heat. *Med Chir Trans* **7**:173–85.

Eaton RG, Crowe JF, Parkes JC. (1980) Anterior transposition of the ulnar nerve using a non-compressing fasciodermal sling. *J Bone Joint Surg* **62**:820–5.

Eisen A, Danon J. (1974) The mild cubital tunnel syndrome. *Neurology* **24**:608.

Feindel W, Stratford J. (1958) The role of the cubital tunnel in tardy ulnar palsy. *Can J Surg* **1**:287–300.

Ferlic DC, Ries MD. (1990) Epineural ganglion of the ulnar nerve at the elbow. *J Hand Surg* **15**:996–8.

Finelli MPF. (1975) Ulnar neuropathy after liquid nitrogen cryotherapy. *Arch Dermatol* **111**:1340–42.

Friedman RJ, Cochran TP. (1986) Anterior transposition for advanced ulnar neuropathy at the elbow. *Surg Neurol* **25**:446–8.

Froimson AI, Zahawi F. (1980) Treatment of compression neuropathy of the ulnar nerve at the elbow by epicondylectomy and neurolysis. *J Hand Surg* **5**:391–5.

Froment MJ. (1918) La paralysie de l'adducteur du ponce et le signe du pounce. *Rev Neurol* **33**:484.

Gabel GT. Amadio PC. (1990) Reoperation for failed decompression of the ulnar nerve at the elbow. *J Bone Joint Surg* **72**:213–9.

Gilliatt RW, Thomas PK. (1960) Changes in nerve conduction with ulnar lesions at the elbow. *J Neurol Neurosurg Psychiatry* **23**:312–30.

Goldberg BJ, Light TR, Blair SJ. (1989) Ulnar neuropathy at the elbow: results of medial epicondylectomy. *J Hand Surg* **14**:182–18.

Harrison MJG, Nurick S. (1970) Results of anterior transposition of the ulnar nerve for ulnar neuritis. *BMJ* **1**:27–9.

Heithoff SJ, Millender LH, Nalebuff EA, Petruska AJ. (1990) Medial epicondylectomy for the treatment of ulnar nerve compression at the elbow. *J Hand Surg* **15**:22–9.

Hodgkinson PD, Mclean NR. (1994) Ulnar nerve entrapment due to epitrochleo-anconeus muscle. *J Hand Surg* **19B**:706–8.

Holtzman RN, Mark MH, Patel MR, Wiener LM. (1984) Ulnar entrapment neuropathy in the forearm. *J Hand Surg* **9**:576–8.

Hong CZ, Long MA, Kanakamedala RV, Chang YM, Yates L. (1996) Slinting and local steroid injection for the treatment of ulnar neuropathy at the elbow: clinical and electrophysiological evaluation. *Arch Phys Med Rehabil* **77**:573–7.

Inhofe PD, Moneim MS. (1996) Compression of the ulnar nerve at the elbow by an intraneural cyst: a case report. *J Hand Surg* **21A**:1094–6.

Kincaid JC, Phillips LH, Daube JR. (1986) The evaluation of suspected ulnar neuropathy at the elbow. *Arch Neurol* **43**:44–7.

King T, Morgan FP. (1950) The treatment of traumatic ulnar neuritis. *Aust NZ J Surg* **20**:33–45.

King T, Morgan FP. (1959) Late results of removing the medial humeral epicondyle for traumatic ulnar neuritis. *J Bone Joint Surg* **41**:51–5.

Kleinman WB, Bishop AT. (1989) Anterior intramuscular transposition of the ulnar nerve. *J Hand Surg* **14**:972–9.

Kline SC, Moore JR. (1992) Intraneural hemangioma: a case report of acute cubital syndrome. *J Hand Surg* **17**:305–7.

Kuschner SH. (1996) Cubital tunnel syndrome: treatment by medial epicondylectomy. *Hand Clin* **12**:411–18.

Laurencin CT, Schwartz JT, Koris MJ. (1994) Compression of the ulnar nerve at the elbow in association with synovial cysts. *Orthop Rev* **23**:62–5.

Learmonth JR. (1942) A technique for transplanting the ulnar nerve. *Surg Gynecol Obstet* **75**:792–3.

Leffert RD. (1982) Anterior submuscular transposition of the ulnar nerves by the learmonth technique. *J Hand Surg* **7**:147–55.

LeRoux PD, Ensign TD, Burchiel KJ. (1990) Surgical decompression without transposition for ulnar neuropathy: factors determining outcome. *Neurosurgery* **27**:709–14.

Lugnegard H, Juhlin L, Nilsson BY. (1982) Ulnar neuropathy at the elbow treated with decompression. *Scan J Plas Reconstr Surg* **16**:195–200.

Mackinnon SE, Dellon AL. (1988) Ulnar nerve entrapment at the elbow. In: *Surgery of the peripheral nerve,* New York: Thieme: 217–73.

Malkawi H. (1981) Recurrent dislocation of the elbow accompanied by ulnar neuropathy. *Clin Orthop Rel Res* **161**:270–4.

Manicol MF. (1979) The results of operation for ulnar neuritis. *J Bone Joint Surg* **61B**:159–64.

Manske PR, Johnston R, Pruitt DL, Strecker WB. (1992) Ulnar nerve decompression at the cubital tunnel. *Clin Orthop Rel Res* **274**:231–7.

Masear VR, Meyer RD, Pichora DR. (1989) Surgical anatomy of the medial antebrachial cutaneous nerve. *J Hand Surg* **14**:267–71.

Matsuura S, Kojima T, Kinoshita Y. (1994) Cubital tunnel syndrome caused by abnormal insertion of the triceps brachii muscle. *J Hand Surg* **19B**:38–9.

McGowan AJ. (1950) The results of transposition of the ulnar nerve for traumatic ulnar neuritis. *J Bone Joint Surg* **32**:293–301.

Messina A, Messina JC. (1995) Transposition of the ulnar nerve and its vascular bundle for the entrapment syndrome at the elbow. *J Hand Surg* **20B**:638–48.

Miller RG, Camp PE. (1979) Postoperative ulnar neuropathy. *JAMA* **242**:1636–9.

Nathan PA, Keniston RC, Meadows KD. (1995) Outcome study of ulnar nerve compression at the elbow treated with simple decompression and an early programme of physical therapy. *J Hand Surg* **20B**:628–37.

Neary D, Eames A. (1975) The pathology of ulnar nerve compression in man. *Neuropath Appl Neurobiol* **1**:69.

Nouhan R, Kleinert JM. (1997) Ulnar nerve decompression by transposing the nerve and z-lengthening the

flexor-pronator mass: clinical outcome. *J Hand Surg* **22**:127–31.

Novak CB, Lee GW, Mackinnon SE, Lay L. (1994) Provocative testing for cubital tunnel syndrome. *J Hand Surg* **19**:817–20.

Ochiai N, Hayashi T, Ninomiya S. (1992) High ulnar nerve palsy caused by the Arcade of Struthers. *J Hand Surg* **17B**:629–31.

O'Driscoll SW, Horii E, Carmichael SW, Morrey BF. (1991) The cubital tunnel. *J Bone Joint Surg* **73B**:613–17.

Odusote D, Eisen A. (1979) An electrophysiological quantitation of the cubital tunnel syndrome. *Le Journal Canadien des Sciences Neurologiques* **6**:403–10.

Ogata K, Manske PR, Lesker PA. (1985) The effect of surgical dissection on regional blood flow to the ulnar nerve in the cubital tunnel. *Clin Orthop Rel Res* **193**:195–8.

Ogata K, Naito M. (1986) Blood flow of peripheral nerve effects of dissection, stretching and compression. *J Hand Surg* **11B**:10–14.

Ogata K, Shimon S, Owen J, Manske PR. (1991) Effects of compression and devascularization on ulnar nerve function. *J Hand Surg* **16B**:104–8.

Ogino T, Minami A, Fukuda K. (1986) Tardy ulnar nerve palsy caused by cubitus varus deformity. *J Hand Surg* **11**:352–6.

O'Hara JJ, Stone JH. (1996) Ulnar nerve compression at the elbow caused by a prominent medial head of the triceps and an anconeus epitrochlearis muscle. *J Hand Surg* **21B**:133–5.

Osborne GV. (1957) Surgical treatment of tardy ulnar neuritis. *J Bone Joint Surg* **39B**:782.

Osterman AL, Kitay GS. (1996) Compression neuropathies: ulnar. In: Peimer C, ed. *Surgery of the hand and upper extremity*. New York: McGraw-Hill.

Panas J. (1878) Sur une cause peu connue de paralysis du nerf cubital. *Arch Gen Med* **2**:5–22.

Payan J. (1970) Anterior transposition of the ulnar nerve: an electrophysiological study. *J Neurol Neurosurg Psychiatry* **33**:157–65.

Pechan J, Julis I. (1975) The pressure measurement in the ulnar nerve. A contribution to the pathophysiology of the cubital tunnel syndrome. *J Biomech* **8**:75–9.

Pechan J, Kredba J. (1980) Treatment of cubital tunnel syndrome by means of local administration of corti-sonoids. *Acta Universitatis Carolinae Medica* **26**:135–40.

Platt H. (1926) The pathogenesis and treatment of traumatic neuritis of the ulnar nerve in the post-condylar groove. *Br J Surg* **13**:409.

Prevel CD, Matloub HS, Ye Z, Sanger JR, Yousif NJ. (1993) The extrinsic blood supply of the ulnar nerve at the elbow: an anatomic study. *J Hand Surg* **18**:433–8.

Race CM, Saldana MJ. (1991) Anatomic course of the medial cutaneous nerves of the arm. *J Hand Surg* **16**:48–52.

Rayan GM. (1990) Recurrent anterior dislocation of the ulnar nerve at the cubital tunnel. *Plast Reconstr Surg* **86**:773–5.

Rayan GM, Jensen C, Duke J. (1992) Elbow flexion test in the normal population. *J Hand Surg* **17**:86–9.

Raynor EM, Shefner JM, Preston DC, Logigian EL. (1994) Sensory and mixed nerve conduction studies in the evaluation of ulnar neuropathy at the elbow. *Muscle Nerve* **17**:785–92.

Renwick SE, Moneim MS. (1993) Cubital tunnel syndrome in a child with hemophilia. *J Hand Surg* **18**:458–61.

Robinson D, Aghasi MK, Halperin N. (1992) Medial epicondylectomy in cubital tunnel syndrome: an electrodiagnostic study. *J Hand Surg* **17B**:255–6.

Rogers MR, Bertfield TG, Aulicino PL. (1991) The failed ulnar nerve transposition. *Clin Orthop* **269**:193–200.

Seror P. (1993) Treatment of ulnar nerve palsy at the elbow with a night splint. *J Bone Joint Surg* **75B**:322–7.

Sheldon WD. (1921) Tardy palsy of the ulnar nerve. *Med Clin North Am* **5**:499–509.

Sherren J. (1908) Remarks on chronic neuritis of the ulnar nerve due to deformity in the region of the elbow joint. *Edinb Med J* **23**:500–9.

Simpson JA. (1956) Electrical signs in the diagnosis of carpal tunnel and related syndromes. *J Neurol Neurosurg Psychiatry* **50**:252–8.

Spinner RJ, Carmichael SE, Spinner M. (1991) Infraclavicular ulnar nerve entrapment due to a chondroepitrochlearis muscle. *J Hand Surg* **16B**:315–7.

St John JN, Palmaz JC. (1986) The cubital tunnel in ulnar entrapment neuropathy. *Musculoskeletal Radiol* **158**:119–23.

Steiner HH, von Haken S, Steiner-Milz HG. (1996) Entrapment neuropathy at the cubital tunnel: simple decompression is the method of choice. *Acta Neurochir (Wien)* **138**:308–13.

Struthers J. (1848) On a peculiarity of the humerus and humeral artery. *Month J Med Sci* **28**:264–7.

Stuffer M, Jungwirth W, Hussl H, Schmutzhardt E. (1991) Subcutaneous or submuscular anterior transposition of the ulnar nerve. *J Hand Surg* **17B**:248–50.

Sugawara M. (1988) Experimental and clinical studies of the vascularized anterior transposition of the ulnar nerve for cubital tunnel syndrome. *J Jpn Orthop Assoc* **62**:755–65.

Tada H, Hirayama T, Katsuki M , Habaguchi T. (1997) Long term results using a modified King's method for cubital tunnel syndrome. *Clin Orthop Rel Res* **336**:107–10.

Taniguchi Y, Yoshida M, Tamaki T. (1996) Cubital tunnel syndrome associated with calcium pyrophosphate dihydrate crystal deposition disease. *J Hand Surg* **21A**:870–4.

Thomsen PB. (1977) Compression neuritis of the ulnar nerve treated with simple decompression. *Acta Orthop Scand* **48**:164–7.

Tsai T, Bonczar M, Tsuruta T, Ahmed Syed S. (1995) A new operative technique: cubital tunnel decompression with endoscopic assistance. *Hand Clin* **11**:71–9.

Vorenkamp SE, Nelson TL. (1987) Ulnar nerve entrap-ment due to heterotopic bone formation after a severe burn. *J Hand Surg* **12**:378–80.

Warner MA, Warner ME, Martin JT. (1994) Ulnar neuropathy: incidence, outcome, and risk factors in sedated or anesthetized patients. *Anesthesiology* **81**(6):1332–40.

Wartenberg R. (1939) A sign of ulnar palsy. *JAMA* **112**:1688–9.

Watchmaker GP, Lee G, Mackinnon SE. (1994) Intraneural topography of the ulnar nerve in the cubital tunnel facili-tates anterior transposition. *J Hand Surg* **19**:915–22.

Werner C, Ohlin P, Elmqvist D. (1985) Pressures recorded in ulnar neuropathy. *Acta Orthop Scand* **56**:404–6.

8
Carpal tunnel syndrome

Philip E. Higgs and Christine J. Cheng

Historical introduction

Medical literature prior to the turn of the century often described symptoms that may be recognized as advanced carpal tunnel syndrome. Termed 'acroparesthesia', the etiology and pathophysiology were poorly understood. In the early twentieth century, a better understanding of the nature of the problem and the exact anatomical considerations were developed (Figure 8.1). These early advances were closely associated with physicians at the Mayo Clinic (Amadio, 1992). While division of the transverse carpal ligament was suggested as early as 1913 by Marie and Foix, the operation was not performed on a regular basis for compressive neuropathy of the distal median nerve until the 1930s, by James Learmonth. By the late 1930s, Morersch was recommending early decompression as treatment (Amadio, 1992; Pfeffer et al., 1988).

Reports of successful decompressions of the median nerve for 'Tardy Median Palsy' were published in the late 1940s by Brain et al. and Cannon and Love (Brain 1947; Cannon 1946). It remained for Phalen to raise awareness of carpal tunnel syndrome and popularize its name and concept (Phalen et al., 1950). In 1966, he reported his experience with diagnosis and treatment in a series of 644 hands (Phalen, 1966). In that report he suggested an occupational association, but also indicated that he believed there were predisposing conditions. Phalen reported good results from division of the transverse carpal ligament. Later publications recommended steroid injection for patients without severe sensory loss or thenar atrophy. Subsequent literature has

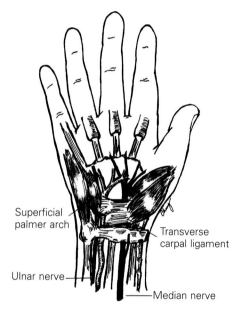

Figure 8.1

Median nerve at the carpal tunnel.

suggested that steroid injection may be useful only for diagnostic purposes. Symptom relief occurs in a high percentage of patients, but recurrence is common within 6 months.

An association between carpal syndrome and work was suggested as early as the 1920s. In the 1970s, strong associations were made between carpal tunnel syndrome and certain highly repetitive tasks (Birkbeck and Beer, 1975; Gainer and Nugent, 1977). Growing awareness of carpal tunnel syndrome and the ability of individuals to obtain coverage of its treatment by the workers' compensation insurance system significantly increased the frequency of diagnosis. The association between heavy loads and highly repetitive jobs, such as meat processing, and carpal tunnel syndrome was extrapolated to almost any job task that required stereotyped movements. This has since been extended even further to include any use of devices such as keyboards as responsible for the development of carpal tunnel syndrome in workers. Widespread 'epidemics' of carpal tunnel syndrome have resulted. Heated controversy over the existence of work-related carpal tunnel syndrome as a real entity still continues today (Hadler, 1997; Mackinnon and Novak, 1997). While the specific etiology is uncertain, there does appear to be an association with high ergonomic demands on the extremity. This is especially true for highly repetitive tasks in cold environments. The use of vibratory tools also seems to be strongly associated. Carpal tunnel syndrome has been linked to a variety of medical problems including diabetes, rheumatoid arthritis, gout, hypothyroidism, uremia, or previous wrist fractures. The presence of any of these medical problems does not establish an etiology, nor does it rule out any other. Rarely, there have been reports in the literature of familial carpal tunnel syndrome in the absence of other associated conditions (Leifer et al., 1992).

Today, carpal tunnel syndrome is one of the most common diagnoses in any hand surgery practice and carpal tunnel decompression is one of the most frequently performed surgical procedures. The cost of carpal tunnel syndrome to industry is approximately US$112 billion in yearly medical fees, compensation and lost productivity (Straaton et al., 1996). The lifetime risk for developing carpal tunnel syndrome is estimated to be 5–10% (Stevens et al., 1988). Regardless of etiology, the symptoms are extremely bothersome and include dense paresthesias and sleep-disturbing nocturnal hand pain. Fortunately, surgical decompression of the carpal canal provides substantial symptom relief in most patients.

Patient evaluation

The diagnosis of carpal tunnel syndrome is made chiefly from the history and physical exam. The malady is characterized by numbness and tingling in the hand and fingers in the median nerve distribution, often accompanied by pain and burning in the hand and wrist. Symptoms can be primarily nocturnal. In fact, being awakened on a nightly basis with pain, numbness and tingling is almost pathognomonic of the condition. Patients may try to relieve the symptoms by shaking the hand or placing it under running water. Symptoms may occur while driving, combing hair, or holding a telephone or newspaper and are often exacerbated by heavy or prolonged use of the hand. Other associated complaints include dropping objects or a sensation of hand 'swelling'. Symptom duration may not correspond with severity. Patients frequently report that their symptoms began just prior to seeking medical evaluation, but when questioned, will give a longer history of nocturnal paresthesias, 'but only after sleeping on the hand "wrong"'.

The physical examination starts with observation. The patient is positioned directly in front of the examiner with both upper extremities exposed. Bilateral comparison is made of the skin color and skin texture. The thenar eminences are examined for muscle wasting. Only patients suffering from severe chronic nerve compression will show prominent differences from side to side. Sensation is tested next. We prefer to evaluate subjective sensation to light touch by stroking the corresponding digits on the right and left hands simultaneously. Comparison is also made between the median and ulnar innervated digits in the same hand. This technique has been shown to be valid and reliable (Strauch et al., 1997) and will quickly produce information that may be missed by more formal methods of testing sensation. Formal testing methods, from a practical standpoint, are limited to two-point discrimination and the use of Semmes–Weinstein monofilaments. Clinics with a special interest may choose to include vibration testing. While vibration is the first sensory mode to show deterioration (Jetzer, 1991), reliably reproducible results require highly trained personnel and consistently calibrated equipment. Absolute norms for vibration sensation are not well established and may depend on a variety of factors such as sex, body mass index or occupation.

The strength of the median and ulnar-innervated intrinsic muscles is evaluated next.

Ulnar intrinsic function is assessed by resisted abduction of all the fingers at once. We find it useful to test both hands simultaneously. An incomplete effort by the patient can often be overcome by alternately testing the right and left hands rapidly. Median motor function is evaluated by resisted palmar abduction of the thumb with the wrist fully supinated. Early changes in pinch and grip strength may be detected using the appropriate dynamometers. However, norms for these tests are not well established for all patient groups either, and changes may be non-specific.

Electrodiagnostic testing is the only available objective means for diagnosing carpal tunnel syndrome. Some authors have suggested that it is unnecessary for making a diagnosis (Glowacki et al., 1996; Tetro et al., 1998), with more than 10% of patients with normal nerve conduction studies responding favorably to surgical decompression (Grundberg 1983; Louis and Hankin, 1987). In contrast, others have obtained poor results in patients, especially workers, with normal or nearly normal electrodiagnostic studies (Harris et al., 1979; Higgs et al., 1995). Comparison between the median and ulnar terminal latencies and conduction velocities is useful, especially when values are close to normal. Electrodiagnostic studies should be performed by an experienced and reliable electroneurographer, as testing technique and temperature need to be well controlled. Electromyograms (EMG) are usually not needed to make the diagnosis of carpal tunnel syndrome. However, they can help to differentiate a compressive neuropathy from an intrinsic or systemic neuropathy. It is important to note that postoperative nerve conduction study values fail to return to normal in a large percentage of patients (Aulisa et al., 1998; Melvin et al., 1968). X-ray or MRI may be used to rule out cervical spine or brachial plexus abnormalities as a cause for distal paresthesias. These tests are usually reserved for situations in which the diagnosis is unclear.

Several authors have used steroid injections for therapeutic and diagnostic purposes (Green, 1984; Phalen, 1966). Owing to the potential for injury to the median nerve from needle laceration or intraneural injection, great care should be taken when injecting the carpal canal. Mackinnon recommends dexamethasone as the injectable

steroid of choice, since it was the only one found to cause minimal nerve damage in an animal model after intrafascicular injection (Mackinnon, 1982). Steroid injections can be highly successful in relieving the symptoms of carpal tunnel syndrome, but relief tends to be temporary (Goodwill, 1965; Wood, 1980). A positive response can help to localize the patient's problem to the carpal canal. Temporary relief may also be a diagnostic indicator for potential response to surgery. Green found those who failed to respond to steroid injection did not fare as well with surgical decompression, although the differences did not achieve statistical significance (14 of 17 v. 77 of 82; Green, 1984).

Conservative management

Activity modification

The specific ergonomic loads or exposures necessary to either cause carpal tunnel syndrome or exacerbate an existing carpal tunnel syndrome are unknown. Several epidemiological studies have associated carpal tunnel syndrome with prolonged, highly repetitive activities. The long list of occupations reported to have high associations include poultry processors (Armstrong et al., 1982), garment workers (Punnett et al., 1985), meat packers (Masear et al., 1986), assembly workers (Feldman et al., 1987), and supermarket checkers (Margolis and Kraus, 1987). Tasks requiring wrist flexion, extension, or deviation, pinching or fine finger motion, and the use of vibratory tools have been implicated. Current recommendations for job modification include identification of occupational risk factors, decreasing exposure by changing the work process, using alternative tools and protective equipment, and job rotation or transfer (Rempel et al., 1992).

Modification of the workstation may help reduce risk as well. Specific suggestions vary, but generally involve comfortable positioning of workspaces to avoid prolonged static postures such as shoulder extension or abduction, and wrist flexion, extension, or deviation. In recent times, attention has shifted to computer use, with video display terminals, keyboards, and the computer mouse all implicated in work-related musculoskeletal complaints. A study of computer-aided design operators, who use a computer mouse for prolonged periods showed an increased prevalence of musculoskeletal symptoms in the upper extremity that is operating the mouse, when compared to the contralateral extremity (Jensen et al., 1998). The arm operating the mouse was found to be flexed and abducted, and the wrist extended and ulnarly deviated more than 90% of the worktime.

Frequent breaks to interrupt prolonged static positions are advised. Measured pressures within the carpal canal have been noted to rise with active wrist flexion and extension, making a fist, and isolated finger flexion against resistance in normal individuals as well as those with carpal tunnel syndrome (Seradge et al., 1995). However, intratunnel pressures in all persons dropped below resting levels after 1 minute of wrist flexion–extension exercises. Some clinicians even recommend hand and wrist exercises to promote nerve and tendon gliding as part of conservative management for carpal tunnel syndrome (Rozmaryn et al., 1998). Further studies, however, are needed to adequately establish the role of exercise as an effective adjunct to treatment.

Prolonged exposure to vibration has been associated with neurovascular abnormalities of the hand. Vasospasm may be associated, so the use of warm clothing and gloves is recommended. Equipment modification to reduce vibration is desirable. If this is not possible, anti-vibration gloves will help to reduce injury to the hands. Structural and functional peripheral nerve changes have been demonstrated in animals and humans exposed to vibration (Stromberg et al., 1996). However, the amount of intrinsic nerve damage versus nerve compression in each individual's combination of symptoms may be difficult to delineate. After evaluating vibratory thresholds, temperature thresholds, and nerve conduction of the median and ulnar nerves in vibration-exposed workers, Stromberg suggested that symptoms could be due to distal receptor pathology, in addition to carpal tunnel syndrome (Stromberg et al., 1999). For this reason, clinical and electrodiagnostic verification of carpal tunnel syndrome is important when treating vibration-exposed patients. Treatment results may be suboptimal if distal neural injury is also present.

Splints

Splints have been one of the keys to conservative treatment of carpal tunnel syndrome. However, there has been controversy regarding the position of splinting, when splints should be used, and whether flexible splints are beneficial. The traditionally recommended splint position has been 20 to 30 degrees of extension. However, pressures within the carpal tunnel were found to be lowest with the wrist in neutral position (Gelberman et al., 1980; Weiss 1995). A prospective, blinded study by Burke et al. found that carpal tunnel syndrome patients reported more symptomatic relief when the wrist was splinted in neutral position, with night splinting more effective than splinting during the day (Burke et al., 1994).

We recommend rigid splints in the neutral position worn only at night. Patients are less likely to comply with rigid splints during waking hours because they are restrictive and can increase stress on the proximal joints. Commercially available splints can be used, but may require straightening of the metal support bar to a wrist neutral position. Soft or flexible wrist supports have been used for symptomatic relief and as a preventative measure for workers in 'high risk' occupations. These splints limit wrist motion, but have no effect on carpal tunnel pressure during repetitive activity (Rempel et al., 1994). Splinting can be quite successful at relieving nocturnal symptoms, but may not affect progression of the syndrome. At 2 months follow-up, 76% of Burkle's patients reported no change or worsened subjective symptoms when compared with follow-up at 2 weeks (Burke et al., 1994).

Non-steroidal anti-inflammatory drugs (NSAIDs)

Non-steroidal anti-inflammatory medication may be useful as a conservative treatment of carpal tunnel syndrome primarily when concomitant swelling or inflammation, such as tenosynovitis, is present. The most common adverse effect related to NSAID use is gastrointestinal toxicity, which ranges from mild gastric irritation to bleeding, ulceration and perforation. Strategies that counteract the gastrointestinal complications, such as protective prostaglandin analogs, add considerably to the treatment cost. In our experience, these drugs have been of limited usefulness. While the newer cyclooxygenase-2 inhibitors seem to be effective in the treatment of osteoarthritis and rheumatoid arthritis, with a marked reduction in associated gastrointestinal side-effects, their efficacy in treating carpal tunnel syndrome has not been studied (Kaplan-Machlis and Klostermeyer, 1999).

Vitamin B$_6$

Deficiencies of vitamins such as thiamine (B$_1$), riboflavin (B$_2$), and pyridoxine (B$_6$) can cause peripheral neuropathy (Kraft, 1980). Several authors have advocated vitamin B$_6$ supplementation as a conservative treatment for carpal tunnel syndrome (Ellis, 1987; Fuhr et al., 1989; Kasdan and James, 1986). Many of these reports (Ellis, 1987; Kasdan and Janes, 1986) have been anecdotal in nature, with no controls, blinding, or statistical analyses. Controlled studies have shown no relationship between pyridoxine levels and the symptoms and electrodiagnostic abnormalities of carpal tunnel syndrome (Byers et al., 1984; Franzblau et al., 1996). Randomized, controlled, double-blinded studies of patients with carpal tunnel syndrome treated for 2–3 months with vitamin B$_6$ in moderate doses (200 mg) have not shown the drug to be efficacious (Spooner et al., 1993; Stransky et al., 1989). Most of these trials have involved relatively small sample sizes.

Although some studies suggest that vitamin B$_6$ improves non-specific subjective pain due to underlying peripheral neuropathy, many factors limit its usefulness. The proposed mechanism of pyridoxine in carpal tunnel syndrome therapy has not been defined. Speculated mechanisms include a diuretic effect (Keniston et al., 1997) and pain threshold modulation (Bernstein and Dinesen, 1993). The biochemical assays used to assess pyridoxine deficiency (erythrocyte glutamic oxalacetic transaminase activity, leukocyte pyridoxal phosphate concentration) are not widely available. 'High' doses (2000 mg/day) of vitamin B$_6$ may cause toxicity, manifested by progressive sensory neuropathy (Copeland and Stoukides, 1994). In addition, the recommended minimal treatment period is long – 10–12 weeks. Until its role is better defined, we cannot recommend vitamin B$_6$ as the sole treatment modality in the conservative management of carpal tunnel syndrome.

Obesity

Nathan first reported an association between slowed median nerve conduction latency and body mass index which suggested that obese individuals are at greater risk of developing carpal tunnel syndrome (Nathan et al., 1992). This was an industrially based population; subsequent studies have examined other groups. A cross-sectional study of hospital electrodiagnostic laboratory patients found obese patients (Body mass index>29) to have a 2.5 relative risk for carpal tunnel syndrome by nerve conduction criteria (Werner et al., 1994). A case–control study of patients referred for independent medical examination in disability or workmen's compensation cases reported an odds ratio of 3.75 for carpal tunnel syndrome in obese subjects (Stallings et al., 1997). A New Zealand population of patients undergoing carpal tunnel decompression was twice as likely to be obese when compared with the general national population (Lam and Thurston, 1998). Adjusting for the confounding factor of older age did not eliminate obesity as a risk factor in these studies. Weight loss in overweight patients is now recommended as a component of conservative treatment. However, the pathophysiologic mechanism has not been defined and it remains to be shown that overweight patients who lose weight have resolution of their carpal tunnel syndrome.

Steroid injection

Steroid injection into the carpal canal has been advocated for several decades. Generally, relief of symptoms is reported in a high percentage of patients, but the recurrence rate is substantial (Dammers et al., 1999; Girlanda et al., 1993; Green 1984; Irwin et al., 1996; Weiss et al., 1994).

When follow-up after steroid injection is extended to 12 months or longer, recurrence rates range from 50% to nearly 90%. Gelberman reported poor long-term results for those with symptoms of greater severity or longer duration (Gelberman et al., 1980), but others have not found these characteristics to be predictive (Irwin et al., 1996).

Care must be exercised when injecting the carpal canal to avoid intraneural injection, which can cause significant injury to the median nerve (Mackinnon et al., 1982). We prefer to inject a water-soluble betamethasone through a 27-gauge needle inserted just ulnar to the palmaris longus tendon at the proximal wrist flexion crease. An explicit description of the needlestick sensation is elicited from the patient to check for associated paresthesias. Any discomfort should be localized to the wrist only, and should not be paresthetic. If insertion of the needle produces any paresthesias, it is withdrawn and repositioned without injecting any of the drug. We abandon the procedure if two attempts at needle placement fail to be free of paresthesias. The patient may experience an initial inflammatory reaction to the steroid, which usually lasts for 24 to 36 hours. This is effectively relieved by non-steroidal anti-inflammatory medications.

Since symptom relief from steroid injection is often temporary, we generally limit its use to diagnostic purposes. However, some patients may still benefit from temporary relief of symptoms while awaiting surgery, or if the condition is expected to resolve, such as in the later stages of pregnancy.

Surgical management

Definitive treatment of carpal tunnel syndrome is surgical decompression of the carpal tunnel using any of a variety of methods. Those currently used include the open technique, the limited open technique, and the endoscopic technique.

Open technique

The open technique is the oldest of the methods currently in use. An incision is made in the proxi-

mal palm, which may be extended proximally into the distal forearm. The palmar fascia and transverse carpal ligament are divided sharply. The recurrent motor branch of the median nerve may be easily identified and decompressed through this incision. This is done only when marked thenar atrophy is present. The carpel ligament and palmar fascia are not re-approximated. A simple skin closure completes the operation. Some authors have recommended internal neurolysis when there is evidence of long-standing or severe carpal tunnel syndrome (Rhoades et al., 1985), although others have reported no difference in results whether internal neurolysis or epineurotomy was performed, even in cases of severe compression (Blair et al., 1996; Mackinnon et al., 1991).

The term 'limited open technique' is a product of semantic manipulation. It typically describes an open carpal tunnel release performed through a shortened incision. The incision is made in the mid-palm or at the wrist flexion crease, and sometimes includes a mid-palmar counterincision (Biyani and Downes, 1993; Lee and Strickland, 1998; Wilson, 1944). The carpel ligament is usually transected under direct vision (Lee and Jackson, 1996). The use of a guarded ligament knife is described, which apparently is done in a relatively blinded fashion (Paine and Polyzoidis, 1983). This method allows only limited inspection of the carpal canal. Advocates recommend that the procedure be converted to the traditional open technique if inspection of the canal is indicated.

Endoscopic technique

The endoscopic technique is the most recently introduced. Though it has been in use for well over a decade now, it still incites a great deal of controversy. An assortment of endoscopic instrumentation has been developed. The most widely used systems are the Agee single portal system (Agee et al., 1994 (Figure 8.2) and the Chow dual portal system (Chow, 1994) (Figure 8.3). Both methods employ an open-roofed trocar, which is inserted into the carpal canal and allows visualization of the deep surface of the transverse carpal ligament through an endoscope. The ligament is transected from below with a

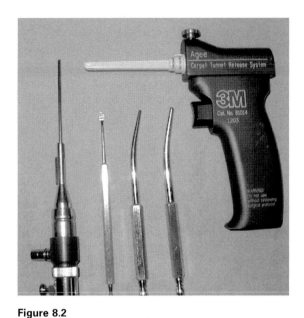

Figure 8.2

Agee single portal endoscopic carpal tunnel release system.

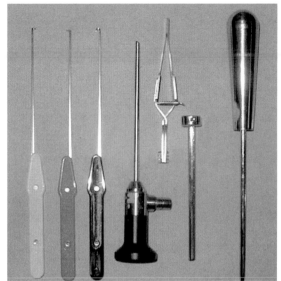

Figure 8.3

Chow dual portal endoscopic carpal tunnel release system.

specially designed blade through the open roof of the trocar. Advocates of this approach report that postoperative patient recovery and return to work are accelerated (Agee et al., 1994; Brown et al., 1993; Jimenez et al., 1998), while detractors believe the procedure is more expensive and carries a higher complication rate, without a substantial improvement in outcomes (Deune and Mackinnon, 1996; Shinya et al., 1995).

Authors' surgical procedure of choice

Our procedure of choice is the open method of carpal tunnel decompression (Figure 8.4). It allows direct visualization of the carpal canal and all of its contents and is generally associated with a lower complication rate. While the overall complication rate associated with endoscopic release is not high, major complications such as injury to the median or ulnar nerve are so serious that we feel a special effort is warranted to avoid them. We divide the entire transverse carpal ligament under direct vision (Figure 8.5). Epineurotomy or specific decompression of the

recurrent motor branch is rarely required. Our carpal tunnel decompressions are performed under tourniquet control, as outpatient procedures with local or regional anesthesia.

Postoperative management is straightforward. Based largely on our personal experience and favorable results reported by Cook regarding early mobilization (Cook et al., 1995), we do not routinely use postoperative splints. The patient is seen in the office 7–10 days after surgery. At the first visit, the original bulky dressing is removed and replaced by a light gauze wrap. Self-performed active finger and wrist range of motion exercises are started. If significant swelling or stiffness is noted at any visit during the postoperative period, the patient is referred to a hand therapist. Formal hand therapy is necessary for only 10–15% of our patients. We recommend light use of the hand for the first 3–4 weeks, which gradually increases over the next 3–4 weeks. At 6–8 weeks postoperatively, patients are released to unrestricted activity. At that time, most will still have some minor incisional tenderness and hand weakness, but will be able to adjust for this at their jobs. Jobs that place very high demands on the hand may require work restrictions for slightly longer periods.

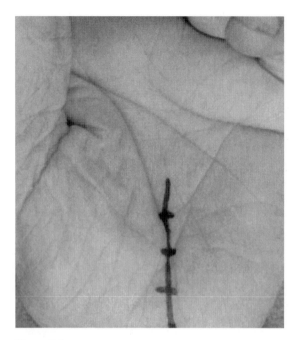

Figure 8.4

Authors' incision for open carpal tunnel decompression.

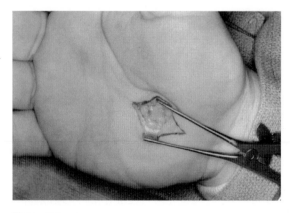

Figure 8.5

Open carpal tunnel decompression.

Complications of surgery

Although reported rates have varied significantly, the overall complication rate for surgical
carpal canal decompression is relatively low,
regardless of technique. Significant complications have been reported with both open and
endoscopic procedures. The extensive list
includes: infection, hematoma, flexor tendon
injury, superficial palmar arch injury, injury to the
median nerve or its recurrent motor branch,
ulnar nerve injury, digital nerve injury, injury to
the palmar cutaneous nerve, incomplete release
of the carpal ligament, and reflex sympathetic
dystrophy. Rarely reported complications include
radial nerve injury and bowstringing of the flexor
tendons.

A recent survey of members of the American
Society for Surgery of the Hand by Palmer and
Toivonen (1999) presented an overview of the
number and magnitude of self-reported surgical
complications. A striking total of 247 median
nerve lacerations, 117 ulnar nerve lacerations,
131 digital nerve lacerations, 155 vessel lacerations, and 88 tendon lacerations were reported.
Both endoscopic and open techniques were
included. The overall incidence of complications
could not be calculated from this report because
the denominator, or total number of carpal
tunnel surgeries performed by survey respon-
dents, was not collected. Although absolute
numbers of these major complications were
higher for endoscopic procedures than for open
procedures, again, incidences for each group
could not be calculated because the total number
of each type was not known.

The need for critical evaluation of endoscopic
versus open carpal tunnel surgery has generated
many attempts at comparing complication rates
between the two methods. Unfortunately, most
of these studies have not been adequate for
definitive conclusions to be drawn and the
group as a whole has been too inhomogeneous
for valid meta-analysis. Complications after
endoscopic release may have been more closely
scrutinized after reports of major complications
such as transection of the median or ulnar
nerves, which have been noted in practice and
also in cadaver studies (Nath et al., 1993;
Rowland and Kleinert, 1994). There does seem to
be a substantial learning curve associated with
endoscopic carpal tunnel surgery (Bozentka and
Osterman, 1995). However, the technique can be
taught safely with adequate instruction followed
by proper initial supervision, even in resident
training programs (Wheatley et al., 1997). The
most commonly reported problems are incomplete release of the ligament (Forman et al.,
1998) and transient paresthesia, especially in the
ring finger distribution (Arner et al., 1994;

Bozentka and Osterman 1995; Jimenez et al., 1998; Rowland and Kleinert, 1994). Some studies found endoscopic carpal tunnel release performed by *experienced* surgeons to have complication rates which were not different from those with open release (Agee et al., 1995; Boeckstyns and Sorensen, 1999). On the whole, complications following carpal tunnel release by any technique are relatively infrequent and can be avoided with thorough knowledge of the anatomy, adherence to proper technique, and careful execution.

Results

Most of the literature considers a resolution *or* reduction in symptoms, along with patient satisfaction as a 'good' result. Among published reports, residual symptoms are common, but they are usually at a low level that is not disturbing to the patient (Aulisa et al., 1998; Higgs et al., 1995). Nocturnal awakening due to paresthesias is frequently relieved, while numbness often persists. In the study by Higgs et al. (1995), up to 50% of all patients reported some residual symptoms even when outcomes were classified as 'excellent' or 'good'.

Patients receiving workers' compensation tend to fare poorly compared to others after carpal tunnel surgery (Higgs et al., 1995; Katz et al., 1998). Higgs et al. reported good results in 95% of non-workers' compensation patients versus only two-thirds of workers' compensation patients. Most patients can be expected to return to unrestricted activity between 2 and 12 weeks after surgery. Recovery time seems to depend on whether the surgery is covered by the workers' compensation system. Longer convalescence is the norm in workers. Although proponents of endoscopic carpal tunnel release tout comparatively earlier return to work times, this is not for workers' compensation patients (Kerr et al., 1994; Nagle et al., 1996; Palmer et al., 1993).

Poorer results have been associated with more advanced cases of carpal tunnel syndrome. As a general rule, symptom duration is thought to be indicative of disease severity. Cseuz et al. reported better results when surgical decompression was performed within 1 year of symptom onset (Cseuz et al., 1966). They also

suggested that results in elderly patients were worse than in younger patients. However, 90% 'good' and 'fair' results were still reported overall. Similarly, more recent reports suggest that better outcomes are achieved when carpal tunnel release is performed within 3 years of diagnosis (DeStefano et al., 1997).

Although results were poorer after carpal tunnel decompression in workers' compensation patients overall in their study, Higgs et al. found that those with significantly abnormal nerve conduction studies achieved results approaching those in the non-workers' compensation population (Higgs et al., 1995). Nerve conduction studies have not been predictive in non-worker populations. In fact, Grundberg reported that 97% of carefully selected patients with *normal* nerve conduction studies benefited from surgical decompression (Grundberg, 1983). Braun and Jackson (1994) and Glowacki et al. (1996) also found nerve conductions tests to be of no predictive value. Up to 12% of patients with significantly symptomatic carpal tunnel syndrome have normal nerve conduction studies (Concannon et al., 1997; Louis and Hankin, 1987). Some authors have suggested that patients with motor abnormalities fared better than those with only sensory abnormalities (Harris et al., 1979), while others have reported consistently good with improvement of both paresthesias and thenar strength (Goodwill 1965; Phalen 1966, 1972). Improvement or resolution of symptoms was achieved in 94–95% of patients in these series.

Results after repeat or secondary carpal tunnel decompression are inferior to those for primary decompression. 'Success' rates of secondary surgery are generally in the range of 50–75% (Cobb et al., 1996; Hulsizer et al., 1998; Strasberg et al., 1994), rather than the 80–90% achieved with primary surgery. The best results are in non-workers' compensation patients (Cobb et al., 1996; Hulsizer et al., 1998; Strasberg et al., 1994), especially when nerve conduction studies are abnormal, and in patients who had endoscopic decompression as their initial procedure (Hulsizer et al., 1998).

Many authors have reported excellent symptom relief and patient satisfaction in more than 90% of non-workers' compensation patients undergoing endoscopic carpal tunnel decompression (Brown et al., 1993; Jimenez et al., 1998;

Straub 1999). Studies comparing open and endoscopic release have reported less early postoperative pain or discomfort, faster recovery of strength, and sooner return to preoperative activities in the endoscopic group (Bande et al., 1994; Brown et al., 1993). A multicenter, randomized, prospective study by Brown and colleagues found that those undergoing endoscopic surgery returned to work in 14 days instead of 28 days for those who had open carpal tunnel surgery (Brown et al., 1993). However, results 6 months after surgery showed no significant differences between the two populations (Bande et al., 1994). In theory, release of the transverse carpal ligament may eliminate its pulley effect on the flexor tendons, weakening grip and pinch strength. Biomechanical cadaver studies suggest that finger flexion becomes less efficient, as greater tendon excursion is required to achieve the same amount of flexion (Brown and Peimer, 2000; Netscher et al., 1997, 1998a). A flap-type reconstruction of the ligament restores normal flexion properties (Netscher et al., 1997, 1998a). The same cadaver studies suggest that endoscopic release may be less disruptive to normal flexor biomechanics (Brown and Peimer, 2000). Clinical studies, however, failed to show any long-term difference in strength between open and endoscopic decompression (Netscher et al., 1998b). By 12 weeks after surgery, pinch and grip strengths were comparable between the two groups. Postoperative grip strength commonly exceeded preoperative grip strength after both procedures. This was noted as early as 12 weeks after surgery (Netscher et al., 1998b), and has been reported to approach 116% of preoperative values between 6 and 12 months postoperatively (Gellman et al., 1998).

Concluding remarks

If similar results are achieved with open and endoscopic carpal surgery, the issue of cost may play a role in determining a physician's procedure of choice. The additional training and equipment required to perform endoscopic carpal tunnel surgery, as well as the early learning curve that has been observed, raises the cost of this technique. Two recent studies have looked specifically at this question of cost-effectiveness.

The results depend heavily on the key factors of complication rates and return to work. Chung et al. found that endoscopic carpal tunnel decompression is cost-effective, as long as the incidence of major complications, such as a median nerve injury, remains at least one per cent less than that associated with open decompression (Chung et al., 1998). Current evidence does not find this to be true. The literature reports major complication rates with endoscopic release to be the same or higher, especially with inexperienced surgeons. Vasen and colleagues determined that endoscopic release is cost-effective if the overall complication rate remains 6.2% or lower, the risk of 'career-ending injury' remains less than 0.001, absence from work following any complication does not exceed 15.5 months, and patients return to work 21 days sooner than those receiving open decompression (Vasen et al., 1999). In workers' compensation patients, however, these differences in complication rates and return to work times must be even greater in order for endoscopic carpal tunnel surgery to be cost-effective. While some issues remain to be resolved, and certain subgroups of patients should be approached with special care, it can be safely stated that overall, carpal tunnel decompression is a safe and effective procedure.

References

Agee JM, McCarroll HR, North ER. (1994) Endoscopic carpal tunnel release using the single proximal incision technique. *Hand Clin* **10**:647–59.

Agee JM, Peimer CA, Pyrek JD, Walsh WE. (1995) Endoscopic carpal tunnel release: a prospective study of complications and surgical experience. *J Hand Surg* **20A**:165–71.

Amadio JC. (1992) The Mayo Clinic and carpal tunnel syndrome. *Mayo Clin Proc* **67**:42–8.

Armstrong TJ, Foulke JA, Joseph BS, Goldstein SA. (1982) Investigation of cumulative trauma disorders in a poultry processing plant. *Am Ind Hyg Assoc J* **43**:103–16.

Arner M, Hagberg L, Rosen B. (1994) Sensory disturbances after two-portal endoscopic carpal tunnel release: a preliminary report. *J Hand Surg* **19A**:548–51.

Aulisa L, Tamburrelli F, Padua R, et al. (1998) Carpal tunnel syndrome: indication for surgical treatment based on electrophysiologic study. *J Hand Surg* **23A**:687–91.

Bande S, DeSmet L, Fabry G, (1994) The results of carpal tunnel releases: open versus endoscopic technique, *J Hand Surg* **19B**:14–17.

Bernstein AL, Dinesen JS. (1993) Brief communication: effect of pharmacologic doses of vitamin B$_6$ on carpal tunnel syndrome, electroencephalographic results, and pain. *J Am Col Nurtr* **12(1)**:73–6.

Birkbeck MQ, Beer TC. (1975) Occupation in relation to the carpal tunnel syndrome. *Rheum Rehab* **14**:218–21.

Biyani A, Downes EM. (1993) An open twin incision technique of carpal tunnel decompression with reduced incidence of scar tenderness. *J Hand Surg* **18B**:331–4.

Blair WF, Goetz DD, Ross MA, Steyers CM, Change P. (1996) Carpel tunnel release with and without epineurotomy: a comparative prospective trial. *J Hand Surg* **21A**:655–61.

Boeckstyns ME, Sorensen AI. (1999) Does endoscopic carpal tunnel release have a higher rate of complications than open carpal tunnel release? An analysis of published series. *J Hand Surg* **24B**:9–15.

Bozentka DJ, Osterman AL. (1995) Complications of endoscopic carpal tunnel release. *Hand Clin* **11**:91–5.

Brain WR, Wright AD, Wilkinson M. (1947) Spontaneous compression of both median nerves in the carpal tunnel: six cases treated surgically. *Lancet* **1**:277–82.

Braun RM, Jackson WJ. (1994) Electrical studies as prognostic factor in the surgical treatment of carpal tunnel syndrome. *J Hand Surg* **19A**(6):893–900.

Brown RA, Gelberman RH, Seiler JG III, et al. (1993) Carpal tunnel release. A prospective, randomized assessment of open and endoscopic methods. *J Bone Joint Surg* **75A**:1265–75.

Brown RK, Peimer CA. (2000) Changes in digital flexor tendon mechanics after endoscopic and open carpal tunnel releases in cadaver wrists. *J Hand Surg* **25A**:112–19.

Burke DT, McHale Burke M, Stewart GW, Cambre A. (1994) Splinting for carpal tunnel syndrome: in search of the optimal angle. *Arch Phys Med Rehabil* **75**:1241–4.

Cannon BW, Love JG. (1946) Tardy median nerve palsy; median neuritis; median thenar neuritis amenable to surgery. *Surgery* **20**:210–16.

Byers CM, DeLisa JA, Frankel DL, Kraft GH. (1984) Pyridoxine metabolism in carpal tunnel syndrome with and without peripheral neuropathy. *Arch Phys Med Rehabil* **65**:712–16.

Chow JC. (1994) Endoscopic carpal tunnel release. Two-portal technique. *Hand Clin* **10**:637–46.

Chung KC, Walters MR, Greenfield JL, Chenow ME. (1998) Endoscopic versus open carpal tunnel release: a cost-effectiveness analysis. *Plast Reconstr Surg* **102**:1089–99.

Cobb TK, Amadio PC, Leatherwood DF, Schleck CD, Ilstrup DM. (1996) Outcome of reoperation for carpal tunnel syndrome. *J Hand Surg* **21**:347–56.

Concannon MJ, Gainor B, Petroski GF, Puckett CL. (1997) The predictive value of electrodiagnostic studies in carpal tunnel syndrome. *Plast Reconstr Surg* **100**:1452–6.

Cook AC, Szabo RM, Birkholz SW, King EF. (1995) Early mobilization following carpal tunnel release. A prospective randomized study. *J Hand Surg* **20B**:228–30.

Copeland DA, Stoukides CA. (1994) Pyridoxine in carpal tunnel syndrome. *Ann Pharmacother* **28**:1042–4.

Cseuz KA, Thomas JE, Lambert EH, Love JG, Lipscomb PR. (1966) Long-term results of operation for carpal tunnel syndrome. *Mayo Clin Proc* **41**:232–41.

Dammers JW, Veering MM, Vermeulen M. (1999) Injection with methylprednisolone proximal to the carpal tunnel: randomised double blind trial. *BMJ* **319**:884–6.

DeStefano F, Nordstrom DL, Vierkant RA. (1997) Long-term symptom outcomes of carpal tunnel syndromes and its treatment. *J Hand Surg* **22A**:200–10.

Deune EG and Mackinnon SE. (1996) Endoscopic carpal tunnel release. The voice of polite dissent. *Clin Plast Surg* **23**(3):487–505.

Ellis JM. (1987) Treatment of carpal tunnel syndrome with vitamin B$_6$. *South Med J* **80**:882–4.

Feldman RG, Travers PH, Chirico-Post J, Keyserling WM. (1987) Risk assessment in electronic assembly workers: carpal tunnel syndrome. *J Hand Surg* **12A**:849–55.

Forman DL, Watson HK, Caulfield KA, et al. (1998) Resistant or recurrent carpal tunnel syndrome following prior endoscopic carpal tunnel release. *J Hand Surg* **23A**:1010–14.

Franzblau A, Rock CL. Werner RA, et al. (1996) The relationship of vitamin B$_6$ status to median nerve functions and carpal tunnel syndrome among active industrial workers. *J Occup Environ Med* **38**(5):485–91.

Fuhr JE, Farrow A, Nelson HS. (1989) Vitamin B$_6$ levels in patients with carpal tunnel syndrome. *Arch Surg* **124**:1329–30.

Gainer JV, Nugent GR. (1977) Carpal tunnel syndrome: report of 430 operations. *South Med J* **30**:325–8.

Gelberman RH, Aronson D, Weisman MH. (1980) Carpal tunnel syndrome. Results of a prospective trial of steroid injection and splinting. *J Bone Joint Surg* **62A**:1181–4.

Gellman H, Kan D, Gee V, Kuschner SH, Botte MJ. (1998) Analysis of pinch and grip strength after carpal tunnel release. *J Hand Surg* **14A**:863–4.

Girlanda P, Dattola R, Venuto C, et al. (1993) Local steroid treatment in idiopathic carpal tunnel syndrome: short- and long-term efficacy. *J Neurol* **240**:187–90.

Glowacki KA, Breen CJ, Sachar K, Weiss AP. (1996) Electrodiagnostic testing and carpal tunnel release outcome. *J Hand Surg* **21**:117–21.

Goodwill CJ. (1965) The carpal tunnel syndrome. Long-term follow-up showing relation of latency measurements to response to treatment. *Ann Phys Med* **8**:12–21.

Green DP. (1984) Diagnostic and therapeutic value of carpal tunnel injection. *J Hand Surg* **9A**:850–54.

Grundberg AB. (1983) Carpal tunnel decompression in spite of normal electromyography. *J Hand Surg* **8A**:348–9.

Hadler NM. (1997) Repetitive upper-extremity motions in the workplace are not hazardous. *J Hand Surg* **22A**:19–29.

Harris CM, Tanner E, Goldstein MN, Pettee DS. (1979) The surgical treatment of the carpal tunnel syndrome correlated with pre-operative nerve conduction studies. *J Bone Joint Surg* **61A**:93–8.

Higgs PE, Edwards D, Martin DS, Weeks PM. (1995) Carpal tunnel surgery outcomes in workers: effect of workers' compensation status. *J Hand Surg* **20A**:354–60.

Hulsizer DL, Staebler MP, Weiss AP, Akelman E. (1998) The results of revision carpal tunnel releases following previous open versus endoscopic surgery. *J Hand Surg* **23A**:865–9.

Irwin LR, Beckett R, Suman RK. (1996) Steroid injection for carpal tunnel syndrome. *J Hand Surg* **21B**:355–7.

Jensen C, Borg V, Finsen L, et al. (1998) Job demands, muscle activity and musculoskeletal symptoms in relation to work with the computer mouse. *Scand J Work Environ Health* **24**(5):418–24.

Jetzer TC. (1991) Use of vibration testing in the early evaluation of workers with carpal tunnel syndrome. *J Occup Med* **33**:117–20.

Jimenez DF, Gibbs SR, Clapper AT. (1998) Endoscopic treatment of carpal tunnel syndromes: a critical review. *J Neurosurg* **88**:817–26.

Kaplan-Machlis B and Klostermeyer BS. (1999) The cyclooxygenase-2 inhibitors: safety and effectiveness. *Ann Pharmacother* **33**:979–88.

Kasdan ML, Janes C. (1987) Carpal tunnel syndrome and vitamin B$_6$. *Plast Reconstr Surg* **79**:456–9.

Katz JN, Keller RB, Simmons BP, et al. (1998) Maine carpal tunnel study: outcomes of operative and nonoperative therapy for carpal tunnel syndrome in a community-based cohort. *J Hand Surg* **23A**:697–710.

Keniston RC, Nathan PA, Leklem JE, Lockwood RS. (1997) Vitamin B$_6$, vitamin C, and carpal tunnel syndrome: a cross-sectional study of 441 adults. *J Occup Environ Med* **39**(10): 949–59.

Kerr CD, Gittins ME, Sybert DR. (1994) Endoscopic versus open carpal tunnel release: clinical results. *Arthroscopy* **10**:266–9.

Kraft GH. (1980) Peripheral neuropathies. In: Johnson EW, ed. *Practical electromyography*. Baltimore: Williams & Wilkins Co: 155–205.

Lam N, Thurston A. (1998) Association of obesity, gender, age and occupation with carpal tunnel syndrome. *Aust NZ J Surg* **68**:190–3.

Lee H, Jackson TA. (1996) Carpal tunnel release through a limited skin incision under direct visualization using a new instrument, the carposcope. *Plast Reconstr Surg* **98**:313–19.

Lee WP, Strickland JW. (1998) Safe carpal tunnel release via a limited palmar incision. *Plast Reconstr Surg* **101**:418–24.

Leifer D, Cros D, Halperin JJ, et al. (1992) Familial bilateral carpal tunnel syndrome: report of two families. *Arch Phys Med Rehabil* **73**:393–7.

Louis DS, Hankin FM. (1987) Symptomatic relief following carpal tunnel decompression with normal electroneuromyographic studies. *Orthopedics* **10**:434–6.

Mackinnon SE, Novak CB. (1997) Repetitive strain in the workplace. *J Hand Surg* **22A**:2–18.

Mackinnon SE, Hudson AR, Gentilli F, Kline DG, Hunter D. (1982) Peripheral nerve injection injury with steroids. *Plast Reconstr Surg* **69**:482–9.

Mackinnon SE, McCabe S, Murray JF, et al. (1991) Internal neurolysis fails to improve the results of primary carpal tunnel decompression. *J Hand Surg* **16A**:211–18.

Margolis W, Kraus JF. (1987) The prevalence of carpal tunnel syndrome symptoms in female supermarket checkers. *J Occup Med* **29**(12):953–6.

Marie P, Foix C. (1913) Atrophie isolée de l'éminence thénar d'origine névritique. Rôle du ligament annulaire antérieur du carpe dans la pathogénie de la lésion. *Revue Neurol* **26**:647–9.

Masear VR, Hayes JM, Hyde AG. (1986) An industrial cause of carpal tunnel syndrome. *J Hand Surg* **11A**:222–7.

Melvin JL, Johnson EW, Duran R. (1968) Electrodiagnosis after surgery for the carpal tunnel syndrome. *Arch Phys Med Rehab* **49**:502–7.

Nagle DJ, Fischer TJ, Harris GD, et al. (1996) A multicenter prospective review of 640 endoscopic carpal tunnel releases using the transbursal and extrabursal Chow techniques. *Arthroscopy* **12**:139–43.

Nath RK, Mackinnon SE, Weeks PM. (1993) Ulnar nerve transection as a complication of two-portal endoscopic carpal tunnel release: a case report. *J Hand Surg* **18A**:896–8.

Nathan PA, Keniston RC, Myers LD, Meadows KD. (1992) Obesity as a risk factor for slowing of sensory conduction of the median nerve in industry: a cross-sectional and longitudinal study involving 429 workers. *J Occup Med* **34**:379–83.

Netscher D, Dinh T, Cohen V, Thornby J. (1998a) Division of the transverse carpal ligament and flexor tendon excursion: open and endoscopic carpal tunnel release. *Plast Reconstr Surg* **102**:773–8.

Netscher D, Lee M, Thornby J, Polsen C. (1997) The effect of division of the transverse carpal ligament on flexor tendon excursion. *J Hand Surg* **22A**:1016–24.

Netscher D, Steadman AK, Thornby J, Cohen V. (1998b) Temporal changes in grip and pinch strength after open carpal tunnel release and the effect of ligament reconstruction. *J Hand Surg* **23A**:43–54.

Paine KW, Polyzoidis KS. (1983) Carpal tunnel syndrome. Decompression using the Paine retinaulatome. *J Neurosurg* **59**:1031–6.

Palmer AK, Toivonen DA. (1999) Complications of endoscopic and open carpal tunnel release. *J Hand Surg* **24A**:561–5.

Palmer DH, Paulson JC, Lane-larsen CL, et al. (1993). Endoscopic carpal tunnel release: a comparison of two techniques with open release. *Arthroscopy* **9**:498–508.

Pfeffer GB, Gelberman RH, Boyes JH, Rydevik B. (1988) The history of carpal tunnel syndrome. *J Hand Surg* **13B**:28–34.

Phalen GS. (1966) The carpal tunnel syndrome. Seventeen years experience in diagnosis and treatment of 654 hands. *J Bone Joint Surg* **48A**:211–28.

Phalen GS. (1972) The carpal tunnel syndrome. *Clin Orthop* **83**:29–40.

Phalen GS, Gardner WJ, La Londe AA. (1950) Neuropathy of the median nerve due to compression beneath the transverse carpal ligament. *J Bone Joint Surg* **32A**:109–12.

Punnett L Robins JM, Wegman DH, Keyserling WM. (1985) Soft tissue disorders in the upper limbs of female garment workers. *Scand J Work Environ Health* **11**:417–25.

Rempel D, Manojlovic R, Levinsohn DG, Bloom T, Gordon L. (1994) The effect of wearing a flexible wrist splint on carpal tunnel pressure during repetitive hand activity. *J Hand Surg* **19**:106–10.

Rempel DM, Harrison RJ, Barnhart S. (1992) Work-related cumulative trauma disorders of the upper extremity. *JAMA* **267**(6):838–42.

Rhoades CE, Mowery CA, Gelberman RH. (1985) Results of internal neurolysis of the median nerve for severe carpal tunnel syndrome. *J Bone Joint Surg* **67A**:253–6.

Rowland EB, Kleinert JM. (1994) Endoscopic carpal tunnel release in cadavers. An investigation of the results of twelve surgeons with this training model. *J Bone Joint Surg* **76A**:266–8.

Rozmaryn LM, Dovelle S, Roghman ER, et al. (1998) Nerve and tendon gliding exercises and the conservative management of carpal tunnel syndrome. *J Hand Ther* **11**:171–9.

Seradge H, Jia Y-C, Owens W. (1995) In-vivo measurement of carpal tunnel pressure in the functioning hand. *J Hand Surg* **20A**:855–9.

Shinya K, Lanzetta M, Conolly WB. (1995) Risk and complications in endoscopic carpal tunnel release. *J Hand Surg* **20B**:222–7.

Spooner GR, Desai HB, Angel JF, Reeder BA, Donat JR. (1993) Using pyridoxine to treat carpal tunnel syndrome: randomized control trial. *Can Fam Physician* **39**:2122–7.

Stallings SP, Kasdan ML, Soergel TM, Corwin HM. (1997) A case-control study of obesity as a risk factor for carpal tunnel syndrome in a population of 600 patients presenting for independent medical examination. *J Hand Surg* **22A**:211–15.

Stevens JC, Sun S, Beard CM, O'Fallon WM, Kurland LT. (1988) Carpal tunnel syndrome in Rochester, Minnesota, 1961 to 1980. *Neurology* **38**:134–8.

Straaton KV, Maisiak R, Wrigley JM, et al. (1996) Barriers to return to work among persons unemployed due to arthritis and musculoskeletal disorders. *Arthritis Rheumatism* **39**:101–9.

Stranksy M, Rubin A, Lava NS, Lazaro RP. (1989) Treatment of carpal tunnel syndrome with vitamin B_6: a double-blind study. *South Med J* **82**:841–2.

Strasberg SR, Novak CB, Mackinnon SE, Murray JF. (1994) Subjective and employment outcomes following secondary carpal tunnel surgery. *Ann Plast Surg* **32**:485–9.

Straub TA. (1997) Endoscopic carpal tunnel release: a prospective analysis of factors associated with unsatisfactory results. *Arthroscopy* **15**:269–74.

Strauch B, Lang A, Ferder MBA, et al. (1997) The ten test. *Plast Reconstr Surg* **99**:1074–8.

Stromberg T, Dahlin LB, Lundborg G. (1996) Hand problems in 100 vibration-exposed symptomatic male workers. *J Hand Surg* **21B**:315–19.

Stromberg T, Dahlin LB, Rosen I, Lundborg G. (1999) Neurophysiological findings in vibration-exposed male workers. *J Hand Surg* **24B**:203–9.

Tetro Am, Evanoff BA, Hollstein SB, Gelberman RH. (1998) A new provocative test for carpal tunnel syndrome. Assessment of wrist flexion and nerve compression. *J Bone Joint Surg* **80B**:493–8.

Vasen AP. Kuntz KM, Simmons BP, Katz JN. (1999) Open versus endoscopic carpal tunnel release: a decision analysis. *J Hand Surg* **24A**:1109–17.

Weiss A-P, Sachar K, Gendreau M. (1994) Conservative management of carpal tunnel syndrome: a reexamination of steroid injection and splinting. *J Hand Surg* **19A**:410–15.

Weiss ND, Gordon L, Bloom T, Yuen S, Rempel DM. (1995) Position of the wrist associated with the lowest carpal-tunnel pressure: implications for splint design. *J Bone Joint Surg* **77A**:1695–9.

Werner RA, Albers JW, Franzblau A, Armstrong TJ. (1994) The relationship between body mass index and the diagnosis of carpal tunnel syndrome. *Muscle Nerve* **17**:632–6.

Wheatley MJ, Hall JW, Pratt D, Faringer PD. (1997) Is training in endoscopic carpal tunnel release appropriate for residents? *Ann Plas Surg* **37**:254–7.

Wilson KM. (1994) Double incision open technique for carpal tunnel release: an alternative to endoscopic release. *J Hand Surg* **19**:907–12.

Wood MR. (1980) Hydrocortisone injections for carpal tunnel syndrome. *Hand* **12**:62–4.

9
Suprascapular nerve entrapment

Thierry Fabre and Alain Durandeau

Introduction

Suprascapular nerve entrapment is one of the diagnoses to be considered for shoulder pain. This syndrome is often mistakenly diagnosed as tendinitis syndrome, rotator cuff tear or cervical disc disease, and treatment is often delayed until the patient has atrophy of the supraspinatus muscle, the infraspinatus muscle, or both. Such delays slow functional recovery of the shoulder after surgery.

Since Koppel and Thompson (1963) described suprascapular nerve compression at the suprascapular notch, many papers concerning this syndrome have been published (Clein, 1975; Cummins et al., 2000; Garcia and McQueen, 1981; Post and Mayer, 1987). The mechanism of the entrapment, clinical picture and diagnosis have all been thoroughly discussed elsewhere (Hadley et al., 1986; Post and Mayer, 1987; Thompson et al., 1982). Rengachary et al. (1979), Mestdagh et al. (1981), and more recently, Bigliani's and Warner's groups have reported well-documented anatomical studies, which have helped clarify the pathogenesis of the entity (Bigliani et al., 1990; Warner et al., 1992). Various repetitive activities (Callahan et al., 1991; Constant and Murley, 1987; Dredz, 1976), among which are many different sports involving various arm movements (Ferretti et al., 1987; Ringer et al., 1990), have been identified as causes of this syndrome. Furthermore, suprascapular nerve entrapment can also be caused by rotator cuff tear or, less often, associated with it (Moore et al., 1997). Västamäki and Goransson (1993) first reported a very large clinical series. Ganzhorm's and Thompson's groups reported cases of compression of the suprascapular nerve by a ganglion cyst (Ganzhorm et al., 1981; Thomson et al.,1982). Since then, many publications on the subject have appeared in the literature thanks to the increasing use of magnetic resonance imaging (MRI) (Aiello et al., 1982; Demaio et al., 1991; Fehrman et al., 1995; Fritz et al., 1992; Ianotti et al., 1991; Yoon, 1981).

Forty-five patients were operated on for suprascapular nerve entrapment in our unit between 1985 and 2000. They were assessed at an average of 28 months after operation using the functional shoulder score devised by Constant and Murley (Constant and Murley, 1987; Conboy et al., 1996). We present here a review of this subject in the light of our experience (Fabre et al., 1999).

Applied anatomy of the suprascapular nerve

Classically, the suprascapular nerve originates from the upper trunk C-5, C-6 or the distal portion of C-5. The nerve normally (Figure 9.1) leaves the upper trunk 3 cm above the clavicle and travels toward the scapular notch. It is located posterior to the omohyoid muscle and close to the superficial transverse cervical vessels. Most cases of entrapment occur when it courses under the transverse scapular ligament. According to Mestdagh (Mestdagh et al., 1981) and Renchagary (Renchagary et al., 1979), the scapular notch may have several forms (four to six). Dorsal to the notch, the nerve gives off a motor ramus to the supraspinatus muscle. This ramus runs medially and penetrates the muscle

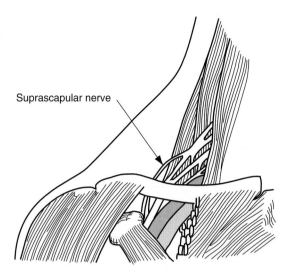

Suprascapular nerve

Figure 9.1

The suprascapular nerve originates at the proximal superior trunk of the brachial plexus.

on its anterior inferior aspect. The lateral branch gives rami to the deep aspect of the acromio-clavicular joint, the subacromial bursa and the dorsal aspect of the gleno-humeral joint.

The nerve then runs obliquely across the supraspinatus fossa toward the rim of the glenoid fossa and enters the infraspinatus fossa around the base of the spine of the scapula beneath the spinoglenoid ligament which determines a fibro-osseous tunnel through which the suprascapular nerve courses (Cummings et al., 1998). The nerve then divides in three to four branches which innervate the infraspinatus. The nerve may give off a dorsal ramus to the skin innervating the posterior aspect of the shoulder medial to the deltoid.

Function of the suprascapular nerve

The role of the suprascapular nerve has been increasingly appreciated recently. Paralysis of the nerve significantly diminishes the power of abduction of the arm (Narakas, 1991). The suprascapular nerve retains 45–55% power of abduc-

tion to 90°. In comparison a complete deltoid paralysis with the suprascapular nerve unaffected permits full elevation of the arm. With a non-functional suprascapular nerve it is more common to have less than 90° of abduction, especially with the humerus in full internal rotation. When the spinatus muscles are paralysed, the power of external rotation (at 0° or 90° of abduction) is significantly decreased compared with the unaffected side.

Pathogenesis

The causes of entrapment include direct injury, traction and repetitive activities, which have led to overuse of the upper limb. Traumatic causes of suprascapular nerve entrapment include scapular fracture (Solheim and Roaas, 1978), shoulder dislocation (Travlos et al., 1990; Zoltan 1979) and massive rotator cuff defects (Bigliani et al., 1990; Warner et al., 1992; Zanotti et al., 1997). We also included in our series patients who had had incomplete injuries to the brachial plexus, which had completely recovered except for the suprascapular branch. The abnormal kinematics of the scapula, caused by temporary palsy of the brachial plexus, were probably responsible for the damage to the suprascapular nerve, explaining the isolated persistence of this deficit. Several authors have reported tethering of the nerve as it passes through the notch beneath the scapular transverse ligament (Rask, 1977; Rengachary et al., 1979; Västamäki and Goransson, 1993). In the spinoglenoid notch, the nerve is compressed in the fibro-osseous tunnel formed by the spine of the scapula and the spinoglenoid ligament (Demaio et al., 1991; Kiss and Komar, 1990; Liveson et al., 1991). Repetitive overhead activities may endanger the nerve. The majority of these injuries occur in athletes who use the upper extremities in an overhead fashion such as professional volleyball players (Ferretti et al., 1987), but also occur in baseball players, tennis players and swimmers (Black and Lombardo, 1990; Cummings et al., 1999; Jackson et al., 1995). Microemboli of the suprascapular vasa nervorum producing nerve ischemia have been suspected (Ringel et al., 1990). A ganglion in the spinoglenoid notch (Aiello et al., 1982; Ganzhorm et al., 1981; Ianotti and Ramsay 1996;

Neviaser et al., 1986; Thompson et al., 1982) more frequently than in the scapular notch (Hadley et al., 1986; Narakas, 1991; Rochwerger et al., 1996; Takakazu and Yoshiharu, 1981) is another cause of entrapment of the suprascapular nerve. Posterior capsular tissue trauma about the shoulder joint may contribute to the formation of a ganglion cyst. Several reports recently focussed on MRI-discovered ganglion cysts and evidence of spinatus muscle atrophy. In certain cases MRI may directly display the nerve with evidence suggesting its involvement such as increase in volume with partial or complete disappearance of the fatty component. Arthroscopic intra-articular findings most often confirmed the posterior capsulolabral tears communicating with ganglion cysts (Fehrman et al., 1995; Tirman et al., 1994).

Clinical evaluation

Patients complain of pain, which is typically lateral on the dorso-lateral aspect of the shoulder exacerbated by repetitive overhead activities. Sometimes a traumatic or an acute event triggered the symptoms. More often the onset of symptoms is insidious, involving the dominant arm in a patient aged between 20 and 50 years. The pain may radiate to the posterior aspect of the arm. With time, the pain may become almost permanent and fatigue may appear. Weakness of abduction or external rotation may be the chief symptom with little or no pain. Atrophy of the muscles may be visible, affecting both the supra- and infraspinatus muscles or only the latter. Patients may be completely asymptomatic and the atrophy of the infraspinatus muscle may be detected as an incidental finding (Ferretti et al., 1987; Steinman, 1988).

Physical examination evaluates the range of motion of the shoulder with special attention to the abduction in the plane of the scapula and the external rotation with the arm at 90° of abduction. Atrophy of the supra- and infraspinatus muscles and tenderness on palpation in the area between the clavicle and the scapular spine or more distally at the spinoglenoid notch may be evaluated. Weakness may be demonstrated on abduction and external rotation. Concerning the abduction, the weakness may become evident by having the patient lift weights in the plane of the scapula as described by Narakas (1991). Weakness in external rotation may be evaluated against manual resistance and compared to the unaffected side. The cross-body test tenses the nerve on the scapular ligament and may increase pain. However the sensitivity of this maneuver is uncertain. Some authors have proposed injections of a local anesthetic into the suprascapular notch as a diagnostic test in producing pain relief.

Electrophysiological studies

Electrodiagnostic studies should always be used when clinical findings suggest entrapment of the suprascapular nerve. Normally, increasing latency on stimulation at Erb's point above 3.3 ms for the supraspinatus and 4.2 ms for the infraspinatus confirm the suprascapular nerve lesion. Electromyography may also demonstrate a decrease in amplitude of motor potential, fibrillations, increase in spontaneous activity and positive sharp waves in denervated muscles. This test can also distinguish between entrapment in the suprascapular notch and the spinoglenoid notch. A compression in the suprascapular notch demonstrates changes in both the supra- and infraspinatus muscles; in contrast a distal injury to the nerve shows changes only in the infraspinatus muscle.

Electromyography provides helpful data when considering differential diagnoses such as C-5, C-6 root compromise, Parsonage–Turner syndrome or degenerative musculotendinous lesions.

Imaging studies

Plain radiography of the shoulder is often the first examination requested. It may rarely show bony erosion due to remodeling of the bone by extrinsic pressure. Various studies indicate that simple films are not helpful in suprascapular nerve disorders, most commonly showing a normal or non-specific aspect (Fritz et al., 1992; Levy et al., 1997).

Ultrasonographic examination is often requested after standard films but it does not appear to be a reliable diagnostic tool in suprascapular nerve lesions (Ogino et al., 1991). Theoretically, it should be contributory in the detection of cysts, which are commonly well delineated as a hypoechoic image with a posterior shadow. Routine sonography may not detect such formations, because of their deep location and the difficult access in certain patients. Furthermore, the labrum cannot be evaluated by sonography.

MRI is the most helpful examination in the suprascapular nerve entrapment. MRI has been demonstrated to be very useful in the diagnosis of a ganglion cyst (Fritz et al., 1992; Ianotti et al., 1991; Takagishi et al., 1991; Tirman et al., 1994). On MRI, these masses typically have clear and regular contours and are rounded and lobulated. They are homogeneous, hypointense on T_1-weighted images and hyperintense on T_2-weighted images (Figure 9.2). MRI shows precisely the extension of the cyst into the supra- or infraspinatus fossa. These cysts, which are remarkably visible on the T_2 images, are easily distinguishable from the other fluid structures of the shoulder. MRI also shows the type and degree of changes in the supra- and infraspinatus muscles secondary to denervation (Kullmer et al., 1998). MRI protocols should include fast spin echo on T_2-weighted images and fat suppression on T_1-weighted images. MRI is able to identify changes in the supra- and infraspinatus muscles secondary to

denervation and help to distinguish between a lesion in the suprascapular or spinoglenoid notches. First changes in supra- or infraspinatus muscles show muscle edema as homogeneous, high signal intensity on T_2-weighted images (Figure 9.3). Fatty infiltration on the spinatus muscles appears for chronic lesions of the nerve on T_1-weighted images and are visualized as hyperintense bands. This lesion most often persists, even after correct treatment has been performed. Muscle atrophy (Figure 9.4) could appear on T_1- or T_2-weighted images and should be reversible after appropriate treatment of the suprascapular nerve entrapment.

MRI has the added advantage compared with other imaging modalities of permitting the detection of associated lesions. Rotator cuff tears are clearly visualized by MRI. These lesions are rarely associated with suprascapular nerve lesion (Brown et al., 2000; Fabre et al., 1999) but should be diagnosed with careful preoperative assessment to repair both lesions during the operative procedure (Drez, 1976). Labral tears are frequently associated with ganglion cysts of the shoulder. MRI may show an area of abnormal signal intensity in the labrum, which can be arthroscopically confirmed (Tirman et al., 1994). But in several case reports, MRI failed to demonstrate a labral tear that was later identified with arthroscopy (Chochole et al., 1997; Ianotti et al.,

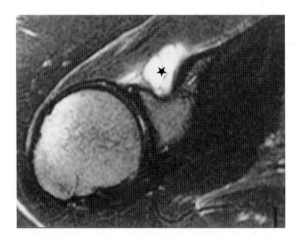

Figure 9.2

T_2-weighted axial image identifies a paralabral cyst in the infraspinatus fossa (asterisk).

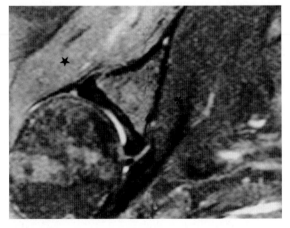

Figure 9.3

The T_2 hyperintense aspect of the infraspinatus muscle (asterisk) shows muscle edema secondary to nerve entrapment. Note that the subscapularis muscle is unaffected.

1991; Moore et al., 1997). Distension of the articulation with MR arthrography permits a more precise analysis of the glenohumeral ligaments. This imaging protocol has been found to show a sensitivity of 91%, a specificity of 93% and an accuracy of 92% (Palmer et al., 1994) for the diagnosis of labral lesions and should be carried out every time a ganglion cyst around the shoulder has been found.

Treatment

There are many opinions concerning the treatment for suprascapular nerve entrapment. Non-operative treatment should be considered for patients who have dysfunction of the nerve without supraspinatus muscular atrophy or evidence of a space-occupying lesion. The initial treatment should include avoidance of performing repetitive activities and lifting objects overhead which exacerbates the symptoms. A progressive program of physical therapy should be prescribed, focussed on increasing the strength of the muscles of the rotator cuff, the deltoid muscle and the periscapular muscles (Martin et al., 1997). If the patient experiences a decrease in pain or increase in strength and the electrophysiologic findings show improvement during the non-operative period, the patient will usually recover spontaneously, particularly if the entrapment follows trauma (Callahan et al., 1991; Vastamäki and Goransson, 1993; Yoon et al., 1981). In a retrospective study (Martin et al., 1997), 12 patients out of 15 avoided operative decompression after a well-conducted non-operative treatment. After 3–4 months, if the symptoms persist, operative decompression of the nerve should be proposed. If there is evidence of muscular atrophy or severe pain that is not controlled by drugs, the operation should not be delayed beyond 3 months. The same treatment should be applied if a ganglion cyst has been diagnosed.

There has been some discussion as to the surgical approach that should be used for decompression of suprascapular nerves. A few authors prefer an anterior approach over the medial aspect of the coracoid process (Murray, 1974; Shupeck and Onofrio, 1990) but we advocate, as others, a posterosuperior approach

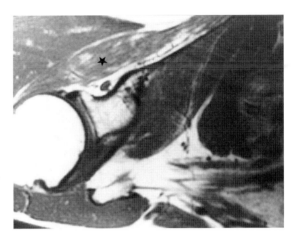

Figure 9.4

T$_2$-weighted axial image shows atrophy of the supraspinatus muscle (asterisk) that is secondary to suprascapular nerve entrapment.

(Callahan et al., 1991; Ficat et al., 1967; Hadley et al., 1986). To release the superior transverse ligament, Post and Mayer (1987) recommended detachment of the trapezius muscle from the scapular spine with a posterior approach. We prefer a posterosuperior approach between the clavicle and the spine of the scapula. The patients were operated on in a semiprone position with the arm draped free and the head turned away. The skin incision was made parallel and slightly proximal to the spine of the scapula. The trapezius was split in the axis of its fibers. The suprascapular muscle was retracted backward with a layer of fatty tissue (Figure 9.4). The index finger was used to locate the suprascapular ligament situated between the superior margin of the scapula and the medial base of the coracoid process. The transverse scapular ligament was then identified and excised with care being taken to avoid injuring the suprascapular artery and vein lying superficial to it. The suprascapular nerve could be identified using electrical stimulation if necessary and was decompressed focally. We do not recommend enlarging the suprascapular notch because the nerve was observed to bulge from the notch after excision of the suprascapular ligament. Active movements within the limit of pain were allowed, beginning on the first day after operation.

With isolated involvement of the infraspinatus muscle we recommend operative decompression of the nerve, both at the suprascapular and spinoglenoid notches. We then prefer a posterior approach as described by Post and Mayer (1987). The insertion of trapezius muscle was released from the spine of the scapula. Then the deltoid muscle was partially detached from the distal part of the spine of the scapula and the supraspinatus muscle was reflected inferiorly to expose the suprascapular notch. The suprascapular ligament was then identified and excised. The nerve was exposed on both sides of the scapular spine at the spinoglenoid notch, reflecting superiorly the supraspinatus muscle and inferiorly the infraspinatus muscle (Figures 9.5 and 9.6). The spinoglenoid ligament was then released. We have never undertaken deepening of the lateral margin of the scapular spine as recommended by others (Aiello et al., 1982; Hama et al., 1993).

When compression of the suprascapular nerve is secondary to compression by a ganglion cyst, ultrasonography or computed tomography-guided aspiration has been proposed (Hashimoto et al., 1994; Tirman et al., 1994). Both methods appear to be effective and are associated with little morbidity. However the patient may be at increased risk for recurrence.

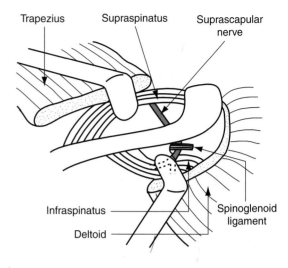

Figure 9.6

Surgical exposure of the spinoglenoid notch. Both the trapezius and the deltoid muscles have been elevated from the scapular spine. The supraspinatus and infraspinatus muscles are retracted superiorly and inferiorly, respectively.

Operative treatments of ganglion cysts of the shoulder according to the preference of the operating surgeon include open and arthroscopic procedures. Open excision of the cyst should be performed with a posterior approach but does not allow the surgeon to identify and treat associated and intra-articular capsulolabral tears. The arthroscopic technique includes a thorough diagnostic shoulder examination. A posterior capsulolabral tear should be visualized and debrided. The ganglion cyst should require careful arthroscopic blunt dissection in the region correlated with the MRI. Care must be taken to avoid dissection beyond 1 cm medial to the superior capsular attachment to protect the suprascapular nerve. Combined arthroscopic and open procedures have been recommended (Moore et al., 1997).

The use of Constant and Murley's scoring system is helpful in the evaluation of suprascapular nerve entrapment. We found it to be simple, reliable, cheap and easy to use in a clinical setting (Fabre et al., 1999). The results of operative treatment regardless of the cause of nerve entrapment are good, resulting in most

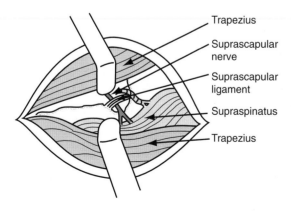

Figure 9.5

Surgical exposure of the suprascapular notch. The trapezius has been split in the axis of its fibers. The supraspinatus muscle has been retracted backward.

cases in rapid disappearance of the pain (Callahan et al., 1991; Post and Mayer, 1987). Muscle strength returned more gradually (Vastamäki and Goransson, 1993). Persistence of atrophy has been noted in several reports (Black and Lombardo, 1990; Clein, 1975; Hadley et al.,1986; Post and Grinblat, 1993), and was more frequent for patients operated on 6 months after the onset of symptoms (Fabre et al., 1999). Atrophy of the infraspinatus muscle was the slowest to improve but does not affect the function of the shoulder (Ferretti et al., 1987). Recurrence of symptoms although uncommon has been reported in some cases after open operative excision of a ganglion cyst (Moore et al., 1997; Skirving et al., 1994).

Conclusion

The syndrome of suprascapular nerve entrapment occurs much more frequently than is reported. It often presents as a chronic pain problem associated with weakness of the spinatus muscles in patients who have over-exerted their shoulder with repetitive active movements. Electrodiagnostic studies should be obtained in patients suspected of having this entrapment neuropathy, to confirm the diagnosis and identify the site of the nerve injury. MRI may allow early recognition of muscle denervation. It may also help to visualize mass lesions or identify labral tears in association with ganglion cysts. A period of 3–4 months of conservative therapy is advocated for most patients. If non-operative treatment does not result in amelioration of symptoms, an operation may be indicated. Surgical decompression should be performed at the site of entrapment and requires an appropriate approach. A ganglion cyst may be treated with open excision or an arthroscopic procedure. The symptomatic and functional outcome in series reported in the literature confirms the usefulness and safety of operative decompression for entrapment of the suprascapular nerve.

References

Aiello I, Serra G, Traina GC, Tugnoli V. (1982) Entrapment of the suprascapular nerve at the spinoglenoid notch. *Ann Neurol* **12**: 225–8.

Bigliani LU, Dalsey RM, McCann PD, April EW. (1990) An anatomical study of the suprascapular nerve. *Arthroscopy* **6**:301–5.

Black KP, Lombardo JA. (1990) Suprascapular nerve injuries with isolated paralysis of the infraspinatus. *Am J Sports Med* **18**:225–8.

Brown TD, Newton PM, Steinmann SP, Levine WN, Bigliani LU. (2000) Rotator cuff tears and associated nerve injuries. *Orthopedics* **23**(4):329–32.

Callahan JD, Scully TB, Shapiro SA, Worth RM. (1991) Suprascapular nerve entrapment. A series of 27 cases. *J Neurosurg* **74**:893–6.

Chochole MH, Senker W, Meznik C, Breitenseher MJ. (1997) Glenoid labral cyst entrapping the suprascapular nerve: dissolution after arthroscopic debridement of an extended SLAP lesion. *Arthroscopy* **13**:753–5.

Clein LJ. (1975) Suprascapular entrapment neuropathy. *J Neurosurg* **43**:337–42.

Conboy WB, Morris RW, Kiss J, Carr AJ. (1996) An evaluation of the Constant and Murley shoulder assessment. *J Bone Joint Surg* **78B**:229–32.

Constant CR, Murley AHG. (1987) A clinical method of functional assessment of the shoulder. *Clin Orthop* **214**:160–4.

Cummins CA, Messer TM, Nuber GW. (2000) Suprascapular nerve entrapment. *J Bone Joint Surg* **82A**: 415–24.

Cummins CA, Anderson K, Bowen M, Nuber G, Roth SI. (1998) Anatomy and histological characteristics of the spinoglenoid ligament. *J Bone Joint Surg* **80A**: 1622–25.

Cummins CA, Bowen M, Anderson K. Messer T. (1999) Suprascapular nerve entrapment at the spinoglenoid notch in a professional baseball pitcher. *Am J Sports Med* **7**:810–12.

Demaio M, Drez D Jr, Mullins RC. (1991) The inferior transverse scapular ligament as a possible cause of entrapment neuropathy of the nerve to the infraspinatus. A brief note. *J Bone Joint Surg* **73A**:1061–3.

Drez D Jr. (1976) Suprascapular neuropathy in the differential diagnosis of rotator cuff injuries. *Sports Med* **4**:43–5.

Fabre T, Piton C, Leclouerec G, Gervais-delion F, Durandeau A. (1999) Entrapment of the suprascapular nerve. *J Bone Joint Surg* **81B**:414–18.

Fehrman DA, Orwin JF, Jennings RM. (1995) Suprascapular nerve entrapment by ganglion cysts: A report of six cases with arthroscopic findings and review of the literature. *Arthroscopy* **11**:724–34.

Ferretti A, Cerullo G, Russo G. (1987) Suprascapular neuropathy in volleyball players. *J Bone Joint Surg* **69A**:260–3.

Ficat P, Mansat C, Roudil J. (1967) Neurolyse du suprascapulaire. *Rev Med Toulouse* **III**: 229–32.

Fritz RC, Helms CA, Steinbach LS, Genant HK. (1992) Suprascapular nerve entrapment: evaluation with MRI imaging. *Radiology* **182**:437–44.

Ganzhorm RW, Hocker JT, Horowitz M, Switzer HE. (1981) Suprascapular nerve entrapment. A case report. *J Bone Joint Surg* **63A**:492–4.

Garcia G, McQueen D. (1981) Bilateral suprascapular nerve entrapment syndrome. *J Bone Joint Surg* **63A**:491–4.

Hadley MD, Sonntag VKN, Pittman HW. (1986) Suprascapular nerve entrapment. A summary of seven cases. *J Neurosurg* **64**:843–8.

Hama H, Ueba Y, Morinaga T, Suzuki K, Kuroki H, Yammamuro T. (1993) A new strategy for treatment of suprascapular entrapment neuropathy in athletes, shaving off the base of the scapular spine. *J Shoulder Elbow Surg* **1**:257–9.

Hashimoto BE, Hayes AS, Ager JD. (1994) Sonographic diagnosis and treatment of ganglion cysts causing suprascapular nerve entrapment. *J Ultrasound Med* **13**:671–4.

Ianotti JP, Ramsey ML. (1996) Arthroscopic decompression of a ganglion cyst causing suprascapular nerve compression. *Arthroscopy* **12**:739–5.

Ianotti JP, Zlatkin MB, Esterhai JL et al. (1991) Magnetic resonance imaging of the shoulder: sensitivity, specificity and predictive value. *J Bone Joint Surg* **73A**:17–29.

Jackson DL, Farrage J, Hynninen BC, Cabom DN. (1995) Suprascapular neuropathy in athletes: case reports. *Clin J Sports Med* **5**:134–7.

Kiss G, Komar J. (1990) Suprascapular nerve decompression at the spinoglenoid notch. *Muscle Nerve* **13**:556–7.

Koppel HP, Thompson WAL. (1963) *Peripheral entrapment neuropathies*. Baltimore: Williams and Wilkins: 131–42.

Kullmer K, Sievers KW, Reimers CD, et al. (1968) Changes of sonographic, magnetic resonance tomographic, electromyographic, and histopathologic findings within a two months period of examination after experimental muscle denervation. *Arch Orthop Trauma Surg* **117**:228–34.

Levy P, Roger B, Rodineau J. (1997) Compression kystique du nerf suprascapulaire. *J Radiol* **78**:123–30.

Liveson JA, Bronson MJ, Pollack MA. (1991) Suprascapular nerve lesion at the spinoglenoid notch: report of three cases and review of the literature. *J Neurol Neurosurg Psychiatry* **54**:241–3.

Martin SD, Warren RF, Martin TL, Kennedy K, O'Brien SJ, Wickiewicz TL. (1997) Suprascapular neuropathy. Results of non-operative treatment. *J Bone Joint Surg* **79A**:1159–65.

Mestdagh H, Drizenko A, Ghestem P. (1981) Anatomical bases of suprascapular nerve syndrome. *Anat Clin* **3**:67–71.

Moore TP, Fritts HM, Quick DC, Buss DD. (1997) Suprascapular nerve entrapment caused by supraglenoid cyst compression. *J Shoulder Elbow Surg* **6**:455–62.

Murray JWG. (1974) A surgical approach for entrapment neuropathy of the suprascapular nerve. *Orthop Rev* **3**:33–5.

Narakas AO. (1991) Compression and traction neuropathies about the shoulder and arm. In: Other AN, Bloggs J, ed. *Operative nerve repair and reconstruction*. Philadelphia PA: JB Lippincott **2**:1151–7.

Neviaser TJ, Ain BR, Neviaser RJ. (1986) Suprascapular nerve denervation secondary to attenuation by a ganglion cyst. *J Bone Joint Surg* **68A**:627–8.

Ogino T, Minami A, Kato H, Hara R, Suzuki K. (1991) Entrapment neuropathy of the suprascapular nerve by a ganglion. *J Bone Joint Surg* **73A**:141–7.

Palmer WE, Brown JH, Rosenthal DI. (1994) Labral-ligamentous complex of the shoulder: evaluation with MR arthrography. *Radiology* **190**:645–50.

Post M, Mayer J. (1987) Suprascapular nerve entrapment. Diagnosis and treatment. *Clin Orthop* **223**:126–36.

Post M, Grinblat E. (1963) Suprascapular nerve entrapment: diagnosis and results of treatment. *J Shoulder Elbow Surg* **2**:197.

Rask MR. (1977) Suprascapular nerve entrapment: a report of two cases treated with suprascapular notch resection. *Clin Orthop* **123**:73.

Rengachary SS, Burr D, Lucas S, Hassanein KM, Mohn MP, Matzke H. (1979) Suprascapular entrapment neuropathy: a clinical, anatomical and comparative study. Parts 1, 2 and 3. *Neurosurgery* **5**:441–7.

Ringel SP, Treihaft M, Carry M, Fisher R, Jacob P. (1990) Suprascapular nerve neuropathy in pitchers. *Am J Sports Med* **18**:80–6.

Rochwerger A, Franceschi JP, Groullier P. (1996) Kyste synovial de l'échancrure coracoidienne à l'origine d'une compression du nerf suprascapulaire chez un sportif. A propos d'un case. Revue de la littérature. *Rev Chir Orthop* **82**:344–7.

Shupeck M, Onofrio BM. (1990) An anterior approach for decompression of the suprascapular nerve. *J Neurosurg* **73**:53–6.

Skirving A, Kozak TK, Davis SJ. (1994) Infraspinatus paralysis due to spinoglenoid notch ganglion. *J Bone Joint Surg* **76B**:588–91.

Solheim LF, Roaas A. (1978) Compression of the suprascapular nerve after fracture of the scapular notch. *Acta Orthop Scand* **49**:338–40.

Steinman I. (1988) Painless infraspinatus atrophy due to suprascapular nerve entrapment. *Arch Phys Med Rehab* **69**:641–3.

Takagishi K, Maeda K, Ikeda T, Itoman M. Yamamoto M. (1991) Ganglion causing paralysis of the suprascapular nerve: diagnosis by MRI and ultrasonography. *Acta Orthop Scand* **62**:391–3.

Takakazu H, Hoshiharu T. (1981) Compression of the suprascapular nerve by a ganglion at the suprascapular notch. *Clin Orthop* **155**:95–6.

Thompson RC, Schneider W, Kennedy T. (1982) Entrapment neuropathy of the inferior branch of the suprascapular nerve by ganglia. *Clin Orthop* **166**:185–87.

Tirman PF, Feller JF, Janzen DL, Peterfy CG, Bergman GA. (1994) Association of glenoid labral cysts with labral tears and glenohumeral instability: radiologic findings and clinical significance. *Radiology* **190**:653–58.

Travlos J, Goldberg I, Boome RS. (1990) Brachial plexus lesions associated with dislocated shoulders. *J Bone Joint Surg* **72B**:68–71.

Västamäki M, Goransson H. (1993) Suprascapular nerve entrapment. *Clin Orthop* **297**:135–43.

Warner JJP, Krushell RJ, Masquelet A, Gerber C. (1992) Anatomy and relationships of the suprascapular nerve: Anatomical constraints to mobilization of the supraspinatus and infraspinatus muscles in the management of massive rotator cuff tears. *J Bone Joint Surg* **74A**:36–45.

Yoon TN, Grabois M, Ouillen, M. (1981) Suprascapular nerve injury following trauma to the shoulder. *J Trauma* **21**:652–55.

Zanotti R, Carpenter JE, Blasier R, Grennfield ML, Adler RS, Bromberg MB. (1997) The low incidence of suprascapular nerve injury after primary repair of massive rotator cuff tears. *J Shoulder Elbow Surg* **6**:258–64.

Zoltan JA. (1979) Injury to the suprascapular nerve associated with anterior abduction of the shoulder: case report and review of the literature. *J Trauma* **19**:203–6.

10
Spontaneous high radial nerve entrapment

Yves Allieu and Bruno Lussiez

Introduction

Isolated damage to the upper radial nerve can occur in various circumstances, with traumas constituting the most common cause. Of the latter cases, 35% are due, according to Seddon (cited in Mackinnon and Dellon, 1988), to a fracture of the humeral diaphysis, followed by balistic trauma (32%) and direct injection of toxic substances.

The second most frequent group of causes includes extrinsic compression of the radial nerve. These are commonly encountered and are related to damage subsequent to prolonged postures as encountered in comas, crush-syndrome, Saturday night palsy and iatrogenic compression (pressure from a tourniquet or the edge of an operating table); then there is the group of compressions caused by neoformations (e.g. lipomas, nodes, etc.) that are seldom found at this level (Barber, 1962).

A final group includes so-called 'spontaneous' damage. A finer classification of this group based upon clinical observation, surgical experience, anatomic and physiopathologic studies of the nerve has led us to identify three factors which can account, either in isolation or in combination, for spontaneous high radial palsies.

- Anatomic factors
- Dynamic factors
  - nerve mobility
  - muscular contractions
- Systemic factors

Anatomic recap

The radial nerve is the continuation, after the circumflex nerve branch, of the posterior secondary truncus in the axillary fossa; it penetrates into the spiral groove of the humerus by the humero-tripital split, with an onset-angle of 10–15°. It travels along this groove for 8–10 cm in direct contact with the humeral diaphysis, then emerges from the posterior compartment of the arm and gradually circumvents from back to front the outside edge of the humerus through the lateral intermuscular septum, roughly 10–12 cm above the epicondyle (Figure 10.1). The nerve then continues at the bottom of the lateral bicipital groove outside the brachialis and the biceps, and inside the beginning of the brachio-radialis muscle 2–3 cm above the epicondyle. It

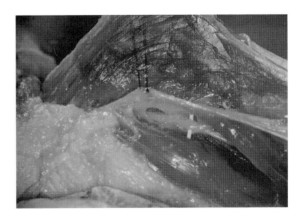

Figure 10.1

Surgical exposure of the radial nerve at the humero-tripital split.

divides above the elbow into two terminal branches: the posterior interosseous nerve and the sensitive anterior branch.

The spiral humeral groove is in fact the bottom of an osteomuscular spiral groove, which is enclosed posteriorly by the long section of the triceps and its lateral head, and is limited proximally by the insertions of the lateral head of the triceps, and distally by the insertions of the medial head. Rouvière (1954) described an inconsistent origin of the lateral head at this level, and variations in this transitional area between the posterior and lateral compartments are commonplace, as we will see later, ranging from a thin and wide intermuscular septum to an orifice which can be more or less closed and narrow (Figure 10.1).

In the groove the radial nerve divides into the posterior brachial cutaneous nerve in its upper section, and the posterior cutaneous nerve of the forearm before entering the groove in 50% of cases, and in the groove in 50%. Finally, the nerve is accompanied by the deep brachial artery and its satellite veins.

Clinical study

The clinical picture varies according to the factors present. Generally speaking, these cases involve middle-aged men (40 years) who present with unilateral high radial palsy which came on more or less quickly (from several hours to several months) and in the absence of all the usual triggering factors listed above.

The presence of pain has been noted by several authors. This can involve either initial pain that reduces or disappears with the onset of palsy; it can also be extremely acute, requiring administration of major painkillers. Pain is located at brachial level and can be referred proximally, but also distally, particularly around the posterior area of the epicondyle, the radial styloid and the back of the hand (Wilhelm, 1931).

Palsy in these cases is generally total sparing only the brachial triceps and affecting the brachioradialis, the extensor carpi radialis longus and brevis, the extensor digitorum communis, the extensor indicis proprius, the extensor digiti minimi, the extensor pollicis longus and brevis and the abductor pollicis longus. Sensitivity

losses usually affect the posterior cutaneous rami of the forearm and/or the upper arm. They can also be totally absent on account of the frequently encountered lack of sensitivity of the autonomous innervation zone of the radial nerve. The most reliable area of hypoesthesia appears to be the dorso-radial face of the second metacarpus.

Lastly, pressure-induced pain and positive Tinel's sign may be encountered opposite the lateral edge of the junction between the medial and the distal thirds of the upper arm.

The work-up includes an electromyography which should be done within several days of the onset of the palsy. This will show the presence of a peripheral neurogenic syndrome (absence of willed activity and of rest potential) affecting the radial nerve around the distal section of the humeral groove and the elbow, combined with signs of distal denervation. While electromyography can quantify the extent of the damage, it cannot, however, specify the nature of the nerve involvement and needs to be repeated during the following weeks (during the third month according to Raimbeau 1996), depending upon the degree of recovery.

Finally, constriction of the nerve may be demonstrated with high-resolution ultrasound.

Factor analysis

Anatomic factors

Anatomic studies of the humeral osteo-muscular groove were performed in the early twentieth century (Bernhardt, 1902; Gerulanos, 1915) and later by Wilhelm (1970) and Lotem et al. (1971), providing a precise description on the basis of cadaver dissections.

Wilhelm observed that, at the distal part of the groove the nerve before entering the hiatus is crossed by the deep tendinous portion of the lateral head of the triceps muscle, which he claims to be a source of compression against the humerus (Figure 10.2). This author found a compression by the lateral head in 13 cases out of 27 cases operated on. Manske (1977) and Mitsunaga and Nakano (1988) each reported a case in which surgical exploration revealed no sign of a fibrous arch but rather compression from lateral head of the triceps.

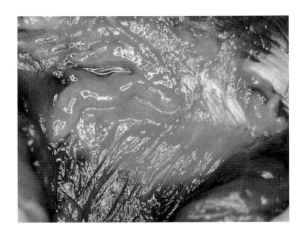

Figure 10.2

Surgical exposure of the radial nerve at the osteo-muscular groove.

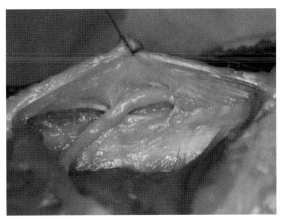

Figure 10.3

Surgical exposure of the fibrous arch of the lateral head of triceps.

Lotem et al. (1971) almost consistently found an arch composed mainly of fibers from the lateral head of the triceps. When the muscle crosses over the spiral groove, some tendinous fibers leave the main band and become inserted in the humerus immediately below the lateral part of the spiral groove. This arch differs from the hiatus of the lateral intermuscular septum which is more distal and thin, and it generally appears to be more conspicuous and stronger in muscular persons.

Lubahn and Lister (1983), Yoshii et al. (1985), then Nakamichi and Tachibana (1991) found a fibrous arch similar to that described by Lotem et al. The present authors (Lussiez and Allieu, 1991) noted the presence of such an arch in two of four operated patients; in a new study (Lussiez et al., 1993) of 20 cadaver upper limbs, they observed the existence of this arch in eight cases out of 20. The arch is located proximal to the hiatus in a latero-frontal plane and possesses a free and generally sharp edge, alongside muscle fibers originating from the arch (Figure 10.3).

These anatomic studies, supplemented by a number of surgical clinical cases, demonstrate that a specific anatomic predisposition of the lower part of the humeral osteo-muscular groove (a fibrous arch and/or the lateral head of the triceps (Figure 10.4) may account for certain cases of 'spontaneous' high radial nerve entrapment.

Dynamic factors

Case reports

The presence of high radial palsy after muscular exertion has been reported by several authors (Baeker, 1955). In 1970, Wilhelm described eight operated cases among manual workers performing repetitive elbow movements. In 1971, Lotem et al. described three non-operated cases which had recovered spontaneously. Several other authors reported similar cases: Manske in 1977 (one case), Allieu in 1980 (three cases), Spinner in 1980 (six cases), Mitsunaga in 1988 (one case), Wilhelm who in 1991 described 13 cases among manual workers (street sweepers, bricklayers, joiners, metal-workers), Lussiez in 1993 who described five cases, four of which required surgery, and lastly Kleinschmidt who reported one case in 2000 at the seventh FESSH Congress.

Analysis of these 30 cases reveals some similarities. The patients are always young, mean age 42 years, and are generally males who, within a few hours of muscular activity of the upper limb of a particularly sustained nature, either by virtue of the duration or of the intensity of the exercise, experienced paralysis of the muscles innervated by the radial nerve, the triceps alone being excepted (Figure 10.4). On the whole, the patients are described as being muscular and the physical exertion involved either repetitive movements of flexion and

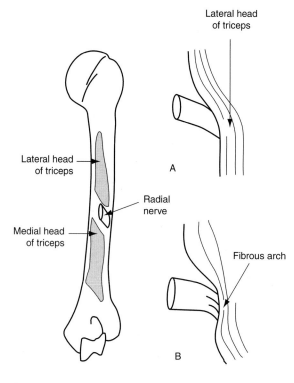

Figure 10.4

Right humerus: compression of the radial nerve by the lateral head of triceps (A) and by the fibrous arch (B). Nagaw A et al. (1996) Spontaneous anterior interosseous nerve palsy with hourglass-like fascicular contribution within the main trunk of the median nerve. *J Hand Surg* **21A**:266–70.

extension of the elbow, such as the loading or carrying of heavy objects, or positions of the arm which had been maintained over a protracted period. These cases can be compared with others involving damage to the posterior interosseous nerve encountered among musicians (Maffulli and Maffulli, 1991), as well as radial palsy caused by ganglions on the anterior aspect of the elbow (Ogino et al., 1991), nine cases out of 30 quoted occurring after intense muscular activity of the upper limb.

In an attempt to explain these phenomena, the present authors (Lussiez et al., 1993) performed a cadaver study of the radial nerve at the level of the posterior humeral groove. Fixed landmarks were placed on the nerve and the effects of contraction of the lateral head of the triceps were simulated. We then observed that the radial nerve was pinched between the humerus and the free edge of the arch (when an arch was found), or between the lateral head of triceps and the lateral edge of the humeral diaphysis (Figure 10.5).

Analysis of these clinical cases and of the cadaver study demonstrated that in this anatomic space, which constitutes a first source of potential compression of the radial nerve, various dynamic phenomena can also be responsible for compression.

Surgical findings

We have noted 19 cases of high operated radial palsy for which we possess a precise surgical description: Manske (1 case); Burns and Lister (3 cases); Wilhelm (8 cases); Mitsunaga and Nakano (1 case); Lussiez et al. (4 cases); and Chesser and Leslie (1 case).

Thirteen cases showed severe constriction of the radial nerve at the lower part of the groove; two cases involved double constriction; two other cases appeared to involve twisting of the radial nerve around its axis (hourglass-like fascicular constriction, Figure 10.6). The last case showed two twists of the nerve several centimeters apart (Figure 10.7). These surgical observations need to be compared with cases of severe compression, constriction and single or double torsion as reported by Hashizume et al. (1996) and Kotani et al. (1995) at the level of the posterior interosseous nerve in cases of non-traumatic paralysis of this nerve, and others reported by Nagano et al. (1996) involving eight cases of spontaneous palsy of the anterior interosseous nerve, and by Nakamura et al. (1992).

These surgical findings call for several comments. The operated cases were those which had not recovered spontaneously; it is not surprising therefore that they include instances of severe compression. In the majority of cases, the macroscopic aspect (constriction, torsion) gave rise to intrafascicular neuromysis involving fascicular bulging adjacent to the constricted area, or intrafascicular scarring within the constricture. In two of 18 cases, a graft resection was performed on account of the almost complete disappearance of nerve tissue at the level of the compression (Figure 10.8).

This analysis of surgical lesions highlights the importance of the severity of the lesions with a quasi-disappearance of the nerve tissue, the

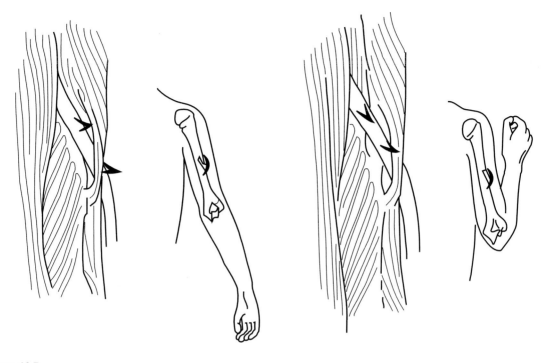

Figure 10.5

Position of the radial nerve in flexion-extension movements of the elbow (in Lussiez et al., 1993).

frequent presence of intraneural (intrafascicular) scarring, the macroscopic aspect of the nerve twisted around its axis, occasionally involving multiple twisting, thus pointing to the presence of combined dynamic factors.

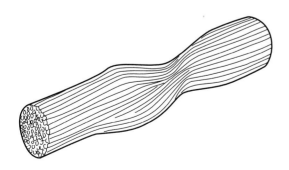

Figure 10.6

Hourglass-like fascicular constriction of the radial nerve.

Systemic factors

In 1983, Palazzi et al. reported four cases of high radial palsy in which the clinical picture differed slightly from the one mentioned above. No dynamic factor was observed but rather a rapid onset of the palsy which was always preceded by acute painful phenomena of the unilateral cervico-brachialgia type. The author suggests a vascular or viral origin. By their mode of onset, these cases can be compared with cases of radial palsy in the Parsonage–Turner syndrome (Parsonage and Turner, 1948), which are unusual (Raimbeau, 1996), and which seem to be of vascular origin. Likewise, radial palsies of vascular origin have been described in rheumatoid arthritis (Chamberlain and Bruckner, 1970), and in periarteritis nodosa (Belsole et al., 1978). Diabetes, sarcoidosis, leprosy, hemophilia and some forms of neurotoxic poisoning (lead, benzol) can also be responsible for peripheral palsies. Lastly, Burns and Lister (1984) described three cases with painful onset, which were

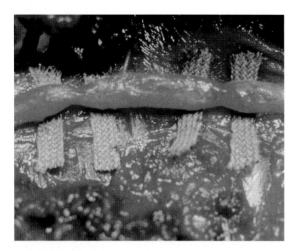

Figure 10.7

Surgical exposure of the level of compression, showing two hour-glass constrictions.

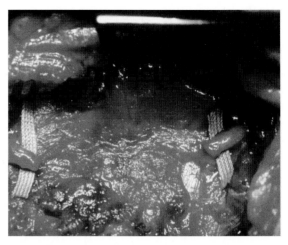

Figure 10.8

Following exploration of the nerve, the damaged tissue was resected. A nerve graft was performed secondarily.

connected with rheumatoid arthritis in one case, allergic angioneuropathy in the second case and spider-bite-poisoning in the third. In the seven operated cases (Burns and Lister 1984; Paluzzi et al., 1983), aspects of major single stenosis of the nerve (six cases) and of double stenosis (one case), located in the proximity of the lower section of the humeral groove have been recorded.

From this analysis one can conclude that some radial palsies can occur in a context of systemic involvement, and that they can be of vascular, inflammatory, toxic or viral origin.

Physiopathology

Even in atraumatic circumstances, and in the absence of obvious extrinsic compression, surgery has revealed aspects of single or double strangulation of the radial nerve, occasionally accompanied by torsion of the nerve around its axis. An understanding of all aspects necessarily involves a study of the physiopatholgy of nerve compression.

According to Lundborg (1988), three factors combining in different ways are required in the mechanics of nerve compression:
- intraneural inflammatory reactions
- stretching
- friction

Intraneural inflammatory reactions are dependent on compression. In the early stage, compression delays the venous flow within the epineurium followed by a decrease in blood flow in the endoneural capillaries and finally, at a later stage, by complete stasis of intraneural circulation. This intraneural microcirculation failure triggers an increase in the permeability to proteins and hence an edema located initially in the epineurium, followed by the endoneurium. This leads to a fully fledged intrafascicular compartment syndrome on account of the barrier placed by the perineurium. In addition, one also encounters direct trauma damage to the intraneural vessels at the edge of the compression, resulting in defective reperfusion of the compressed segment. This intra- and extrafascicular edema gives rise to an invasion of fibroblasts and later to irreversible intraneural scarring.

Stretching of a nerve can occur when the nerve, which can normally slide several millimeters to accompany the movements of the limbs thanks to a sliding mechanism around and within the nerve (Millesi et al., 1990), is prevented from doing so by some external cause. This produces stretching of the affected area and results in edema, microbleeding and, subsequently neural scarring. Finally, **friction** of the nerve occurs when shearing forces give rise to redistribution of tissue from compressed to non-compressed areas.

This analysis demonstrates that any external compression, depending upon its severity and duration, can trigger intraneural circulation disruptions which can lead occasionally to severe peri- and intraneural scarring and to adherence between the nerve and its environment, thus causing additional lesions in the neighboring areas.

Conclusion

Spontaneous high radial palsies are rare as compared with the usual etiologies (fractures, external compression, injections). It appears that the two essential factors are anatomic and dynamic, with sometimes a context of infectious or inflammatory disease.

Reported surgical aspects of severe constriction, twisting of the nerve, or total damage of the nerve are explained by these two factors.

Their treatment is initially conservative, with clinical and electromyographical survey; but it seems it is better to operate at the beginning of the second month, in case of non-recuperation, in regard of the severity of the surgical aspects, as we said; the neurolysis has to be extra- and intraneural; it must be associated with the resection of the lateral intermuscular septum, of the fibrous arch when it exists, and of a partial resection of the lateral head of the triceps when its volume seems to be a potential source of compression. Lastly, in case of complete disappearance of the nerve, a graft is necessary after resection.

References

Allieu Y. (1980) Radial nerve entrapments. Communication at The First Congress of the IFSSH, Rotterdam, 1980.

Baeker AB. (1955) *Clinical neurology*. New York: Hoeber Harper.

Barber KW. (1962) Benign extra-neural soft tissue tumors of the extremities causing compression of nerves. *J Bone Joint Surg* **44A**:98–106.

Belsole RJ, Lister GD, Kleinert HE. (1978) Polyarteritis: a cause of nerve palsy in the extremity. *J Hand Surg* **3**:320–5.

Bernhardt H. (1902) Erkranbrungun des peripheren Nerven. Vienna: Hölder-Verlag.

Birch R. (1990) A new type of peripheral nerve lesion. *J Bone Joint Surg* **72B**:312–13.

Burns J, Lister GD. (1984) Localized constrictive neuropathy in the absence of extrinsic compression: three cases. *J Hand Surg* **9A**:99–103.

Chamberlain MA, Bruckner FE. (1970) Rheumatoid neuropathy: clinical and electrophysiological features. *Ann Rheum Dis* **20**:609–15.

Chesser TJ, Leslie IJ. (2000) Radial nerve entrapment by the lateral intramuscular septum after trauma. *J Orthop Trauma* **14**:(1)65–6.

Gerulanos M. (1915) Uber muskelüberpflanzungen am Schultergürtel. Langenbecks *Arch Klin Chir S* 107–59.

Hashizume H, Nishida K, Nanba Y, Shigeyama Y, Inoue H, Morito Y. (1996) Non-traumatic paralysis of the posterior interosseous nerve. *J Bone Joint Surg (Br)* **78B**:771–6.

Kotani H, Takaaki M, Senzoku F, Nakagawa Y, Ueo T. (1995) Posterior interosseous nerve paralysis with multiple constrictions. *J Hand Surg* **20A**:15–17.

Lotem M, Fried A, Levy M, et al. (1971) Radial palsy following muscular effort. *J Bone Joint Surg*, **53B**:500–6.

Lubahn JD, Lister GD. (1983) Familial radial nerve entrapment syndrome. A case report and literature review. *J Hand Surg* **8**:297–9.

Lundborg G. (1988) Compression and stretching. In *Nerve injury and repair*, Edinburgh: Churchill Livingstone: 64–101.

Lussiez B, Allieu Y. (1991) Paralysies du nerf radial au bras après effort musculaire. In: Tubiana R, ed. *Chirurgie de la Main*, vol 5. Paris: Masson: 645–68.

Lussiez B, Courbier R, Toussaint B, Benichou M, Gomis R, Allieu Y. (1993) Paralysie radiale au bras après effort musculaire – A propos de quatre cas. *Ann Chir Main (Ann Hand Surg)* **12**(2):130–35.

Mackinnon SE, Dellon AL. (1988) Radial nerve entrapment in the proximal forearm and brachium. In: *Surgery of the peripheral nerve*. New York: Thieme: 289–97.

Maffulli N, Maffulli F. (1991) Transient entrapment neuropathy of the posterior interosseous nerve in violin players. *J Neurol Neurosurg Psychiatry* **54**:65–7.

Manske PR. (1977) Compression of the radial nerve by the triceps muscle. *J Bone Joint Surg* **59A**:835.

Millesi H, Zöch G, Rath Th. (1990) The gliding apparatus of peripheral nerve and its clinical significance. *Ann Hand Surg* **9**(2):87–97.

Mitsunaga MM, Nakano K. (1988) High radial nerve palsy following strenuous muscular activity. *Clin Orthop* **234**:39–42.

Nagano A, Shibata K, Tokimura H, Yamamoto S, Tajiri Y. (1996) Spontaneous anterior interosseous nerve palsy with hourglass-like fascicular constriction within the main trunk of the median nerve. *J Hand Surg* **21A**:266–70.

Nakamichi K, Tachibana S. (1991) Radial nerve entrapment by the lateral head of the triceps. *J Hand Surg* **16A**:748–50.

Nakamura M, et al. (1992) A case report of the anterior interosseous nerve palsy in which one of the two funiculi was found twisted at about 5 cm proximal to the elbow. *J Jpn Soc Surg Hand* **8**:986–9.

Ogino T, Minami A, Kato H. (1991) Diagnosis of radial nerve palsy caused by ganglion with use of different imaging techniques. *J Hand Surg* **16A**:230–5.

Palazzi S, Palazzi C, Raimondi P, Aramburo F. (1983) Paralysie radiale idiopathique In: Souquet R, ed. *Syndromes canalaires du membre supérieur.* Monographies GEM. Paris, Expansion Scientifique Française: 46–50.

Parsonage MJ, Turner JWA. (1948) Neuralgyamyotrophy: the shoulder girdle syndrome. *Lancet* 973–78.

Raimbeau G. (1996) Paralysie radiale basse. In *Cahier d'enseignement de la Société Française de Chirurgie de la Main.* Paris: 37–51.

Rouvière. (1954) *Anatomie humaine.* Masson: Paris.

Spinner M. (1980) *Management of peripheral nerve problems.* Philadelphia, London, Toronto: WB Saunders: 569–92.

Wilhelm A. (1970) Das Radialisirritationssyndrom. *Handchirurgie* **2**:139.

Wilhelm A. (1991) Compression proximale du nerf radial. In: Tubiana R, ed. *Chirurgie de la main,* Vol 5. Paris: Masson: 455–65.

Yoshii S, Urushidani H, Yoshikawa K, et al. (1985) Radial nerve palsy related to a fibrous arch of the lateral head of the triceps: a case report. *Cent Jpn J Traumatol* **28**:798–9.

11
Radial nerve compression at the elbow

Guy Raimbeau

Introduction

Compression of the radial nerve at the elbow is uncommon compared with carpal tunnel syndrome, except for cases of acute trauma. Two different manifestations of compression may be seen:

- Radial tunnel syndrome, which is manifested by pain.
- Posterior interosseous nerve syndrome, which is manifested by painless paralysis.

Despite the difference between these two clinical forms, the anatomical origin, which is compression of the radial nerve in the radial tunnel, is the same.

Anatomic predisposition

From the lateral bicipital sulcus, between the brachialis and the brachioradialis and extensor carpi radialis longus muscles, the radial nerve enters the radial tunnel and divides into two branches: the superficial and deep branches. The point at which the nerve divides is variable (Fuss and Wurzl, 1991; Rath et al., 1993). According to Lister, the division takes place from 3 cm proximal to 3 cm distal to the radiohumeral joint. The superficial branch follows the brachioradialis, while the deep branch goes toward the supinator which it enters between its superficial and deep heads. Roles and Maudsley (1972) define three regions of the radial tunnel: the superior region up to the top of the condyle, the middle region to the distal margin of the radial head, and the

distal region between the heads of the supinator. Lister holds that the radial tunnel begins at the radiohumeral joint line, and speaks of a length of 5 cm (Lister et al., 1979). This part is the narrowest, as in the more proximal part of its course the nerve has ample room.

In the proximal part of the tunnel, the radial nerve gives off a branch to the brachioradialis (5–6 cm above the epicondyle), then 2 cm distally, a branch or branches to the extensor carpi radialis longus (ECRL), and small branches to the lateral aspect of the elbow joint. In the middle region, the extensor carpi radialis brevis (ECRB) crosses over the nerve (Laulan et al., 1994), and may come in contact with it in full pronation (Spinner, 1968). The contact may be with a thickening of the tendon of the ECRB or with a fibrous arcade from the ECRB to the flexor aponeurosis. The nerves supplying the ECRB are variable. The most common is a branch from the deep branch of the radial nerve, but in 15% (Fuss and Wurzl, 1991), 43% (Prasartritha et al., 1993), or 75% (Laulan et al., 1994) of cases, this branch comes from the superficial division of the radial nerve, or from a trifurcation. The supinator receives several motor branches. In the distal part of the tunnel, the nerve goes between the two heads of the supinator, and is quite close to the radial head. In 30% of cases, according to Spinner (1968), 40% according to Laulan et al. (1994), and 57% according to Prasartritha et al. (1993), the proximal margin of the superficial head is fibrous. We believe that the terms arcade of Frohse and of Fränkel (in Spinner, 1968) should be reserved for the fibrous bands. This arcade is not pathologic and is not present at birth. Bonnel et al. (1982) have demonstrated the presence of several venous plexuses in contact with the nerve in the supinator, an exceptional finding for a peripheral nerve. In its intra-muscular course, the nerve is flattened, like a bookmark between the two muscular 'pages' of the supinator.

In this region, the nerve is tethered in two places: (i) in the arm, at the level where the nerve enters the lateral compartment, and (ii) at the point where the deep branch enters the supinator. The nerve moves as in a half rotation of a jump rope, as it follows the pronation and supination of the forearm, like a 'jerky action' (Winckworth, 1883). In pronation, the nerve is relaxed and moves away from the head of the radius, but the supinator presses down on it owing to the passive tension on its muscle fibers. In supination, the nerve is stretched to the maximum of its elastic reserve. It is under tension and is flattened by the contraction of the supinator.

The deep branch of the radial nerve is accompanied by a descending branch of the anterior recurrent radial artery. Arterio-venous arcades frequently cross the nerve below the supinator.

It is important to know the branching of the deep branch as it emerges from under the supinator in order to understand the signs and symptoms of the paralyses that may occur (Figure 11.1). Two muscle groups may be distinguished. The superficial group is composed of the extensor digitorum, the extensor digiti minimi, and the extensor carpi ulnaris. This group is innervated by a posterior branch, while the deep group, composed of the extensor pollicis longus, the extensor indicis proprius, and the abductor pollicis longus, is innervated by a more anterior branch. The third terminal branch is, in fact, the continuation of the deep branch and represents the posterior antebrachial interosseous nerve which passes between the extensors pollicis longus and brevis, and descends behind the interosseous membrane to the dorsal surface of the carpus, which it innervates, accompanied by nutrient arteries.

In contrast to the deep branch which is rolled up with the supinator, the superficial branch has a direct course under the brachioradialis. It descends toward the dorso-lateral surface of the wrist to innervate the dorsal surface of the first web space.

Radial tunnel syndrome

The painful syndrome described by Roles and Maudsley (1972) corresponds to the compression of the deep branch of the radial nerve. More than 100 years ago, Winckworth (1883) attributed certain pains on the lateral side of the elbow and forearm to radial neuropathy. This compression syndrome must be differentiated from the paralytic syndrome of the posterior interosseous nerve. The confusion between these two syndromes is due to the fact that the same

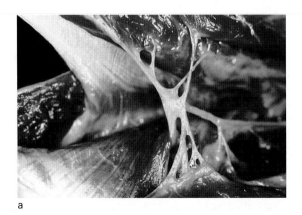
a

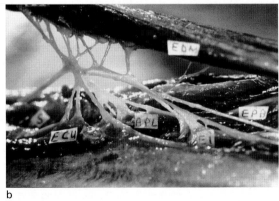
b

Figure 11.1

Views of specimen – right elbow (Dr Ph. Bellemere). (a) The radial nerve as it emerges from the distal side of the supinator muscle. (b) Terminal branches (supinator excised).

structures are involved in the same location in both syndromes. The painful syndrome is classified with epicondylitis by many authors. In the late seventies, Hagert, then Werner, published large studies (Hagert et al., 1977; Werner et al., 1979). Narakas and Comtet emphasized the symptoms and signs of these syndromes (Comtet et al., 1976; Narakas, 1974). We ourselves are quite familiar with these syndromes, as we practice in a region where there are major textile and shoe industries.

This compression syndrome is related to the movement of the elbow, which permits flexion–extension and pronation–supination at the same time. From the anatomical point of view, conditions are set for restriction of movement of the deep branch of the radial nerve, which should follow the movements of pronation and supination of the forearm. The arc of motion of the radius is imposed on the nerve, which is confined between the two muscular layers of the supinator. In addition to the elasticity which all peripheral nerves possess, the radial nerve has a reserve connective structure in axial torsion. The sensory branch is not subject to such stresses in the proximal third of the forearm, because it follows the course of the brachioradialis.

In the radial tunnel, three possible sources of compression were described by Roles and Maudsley (1972) in their first description, and Lister et al. (1979) added a fourth. These four elements have become classic: fibrous bands in front of the radiohumeral capsule; the leash of vessels from a branch of the anterior recurrent radial artery; the tendinous proximal edge of the extensor carpi radialis brevis; and the proximal margin of the supinator. A fifth source, rarely a problem, is the distal edge of the supinator. Compression at this point was described by Sponseller and Engber (1983).

Compression of the superficial branch at the elbow is relatively rare, but it was noted by Moss and Switser (1983), who reported this finding in four patients in their series of 15 cases of radial tunnel syndrome. These four patients were relieved of their symptoms by neurolysis of the two branches of the radial nerve. In one of these four cases, the tendon of the extensor carpi radialis brevis was the source of compression. In this form of the syndrome, the pain radiates distally, and may extend all the way to the first

web space and even to the thumb and index finger. Palpation of this branch is painful well proximal to the localization of Wartenberg's symptom.

Diagnostic criteria

The signs and symptoms of the radial tunnel syndrome rest on the study of the pain, which may be spontaneous or provoked. This pain is easily recognized by those who have experience of the syndrome. The spontaneous pain is located distal to the epicondyle, on the lateral side of the forearm, radiating down the course of the radial nerve, most often descending toward the dorsum of the wrist, without ever going beyond the metacarpophalangeal joints of the central digits. Spontaneous ascending pain may also occur, especially at night. The usual nocturnal pattern is typical of the compression neuropathies, but the nocturnal pain may be inconstant and transient at first, becoming more cyclical in the chronic stages. The pain is usually relieved by shaking the hand or moving the elbow. Repetitive movements, especially those related to work, exacerbate the pain which may become permanent and may occur with activities of daily living such as pouring water or shaking hands. There is often the feeling of weakness associated with the syndrome.

Palpation along the course of the nerve or putting the nerve under tension in the radial tunnel by different maneuvers can elicit pain which reproduces and exacerbates the spontaneous pain. At the radial point, 3–5 cm distal to the lateral epicondyle, pressure should be carefully applied by the examiner's finger and the degree of tenderness should be compared to the opposite side (Figure 11.2). We prefer to do this provocative test towards the end of the examination. This sign is relatively sensitive and should be combined with palpation of the nerve along its course from the lower third of the arm to the lower third of the forearm. The study of resisted active motions is important. It is above-all resisted active supination that gives rise to the pain. We carry out this test in two stages. First, with the flexed elbow supported on the table, the patient attempts to supinate from a position of full pronation, while the examiner

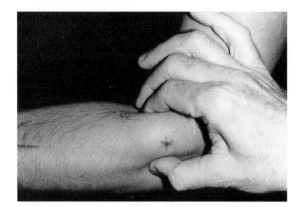

Figure 11.2

Local tenderness on palpation 3–5 cm distal to the lateral epicondyle.

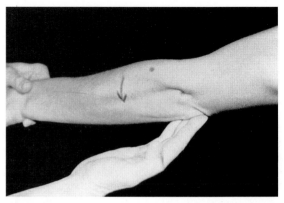

Figure 11.3

Location of the radial point and the specific test which brings out the pain on attempts at active supination, while the examiner holds the forearm to prevent the motion (resisted active motion).

holds the forearm to prevent this motion. This test is then repeated with the elbow in complete extension so that the nerve is under more tension (Figure 11.3). Finally, the examiner puts the supinator under tension by passively extending the elbow while passively pronating the forearm and flexing the wrist. These maneuvers, one passive with maximum tension on the nerve, the other active, are designed to flatten the arcade of the supinator on the radial nerve. In contrast, the pain on resisted extension of the middle finger while the elbow and wrist are extended, or Roles' sign (Roles and Maudsley, 1972), does not seem to us to be specific for the radial tunnel syndrome, as it is frequently positive in cases of lateral epicondylitis. Some authors have recommended the use of local anesthetics to block the radial nerve at the elbow (Ritts et al., 1987; Young and Moise, 1994). Motor weakness of the extensors, which might in principle be expected, is absent in the pure form of radial tunnel syndrome.

Conservative treatment

We recommend conservative treatment for 3–6 months, with limitation of those activities which exacerbate the pain, especially frequent and forceful pronation and supination. We do not recommend steroid injections. In addition to

medical treatment with systemic anti-inflammatory medications, we recommend a rehabilitation program to aid the patient in achieving a balance between the flexor and extensor forces exerted during certain actions, especially those requiring forceful grip. We find that it is common for patients with these syndromes to exert much more gripping force than is necessary to carry out the intended task.

Surgical treatment

The operative treatment must be carried out carefully. The operation should be done in a facility that is equipped to treat peripheral nerve injuries and includes magnifying loupes or an operating microscope. The operation should be done under general or regional anesthesia. We recommend that the pneumatic tourniquet be inflated to 20–25 cmHg above the systolic blood pressure, and the arm not be fully exsanguinated, so that one can identify more easily engorged blood vessels which may contribute to nerve compression. Our approach is the longitudinal dorso-lateral incision recommended by Hagert, which permits an excellent exposure of the radial tunnel and does not leave a bad scar (Hagert et al., 1977).

The incision is made on a line drawn from the lateral epicondyle to the radial styloid process

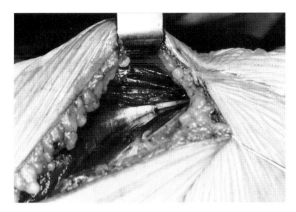

Figure 11.4

Intraoperative view – right elbow; dorso-lateral approach. The key point for entry into the inter-muscular space is the ribbon-like aspect of the tendon of the ECRL.

while the elbow is in 80 degrees of flexion and the forearm is in slight pronation. The usual incision is about 6–10 cm long, depending on the size of the patient and the experience of the surgeon. In the distal part of the incision, especially if it is rather long, one must identify and preserve a cutaneous sensory branch, which is a branch of the posterior antebrachial cutaneous nerve. In the distal part of the incision, one must identify the ribbon-like aspect of the tendon of the extensor carpi radialis longus, which is the key point to enter the inter-muscular space between the two radial extensors of the wrist (Figure 11.4). By developing this inter-muscular space proximally, one opens up the area of the radial tunnel and encounters fatty perineural tissue and an arterio-venous leash across the deep branch of the radial nerve. It is sometimes difficult to find the proper space. One often searches too far posterior, but in some cases there is some degree of fusion between the muscle bellies of the ECRB and the ECRL. In this case, it may be necessary to work from proximal to distal in developing this interval, beginning near the epicondyle and exposing the tendinous portion of the ECRB by dividing muscle fibers and ligating vessels as needed. Decompression of the nerve is accomplished by leaving it in its bed and incising, or sometimes excising, several centimeters of the proximal part of the superficial head of the supinator. In

the absence of signs of compression of the nerve, the neurolysis should be continued as far as the distal part of the supinator. The medial border of the tendon of the ECRB is excised as needed, if it gets in the way. Rarely, one encounters a fibrous band between the ECRL and the arcade of the flexor digitorum superficialis. If found, this band should be resected. We do not consider an arcade of Frohse to be present unless the proximal edge of the supinator is fibrous for several millimeters.

The exploration of the deep branch of the radial nerve should be methodical and systematic, not only at the proximal edge of the supinator, but also anterior to the radiohumeral joint, where fibrous bands may sometimes be found. Flexion of the elbow permits sufficient proximal exposure. One must be sure that the deep branch of the radial nerve is completely free during both flexion–extension and pronation–supination motions of the elbow. The anatomic lesions of the nerve will be even more visible if magnification is used (Capener, 1966). In this way, the surgeon can note whether there is simply a change in color of the nerve due to impaired microcirculation, or a loss of the transverse striations (Werner, 1979), or a post-strictural dilation or even a neuroma in continuity in chronic cases (Figures 11.5–11.7).

We have noted the nerve to be attached by fibrous bands to the floor of the radial tunnel (due to postinflammatory thickening), or constricted by a loop of vessels proximal to the supinator, or compressed by the proximal edge of the supinator, with or without an arcade of Frohse, or by the medial edge of the ECRB, or by a fibrous arcade at the distal margin of the supinator. Sometimes, the syndrome is purely dynamic in nature, due to increased intramuscular pressure. Werner (1979) has shown very high pressures (in the order of five times normal) during tetanic contractions of the supinator. A number of forces act on the nerve as it traverses the supinator, and a histologic study (Rath et al., 1993) has shown a significant increase in fibrous tissue in the epineurium and interstitial connective tissue in this segment of the nerve. The edge of the ECRB can cause compression, either directly in pronation only (Spinner, 1968) as it crosses over the nerve, or indirectly by putting pressure on the supinator, which in turn exerts pressure on the nerve.

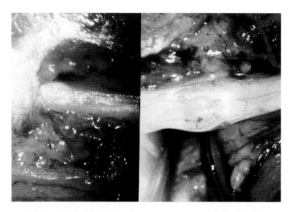

Figure 11.5

Views through operating microscope – left elbow. The radial nerve and the edge of the supinator muscle. After excision, the nerve deformation with the post-stenotic dilatation is clear.

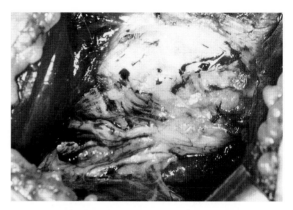

Figure 11.6

Pseudoneuromatous appearance of the radial nerve; intra-operative view – right elbow. After excision of the superficial head of the supinator muscle.

If pathological conditions of the elbow joint or of a tendon are found in addition to a neuropathy, surgical measures to address these problems are carried out at the same operation, but the postoperative care may be different, with a period of immobilization of about 2 weeks after any operation on a tendon. When only neurolysis is done, mobilization is begun immediately.

Henry's classic approach is anterior, between the brachioradialis and the brachialis, but Roles and Maudsley (1972) and Lister et al. (1979) recommend separation of the brachioradialis muscle. This approach has the disadvantage of leaving a scar that is sometimes cosmetically displeasing, even if one uses the 'Lazy S' advocated by Lister. In order to avoid this problem, Crawford (1984) has proposed using Henry's approach, but making a transverse skin incision. Posterior approaches give results that are more cosmetically pleasing. Capener (1966) goes between the ECRB and the extensor digitorum communis (EDC). We believe that this approach limits the exposure of the superficial branch of the radial nerve distal to the elbow. Hybrid approaches do not appear useful to us, as the posterior lateral approach that we use permits us to deal with all of the regional pathology (Hagert et al., 1977; Raimbeau et al., 1990; Werner, 1979).

The published results of surgical treatment are variable (Atroshi et al., 1995). Roles and Maudsley (1972) reported 92% good and excellent results,

while Ritts reported only 51% of his results to be as good (Ritts et al., 1987). The criteria of Roles and Maudsley are strict and should serve as a reference. We published a series of 35 cases in 1990, with 71% good or excellent results (Raimbeau et al., 1990). The worst results were found in patients who had a long history of epicondylitis, especially in the context of a work related condition. Nevertheless, Lawrence et al. (1995) recommended surgical treatment, since they found 66% good results of surgical treatment for patients in this category.

Radial tunnel syndrome in cases of epicondylitis

Pain on the lateral side of the elbow may be caused by referred or radicular pain of cervical origin, by early arthritis of the radiohumeral joint, by inflammation or micro ruptures of the common extensor origins, or by radial tunnel syndrome. These last two conditions are frequently difficult to differentiate preoperatively, but it is at this stage that one must try to separate the two diagnoses. Epicondylitis is more common in athletes or manual workers. In this condition, the pain is behind or on the epicondyle, and medical treatment, particularly local injections, gives temporary relief of

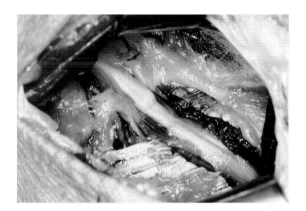

Figure 11.7

Intraoperative view – right elbow. Imprint at the proximal edge of supinator muscle. The muscle is cut straight above the nerve.

symptoms. In the radial tunnel syndrome, it is a matter of dynamic pathology. The pain is worse in the muscular mass of the muscles which originate on the epicondyle, and along the course of the radial nerve. Pain at rest is much more common in the radial tunnel syndrome than it is in epicondylitis. Other areas of nerve symptoms are not rare. After a long history of discomfort, the distinction between the signs and symptoms of these two syndromes becomes less marked, and we must look elsewhere for clues to enable us to distinguish between them. We believe that an inflammatory reaction in the area of the epicondyle which persists for several months can bring about a secondary reaction of the radial nerve by modifying the epineural environment of the nerve. Less that 10% of cases of epicondylitis cause irritation of the radial nerve – Werner (1979) found 5%. If lengthening of the conjoined tendon can relieve pressure on the supinator muscle, the effect on the nerve is far from being constant. Of Werner's cases, 12 had previous surgery for epicondylitis. On the other hand, neurolysis alone will not relieve the symptoms of epicondylitis (10% reoperation rate in Werner's series), except in rare cases by relief of proximal tension on the tendon of the supinator. Heyse-Moore (1984) concluded that one might treat epicondylitis either by lengthening of the ECRB or by opening up the arcade of the supinator. We believe, as Van Rossum does (Van

Rossum et al., 1978), that the radial tunnel syndrome does not cause epicondylitis, and we agree with Hagert et al. (1977) and Crawford (1984) that the two conditions may coexist, especially in those who do forceful repetitive motions.

Electrodiagnostic studies

Considering that the diagnosis of radial tunnel syndrome is made primarily on the basis of symptoms, with few objective confirmatory signs, it seemed to us essential to make use of electrodiagnostic studies. We did not perform surgery on any patient in our series of 250 operations without utilizing these diagnostic tests. The use of electromyography is controversial in this syndrome. Because it is often normal or shows only minor abnormalities, it appears unreliable (Comtet et al., 1985; Jalovaara and Lindholm, 1989; Ritts et al., 1987; Van Rossum et al., 1978; Verhaar and Spans, 1991; Young and Moise, 1994). The examination is long and difficult, often lasting as long as an hour, and it requires an experienced examiner. The examination may be normal in the early stages of the evolution of the syndrome, and it may be necessary to repeat the examination in 4–6 months if there is doubt. The examination should be done in a room at 23°C (82°F). The patient lies down with the forearm pronated, according to the protocol of Pelier-Cady (Table 11.1). This examination includes needle electromyography, motor nerve conduction study by two techniques, and sensory conduction study of the anterior sensory branch which is, in general, normal. Studies of the median nerve at the wrist and the ulnar nerve at the elbow are often done in order to look for evidence of other compression neuropathies.

A. Bipolar needle examination of at least three muscles innervated by the deep branch of the radial nerve is always done. These are: extensor digitorum (ED), extensor pollicis longus (EPL), and extensor indicis proprius (EIP) innervated by the branch of the deep layer. Given that neurologic abnormalities are more pronounced further distally, we have chosen the last two muscles for study. The ED is superficial and easy to explore,

Table 11.1 Protocol for electrodiagnostic study of radial tunnel syndrome (*Marie-Christine Pelier-Cady, MD*)

A – Electromyography

Extensor digitorum communis :   E.D.C.
Extensor pollicis longus :   E.P.L.
Extensor indicis proprius :   E.I.P.

Recruitment of action potentials:

6 – full recruitment	3 – markedly reduced recruitment
5 – slightly reduced recruitment	2 – few units
4 – reduced recruitment	1 – single unit

B – Motor conduction studies

1. Distal latencies

Stimulation at elbow	Distal latencies in ms.
Recorded E.D.C.	3,12 ms +/- 0,32
Recorded E.P.L.	4,04 ms +/- 0,22
Recorded E.I.P.	5,06 ms +/- 0,26

2. Motor conduction velocity

	M.C.V. meters/second	Amplitude in millivolts
H.G. – L.B.S.	69,8 +/- 6,2	
L.B.S. – ½ A.B.	61,4 +/- 5,4	5,7 +/- 3,7

H.G = humeral gutter
L.B.S. = lateral bracial sulcus

C – Sensory conduction velocity

D – Systematic study

Extensor carpi radialis longus (ECRL)	C 6 → Biceps
	C 7 → Triceps
	C 8 → First dorsal interosseous

about 13 cm from the lateral brachial sulcus. The extensors of the thumb and index have long muscle bellies which permit the examiner to insert the electrodes at distances of 16 cm and 20 cm respectively. In order to eliminate the possibility of a more proximal injury to the nerve, the test is completed by a study of the ECRL and the brachioradialis. Motor activity is classified into six categories according to the number of motor unit potentials recruited. This scheme permits the recording of information into a computer so that pre- and postoperative findings may be compared. This may appear subjective, but more than 20 years' experience allows us to affirm the reproducibility of our data. The motor activity is classified as follows:

6 – full recruitment
5 – slightly reduced recruitment
4 – reduced recruitment
3 – markedly reduced recruitment
2 – few units
1 – single unit

B. Motor conduction studies of the deep branch

1. *Distal latencies*

This study is carried out by stimulating the nerve at the level of the lateral brachial sulcus and reading the responses by means of a needle electrode in the three muscles ED, EPL and EIP, at fixed distances of 13 cm, 16 cm and 20 cm, according to our anatomical studies. The values in milliseconds are: ED 3.12 ± 0.32; EPL 4.04 ± 0.22; and EIP 5.06 ± 0.26.

2. *Motor conduction velocities of the radial nerve*

The reading is made by surface electrode on the EIP muscle. The nerve is stimulated by a surface electrode applied at the level of the lateral humeral gutter, then at the lateral brachial sulcus, then in the forearm halfway between the epicondyle and the wrist, where the nerve is stimulated more easily. The normal is 61.4 m/s $\pm$ 5.4 at the elbow. A velocity of less than 50 m/s is definitely pathologic. Between 50 and 60 m/s is borderline. It may be necessary to use the opposite arm as a control. A difference of more than 5 m/s between the two sides may indicate an abnormality of conduction velocity.

C. Sensory conduction velocity is calculated either by the classical orthodromic method, from the first web space to the distal third of the forearm, or by Schirali and Sanders' antidromic method, stimulating the nerve in the distal third of the arm and recording in the distal third of the forearm.

D. Systematic study of other muscles is carried out to detect either a lesion higher up the trunk (ECRL) or a lesion of the C-7 nerve root (triceps). A study of the biceps (C-6) and the first dorsal interosseous is often carried out to check the other nerves' roots.

• abnormalities on EMG in the three muscles

mentioned above, while all other muscles are normal, or

- significant slowing of motor nerve conduction, or
- an association of several abnormalities.

It is important to study the C-7 nerve root in a systematic manner. The dynamic tests have been progressively abandoned because of technical problems and the pain that they often cause the patient. We currently prefer to have the electrodiagnostic tests done after the patient has worked all day. We insist that the protocol be rigorously followed, in spite of the fact that a complete examination may be difficult in a patient who fails to cooperate fully for a variety of reasons.

Postoperative electrodiagnostic studies done in over 90 cases have given us objective evidence of a favorable evolution of the neuropathy. Only four cases failed to show evidence of improvement. The persistent symptoms in these patients were thought to be due to continuing nerve symptoms, and not due to persistent epicondylitis. Persistence of clinical signs of the syndrome demonstrate the complexity of the problem, especially as there were no failures due to epicondylitis. One must consider the duration of symptoms, the workers' compensation aspects, and also the presence or absence of C-7 radiculopathy. The development of radial tunnel syndrome is probably related to susceptibility of the radial nerve, peculiar to the individual (Ritts et al., 1987; Werner, 1979) and associated with repetitive motions.

Electrodiagnostic studies of a peripheral nerve may demonstrate lesions of myelin or axons. Lesions of myelin are more frequent than axonal abnormalities in compression syndromes and are manifested by a slowing of conduction velocity. We have been struck by the very great frequency of axonal abnormalities in the radial tunnel syndrome. This explains the lesions found on EMG examination in the absence of abnormalities on the nerve conduction tests. The radial tunnel syndrome is, then, a peculiar nerve compression syndrome and cannot be compared to the carpal tunnel syndrome. We are convinced that this syndrome is caused by forces of axial torsion which first disturb both antegrade and retrograde axonal transport, without the reaction of the myelin which often occurs in compression syndromes of the median or ulnar nerves. One

must recall that only half the cases of ulnar nerve compression at the elbow show significant slowing of nerve conduction velocity (Dawson et al., 1990).

Low radial nerve palsy

Except for traumatic lesions of the nerve, radial nerve palsy at the elbow is often incomplete. It is defined as a low radial palsy when the ECRB, ECRL and supinator are spared. The localization of the compression is defined by the specific motor deficits. Weakness of the extensor carpi ulnaris causes extension of the wrist to be accompanied by radial deviation. Impaired function of the extensor digitorum causes loss of active extension of the metacarpophalangeal joints. Extension of the interphalangeal joints of the fingers and the thumb remains possible because of the innervation of the interossei and the lumbricals by the median and ulnar nerves. Careful examination of active extension of the fingers should be an integral part of the investigation in cases of painful syndromes on the lateral side of the elbow. These active motions should be studied first with the wrist in neutral position, then with it in slight extension, in order to negate the tenodesis effect which permits some extension of the metacarpophalangeal joints when the wrist drops into flexion. This is even more important in examining active extension of the thumb. Finally, active finger extension is checked with the wrist in full extension. This is Comtet's sign (Comtet et al., 1976).

Deficits of motor function are variable, and can at first be confused with tendon ruptures, particularly at the wrist. The onset of symptoms in the low radial nerve palsy may be abrupt or slow, but most importantly, the condition is painless, except for the first few days.

Extrinsic compression is the most important etiology, and, in particular, that caused by a lipoma. The first description of this occurrence was in 1953 by Richmond (cited in Bieber et al., 1986). A review of 48 tumors published in 1991 reported on 35 of them (Werner, 1991). A painless, sometimes palpable, mass develops on the dorso-lateral aspect of the elbow. At present, a magnetic resonance image would enable us to see the extent of the mass. A lipoma may attain

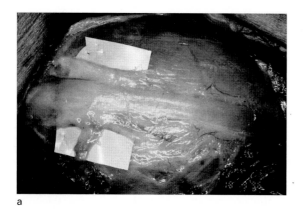
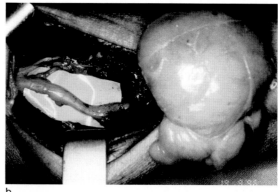

a   b

Figure 11.8

Intraoperative view – right elbow; dorso-lateral approach. (a) The radial nerve is squeezed by a lipoma. (b) After the excision, the constriction of the radial nerve is clear.

a size of 6–8 cm in diameter (Figure 11.8), and may be multilobulated. Excision of the mass and decompression of the radial nerve usually results in complete recovery of function in a few months (Bieber et al., 1986; Capener, 1966; Durandeau and Geneste, 1988; Werner, 1991).

Synovial cysts present a more difficult problem (Bowen and Stone, 1966), as do bursae of the bicipital tuberosity. In spite of the frequency of rheumatoid arthritis, development of synovial cysts causing compression of the radial nerve are relatively rare (Millender et al., 1973).

Idiopathic paralysis, which occurs in the absence of intrinsic or extrinsic compression, is often preceded by a short period of pain, while the paralysis persists and worsens. It is often related to forceful repetitive motion, with constriction of the nerve at the proximal edge of the supinator. In this case, it often is a matter of a true arcade of Frohse. The first description of this anatomical structure was given in 1905 by Guillemain and Courtellemont (cited in Comtet and Chambaud, 1975). The case was that of an orchestra conductor, but one can find this syndrome also in violinists, pianists, corsetieres, or other occupations that require forceful repetitive work in pronation and supination coupled with flexion and extension of the elbow. Sharrard (1966) thought that capsular lesions might cause problems in full extension because he had found adhesions around the nerve. One case of dynamic paralysis in pronation due to a fibrous band just proximal to the supinator has

been reported (Derkash and Niebauer, 1981). The first surgical excision of the arcade was done by Capener (1966) for the relief of pain, but it was Sharrard (1966) who made the first observations of paralysis not due to tumor.

In 1975, Comtet discovered a double constriction of the nerve before it entered the supinator, as if one had put two ligatures around the nerve at 1 cm intervals (Comtet and Chambaud, 1975). Kotani recently reported four cases (Kotani et al., 1995). The constrictions found, with or without arcade of Frohse, show that the nerve moves and that any anatomic anomaly in the radial tunnel can cause single or double constriction.

Electrodiagnostic studies nearly always show abnormalities that correlate well with the clinical findings. There is prolongation of the distal motor latency on conduction studies, and evidence on EMG studies of denervation of the extensor digitorum, extensor indicis proprius, and extensor digiti minimi, while the muscles which are more proximally innervated are spared, and the superficial branch remains normal.

The treatment is surgical for all the compression syndromes caused by an expansile lesion, but in the absence of a mass, surgery should be deferred for two or three months to allow for spontaneous recovery. However, it is early decompression that brings about complete muscular recovery (Nielsen, 1976). The surgical approach is, for us, dorso-lateral unless there is an anterior lesion.

Conclusion

Non-traumatic compression of the radial nerve at the elbow was first noted in its context as a paralytic lesion, usually manifested as an incomplete low radial palsy. The radial tunnel syndrome remains controversial because it evolved in the context of chronic epicondylitis. We believe that confirmation of a neurologic source of symptoms in painful syndromes around the lateral aspect of the elbow requires electrodiagnostic studies, which, unfortunately, are difficult to perform and interpret, and which remain controversial. In its position at the elbow, the radial nerve presents two different compression syndromes, one paralytic and the other painful, both of which involve the same anatomical structures and the same mechanical forces. It seems that slow but constant compression leads more often to the paralytic syndrome, while the intermittent compression leads more often to a painful syndrome. Further advances in neurophysiology may clarify this point for us.

Acknowledgement

Thanks are due to Dr F.E. Jones, Nashville, Tennessee for his help with the translation of this manuscript from French to English.

References

Atroshi I, Johnsson R, Ornstein E. (1995) Radial tunnel release. *Acta Orthop Scand* **6**:255–7.

Bieber EJ, Russel Morre J, Weiland AJ. (1986) Lipomas compressing the radial nerve at the elbow. *J Hand Surg* **11A**:533–5.

Bonnel F, Mansat M, Villa MA, Rabischong P, Allieu Y. (1982) Anatomical and histological basis of surgery to the radial nerve. *Anat Clin* **3**:229–38.

Bowen TL, Stone KH. (1966) Posterior interosseous nerve paralysis caused by a ganglion at the elbow. *J Bone Joint Surg* **48B**:774–6.

Capener N. (1966) The vulnerability of the posterior interosseous nerve of the forearm. A case report and an anatomical study. *J Bone Joint Surg* **48B**:770–3.

Comtet JJ, Chambaud D. (1975) Paralysie «spontanée» du nerf interosseux postérieur par lésion inhabituelle. *Rev Chir Orthop* **61**:533–41.

Comtet JJ, Chambaud D, Genety J. (1976) La compression de la branche postérieure du nerf radial. *Nouv Presse Méd* **5**:1111–14.

Comtet JJ, Lalain JJ, Moyen B, Genety J, Brunet-Guedj E., Lazo-Henriquez R. (1985) Les épicondylalgies avec compression de la branche postérieure du nerf radial. *Rev Chir Ortho* **71**:Suppl. II, 89–93.

Crawford GP. (1984) Radial tunnel syndrome (letter to the editor). *J Hand Surg* **9**:451–2.

Dawson DM, Hallett M, Millender LH. (1990) *Entrapment neuropathies*. Boston, MA: Little, Brown and Co.

Derkash RS. Niebauer JJ. (1981) Entrapment of the posterior interosseous nerve by a fibrous band in the dorsal edge of the supinator muscle and erosion of a groove in the proximal radius. *J Hand Surg* **6A**:524–6.

Durandeau A, Geneste R. (1988) Un syndrome canalaire rare: la paralysie du nerf interosseux postérieur. *Rev Chir Orthop* Supp. II, **74**:156–8.

Fuss FK, Wurzl GH. (1991) Radial nerve entrapment at the elbow: surgical anatomy. *J Hand Surg* **16A**:742–7.

Hagert CG, Lundborg G, Hansen T. (1977) Entrapment of the posterior interosseous nerve. *Scand J Plast Reconstr Surg* **11**:205–12.

Heyse-Moore GH. (1984) Resistant tennis elbow. *J Hand Surg* **9B**:64–6.

Jalovaara P, Lindholm RV. (1989) Decompression of the posterior interosseous nerve for tennis elbow. *Arch Orthop Trauma Surg* **108**:243–5.

Kotani H, Miki T, Senzoku F, Nakagawa Y, Ueo T. (1985) Posterior interosseous nerve paralysis with multiple constrictions. *J Hand Surg* **20A**:15–17.

Laulan J, Daaboul J, Fassio E, Favard L. (1994) Les rapports du muscle court extenseur radial du carpe avec la branche de division profonde du nerf radial. Intérêt dans la physiopathologie des épicondylalgies. *Ann Chir Main* **13**:366–72.

Lawrence T, Mobbs P, Fortems Y, Stanley JK. (1995) Radial tunnel syndrome. A retrospective review of 30 decompressions of the radial nerve. *J Hand Surg* **20B**:454–9.

Lister GD, Belsole RB, Kleinert HE. (1979) The radial tunnel syndrome. *J Hand Surg* **4**:52–9.

Millender LH, Nalbuff EA, Holdsworth DE. (1973) Posterior interosseous nerve syndrome secondary to rheumatoid synovitis. *J Bone Joint Surg* **55A**:375–7.

Moss SH, Switzer HE. (1983) Radial tunnel syndrome: A spectrum of clinical presentations. *J Hand Surg* **8A**:414–23.

Narakas A. (1974) Epicondylite et syndrome compressif du nerf radial. *Med Hyg* **32**:2067–70.

Nielsen HO. (1976) Posterior interosseous nerve paralysis caused by fibrous band compression at the supinator muscle – a report of four cases. *Acta Orthop Scand* **47**:304–7.

Prasartritha T, Liupolvanish P, Rojanakit A. (1993) A study of the posterior interosseous nerve and the radial tunnel in 30 Thai cadavers. *J Hand Surg* **18A**:107–12.

Raimbeau G, Saint-Cast Y, Pelier-Cady MC. (1990) Radial tunnel syndrome: a study of a continuous and homogenous series of 35 cases. *French J Orthop Surg* **4**:159–65.

Rath AM, Perez M, Mainguene C, Masquelet AC, Chevrel JP. (1993) Anatomic basis of the physiopathology of the epicondylagias: a study of the deep branch of the radial nerve. *Surg Radiol Anat* **15**:15–19.

Ritts GD, Wood MB, Linscheid RL. (1987) Radial tunnel syndrome: a ten-year surgical experience. *Clin Orthop* **219**:201–5.

Roles NC, Maudsley R. (1972) Radial tunnel syndrome: Resistant tennis elbow as a nerve entrapment. *J Bone Joint Surg* **54B**:499–508.

Sharrard WJ. (1966) Posterior interosseous neuritis. *J Bone Joint Surg* **48B**:777–80.

Spinner M. (1968) The arcade of Frohse and its relationship to posterior interosseous nerve paralysis. *J Bone Joint Surg* **50B**:809–12.

Sponseller PD, Engber WD. (1983) Double-entrapment radial tunnel syndrome. *J Hand Surg* **8A**:420–3.

Van Rossum J, Buruma OJS, Kamphuisen HAC, Onvlee GJ. (1978) Tennis elbow – a radial tunnel syndrome? *J Bone Joint Surg* **60B**:197–9.

Verhaar J, Spaans F. (1991) Radial tunnel syndrome. An investigation of compression neuropathy as a possible cause. *J Bone Joint Surg* **73A**:539–44.

Werner CO. (1979) Lateral elbow pain and posterior interosseous nerve entrapment. *Acta Orthop Scand Suppl* **174**:1–62.

Werner CO. (1991) Radial nerve paralysis and tumor. *Clin Orthop* **268**:223–5.

Winckworth CE. (1983) Lawn-tennis elbow. *BMJ* 1883, **II**:708.

Younge DH, Moise P. (1994) The radial tunnel syndrome. *Int Orthop* **18**:368–70.

12
Radial sensory nerve entrapment (Wartenberg's syndrome)

Guy Foucher and Giorgio Pajardi

Introduction

Entrapment of the sensory branch of the radial nerve (SBRN) in the forearm, originally described by Matzdorff (1926), bears the name of Robert Wartenberg who reported on four cases (Wartenberg, 1932). Among the numerous synonyms used in the literature are: Wartenberg's syndrome (WS) (Lanzetta and Foucher, 1993; Sprofkin, 1954), cheiralgia paraesthetica (cheiralgia means hand pain) (Chodoroff and Honet, 1985; Ehrlich et al., 1986; Massey and Pleet, 1978), handcuff neuropathy, wristlet watch neuritis (Stopford, 1922), watch-band or wrist-watch syndrome (Bierman, 1959; Dorfman and Jayaram, 1978; Smith, 1981), superficial radial neuropathy (Braidwood, 1975; Rask, 1978), or superficial radial neurapraxia (Rask, 1979).

WS has received scant notice in the literature; it has not been mentioned in the major works on peripheral nerve entrapment, and has been presented as 'exceptionally rare' in some classic neurological textbooks (Wilson, 1941); its description by Eversmann (1982) and more recently the English translation of Wartenberg's original German article (Ehrlich et al., 1986) and a report of 58 cases by Dellon and Mackinnon (1986) drew attention to this disease. We reported successively 22 cases of WS in 1991 (Foucher et al. 1991) and 52 cases in 1997 (Lanzetta and Foucher, 1993; Foucher, 1996). The present review concerns 78 cases of WS to characterize the diagnosis and management of this condition.

Clinical presentation

The frequency of the syndrome has not been estimated in the literature. In a previous study we found an incidence of 0.82% of the total number of patients seen in our Unit during a period of 6 years (Lanzetta and Foucher, 1993). The syndrome is more frequent in women than in men with a ratio of 4 : 1, and occurs in middle age (mean 44 years). The condition is rarely work-related (11%) but a traumatic agent is more frequently found (39%) including wrist-watch compression, tight plaster, splint, dressing or a scar due to previous surgery.

Associated pathology is frequent: diabetes has been found in 4% of cases, carpal tunnel syndrome in 15%, ganglion of the first dorsal compartment in 2%. De Quervain's disease deserves a special mention as it is recorded in 42% of WS cases.

The main complaint is undefined pain, numbness, tingling or dysesthesia in the first three digits mimicking a carpal tunnel syndrome but when asked the patient tends to feel that it involves the dorso-radial part of the hand. These symptoms are frequently triggered by prono-supination and ulnar tilting of the wrist. The area of sensory loss or perturbation is variable, from the ulnar aspect of the thumb only, to the whole classical SBRN area. Patients are limited in their daily or professional activities much more by pain than by alteration of sensation.

A pseudo-Tinel sign is elicited at a variable level, the most frequent one being at the classical entrapment site on the radial border of the forearm, just distally to the brachioradialis muscle belly, at a mean distance 8.8 cm proximal to the radial styloid process. In other cases it is found anywhere over the course of the SBRN with predilection at two levels:

- at the radial styloid level (mainly when associated with de Quervain's disease);
- at the wrist-watch level or at the level of a tight plaster, bandage or splint (Velcro straps).

A double Tinel's sign is also frequently found in the case of distal scar (due to previous release of the first compartment for de Quervain's disease) leading to a 'double crush' entrapment syndrome (Dahlin and Lundborg, 1990). It is sometimes difficult to distinguish between two sites of compression and a single compression with progressive regeneration of the nerve distal to it. Distinction between the site of compression and level of fibers regeneration is easily evaluated at two successive consultations, the peripheral Tinel's sign migrating distally with time.

The Finkelstein's test is positive in all patients presenting an association to De Quervain's disease. In 12% of patients a 'false positive' test is found, with a typical WS without first compartment tenoviginitis.

A provocative test (Dellon and Mackinnon, 1986) consists of maintaining the upper extremity extended along the body, rotated in hyper-pronation with ulnar wrist deviation; paresthesia in the radial territory occurs in less than 30 seconds. This test is positive in 96% of our cases.

Paraclinical examination

Electromyographic diagnostic studies may be carried out. In our experience of 16 cases, the results were considered as normal in 8 cases, while in 4 cases a decreased sensory conduction velocity was found; in 2 cases there was no sensory recording available, and in 2 cases there was evidence of an underlying polyneuropathy.

Diagnostic nerve blocking is usually unnecessary. However, innervation by the lateral antebrachial cutaneous nerve may overlap that of the SBRN on the dorso-radial aspect of the hand, or even completely replace it (Mackinnon and Dellon, 1985). In such cases, diagnostic nerve blocks of the antebrachial cutaneous nerve and/or SBRN could be helpful.

Recently we have used MRI, in four cases, to try to demonstrate the entrapment without success.

Treatment

Conservative treatment is always tried, except in severe forms for which surgery is proposed. Most patients suffering from external compression of the SBRN (watchband, plaster, splint or dressing) have been treated conservatively, surgical treatment being reserved for those cases in which the compression was judged to be long-standing, without distal progression of Tinel's sign.

Non-operative management included removal of any external compression, change in manual activity, rest, splinting and corticosteroid injection at the entrapment site. Injection could be useful but our experience is limited, and we fear skin atrophy and vascular skin changes in such a superficial location. We favor a loose and well padded splint, worn at night, maintaining the wrist in slight radial inclination and the thumb in full abduction. We are reluctant to include the elbow to block the prono-supination. This conservative treatment has been effective in 94% of the patients.

Surgical treatment was always carried out under axillary block, tourniquet and loupe magnification. None of the patients needed hospitalization. The mean operative time for isolated neurolysis of SBRN was 12 minutes. At 9 cm from the radial styloid, the nerve could be palpated on the radial border of the radius. It is exposed through a 3 cm longitudinal incision. The cephalic vein is gently retracted and the nerve is found between the two tendinous 'blades' of the extensor carpi radialis longus posteriorly and the brachioradialis anteriorly. A fascia is frequently found, uniting these two tendons, or more rarely a penetration of the SBRN through the brachioradialis tendon; resection of the fascia or tendon slip exposes the SBRN immediately. After neurolysis we always removed the posterior border of the tendon of the brachioradialis to give more room to the nerve, controlling perioperatively the disappearance of the scissoring effect of the two tendons. No microsurgical internal neurolysis is performed. After careful hemostasis with a bipolar coagulation, the wound is closed without drainage. Postoperatively the patients are encouraged to move early without restriction to avoid adhesion of the nerve and secondary lesion by traction.

In 9 out of 36 operated hands, a de Quervain release was performed at the same stage. In six patients who presented with de Quervain's disease and contiguous SBRN irritation, a simple first dorsal compartment release and tenosynovectomy were performed, without neurolysis, avoiding any traction on the nerve.

Results

Of the 71 patients (78 cases) treated, 54 patients (58 hands) were reviewed with a mean follow-up of 2 years. Pain relief, especially during daily and professional activities, was assessed on a visual analogic scale of 10 points and used as the main criterion to differentiate between 'excellent', 'good', 'fair' or 'poor' results. Sensation recovery was not judged to be a critical factor in follow-up examination, as often patients reported an excellent subjective result, even if sensation was not completely restored. Conservative treatment gave excellent results in 58%, good in 20%, fair in 10% and poor in 12% of the cases. Patients giving a poor result were operated on. Surgical treatment gave excellent results in 71%, good in 19%, fair in 7% and poor in 3% of the cases. The only poor result is due to a reflex sympathetic dystrophy in a case where a Bower's hemi-resection arthroplasty of the ulnar head was associated.

In one of the WS cases associated to de Quervain's disease, where only the first extensor compartment release was performed, the patient recovered completely from the symptoms postoperatively, showing a positive Tinel's sign progressively migrating distally and finally disappearing. Four months later she complained of recurrent paresthesia on the dorsum of the hand. A positive Tinel's sign was found this time at the mid-forearm level. An EMG study showed 'no sensory recording' at the upper third of the forearm after thumb stimulation, indicating an entrapment at the mid-forearm level. She recovered completely in 10 weeks of conservative measures, including rest and splinting.

Discussion

Entrapment of the SBRN at the forearm is not as rare as one might think, given the scarce literature on the subject. The diagnosis is frequently overlooked, mainly when associated with carpal tunnel syndrome or de Quervain tenovaginitis. In its classical presentation, the WS is manifested by tingling in the SBRN territory and a pseudo-Tinel's sign elicited in the forearm at an average of 8.8 cm proximal to the radial styloid. At this level the entrapment is due to a 'scissoring' effect of the tendons of the extensor carpi radialis longus and brachioradialis during pronosupination; another mechanism could be a traction lesion of the SBRN, tethered by the fascia uniting the two tendons during repeated ulnar inclination of the wrist.

When the pseudo-Tinel's sign is elicited more distally, different hypotheses should be considered: external compression (wrist-watch, plaster, splint or dressing), contiguous pathology like de Quervain tenovaginitis with a Tinel's sign at the styloid level or progression of regenerating fibers during spontaneous recovery of a classical WS. In such cases, removal of any external compression, conservative treatment of associated pathology, decreased frequency of the offending manual activity and a well padded splint worn at night are to be recommended. Successive consultation will demonstrate distal progression of the pseudo-Tinel's sign, reassuring the prognosis.

In some cases a distal Tinel's sign is combined with a more proximal one; it is a form of the so-called 'double crush syndrome', where a slight compression due, for example to a wrist-watch, can decompensate the state of a proximally entrapped nerve (Upton and McComas, 1973; Wilgis and Murphy, 1992). It has been hypothesized that the opposite may also occur (Dahlin and Lundborg, 1990). A distal entrapment of the nerve would then impair retrograde transport of trophic substances to the nerve cell body. The neuron will then decrease the production and transport of essential material to the axon (antegrade transport), which may make the proximal part of the nerve more vulnerable to compression.

In a previous study (Lanzetta and Foucher, 1993), de Quervain's disease was associated in

50% of WS, a high percentage, close to the presently reported 42%, much higher than the 17% reported in another series (Dellon and MacKinnon, 1986). Three hypotheses could be advanced for such an association. First, both pathologies have a common mechanism and repeated ulnar inclination of the wrist is followed by both entities. Second, de Quervain's disease precedes the WS, which is due to the reaction of surrounding tissue over the radial styloid entrapping the SBRN; then ulnar inclination of the wrist is followed by traction lesions of a nerve fixed at two points. Finally the 'double crush' hypothesis could also explain the frequency of the association with distal (or proximal) decompensation of an already sensitized nerve.

Useful indications when planning a treatment can be obtained by systematic research of one or more Tinel's signs at the time of clinical examination. The recovery of the nerve showed by distal migration of the Tinel's sign can be tested periodically and surgical treatment delayed accordingly.

Preoperative identification of any compression of the SBRN is mandatory when performing a de Quervain's release or removal of ganglions of the first dorsal extensor compartment; incomplete recovery, persistence of pain, paresthesia or Tinel's sign might be attributed to a neuroma due to an introgenic surgical lesion rather than a preexisting condition, with all the medico-legal problems that this implies. The same care also needs to be taken at the time of injection of the first compartment for de Quervain's disease and in case of association it is relevant to clearly inform the patient.

From our experience it appears evident that conservative means can be successful when indicated. A review of the previously reported cases reveals similar results. We might suggest that when the Tinel's sign is at the radial styloid level and the cause of compression is evident (watchband, handcuffs, plaster, splint or dressing), and when the onset of the symptoms occurred within 3–6 months, a conservative treatment consisting of change in manual activity, rest and splintage can frequently provide very satisfactory results.

When pain and neurological symptoms are more severe and have been constant, without progression of the Tinel's sign, for more than 6 months, recovery by conservative treatment is usually slow and incomplete, leading to an unsatisfactory result. If two distinct Tinel's signs are found (radial styloid level and mid-forearm), and no signs of nerve recovery are present, surgery usually becomes mandatory and proximal neurolysis is recommended. Proximal neurolysis and first compartment release may be suggested in the case of double Tinel's sign in association with de Quervain's disease. Failure to associate the two operations could decompensate the WS due to the scar at the styloid level.

On the contrary, as already reported by Rask in two cases (Rask, 1978), when there is an association of de Quervain's disease and a contiguous irritation or compression of the SBRN, a simple release of the first extensor compartment usually leads to a total and permanent recovery of the neurological symptoms.

Prompt recognition of this entrapment, and careful clinical assessment at successive consultations allows choice of the appropriate treatment and avoidance of surgical and medico-legal pitfalls.

References

Bierman HR. (1959) Nerve compression due to tight watchband. *New Engl J Med* **261**:237–8.

Braidwood AS. (1975) Superficial radial neuropathy. *J Bone Joint Surg* **57B**:380–3.

Chodoroff G, Honet JC. (1985) Cheiralgia paresthetica and linear atrophy as a complication of local steroid injection. *Arch Physical Med Rehabil* **66**:637–9.

Dahlin LB, Lundborg G. (1990) The neurone and its response to peripheral nerve compression. *J Hand Surg* **15B**:5–10.

Dellon AL, Mackinnon SE. (1986) Radial sensory nerve entrapment in the forearm. *J Hand Surg* **11A**:199–205.

Dorfman LJ, Jayaram AR. (1978) Handcuff neuropathy. *JAMA* **239**:957.

Ehrlich W, Dellon AL, Mackinnon SE. (1986) Cheiralgia parestetica (entrapment of the radial sensory nerve). *J Hand Surg* **11A**:196–8.

Eversmann WH Jr. (1982) Entrapment and compression neuropathies. In: Green DP, ed. *Operative Hand Surgery*. New York: Churchill Livingstone: 990–2.

Foucher G, Greant P, Sammut D, Buch N. (1991) Nevrites et névromes des branches sensitives du nerf radial. A propos de quarante-quatre cas. *Ann Chir Main* **10**(2):108–12.

Foucher G. (1996) Le syndrome de Wartenberg: une compression méconnue du nerf radial. *Rhumatologie*, **48**(9–10):321–3.

Lanzetta M, Foucher G. (1993) Entrapment of the superficial branch of the radial nerve (the Wartenberg's syndrome). A report of 52 cases. *Int Orthop* **17**:342–5.

Mackinnon SE, Dellon AL. (1985) The overlap pattern of the lateral antebrachial cutaneous nerve and the superficial radial nerve. *J Hand Surg* **10A**:522–6.

Massey EW, Pleet AB. (1978) Handcuffs and cheiralgia parestetica. *Neurology* **28**:1212–3.

Matzdorff P. (1926) Zwei seltene Falle von peripherer sensibler Lahmung. *Klin Wochenschr* **5**:1187.

Rask MR. (1978) Superficial radial neuritis and De Quervain's disease. Report of 3 cases. *Clin Orthop* **131**:176–8.

Rask MR. (1979) Watchband superficial radial neurapraxia. *JAMA* **241**:2702.

Smith MS. (1981) Handcuff neuropathy. *Ann Emerg Med* **10**:668.

Sprofkin RE. (1954) Cheiralgia parestetica – Wartenberg's disease. *Neurology* **4**:857–62.

Stopford JSB. (1922) Neuritis produced by a wristlet watch. *Lancet* **1**:993–4.

Upton ARM, McComas AJ. (1973) The double crush nerve entrapment syndromes. *Lancet* **2**:359–61.

Wartenberg R. (1932) Cheiralgia Parestetica (Isolierte Neuritis des Ramus superficialis nervi radialis). *Z Ger Neurol Psychiatr* **141**:145–55.

Wilgis EFS, Murphy R. (1992) The significance of longitudinal excursion in peripheral nerves. *Hand Clin* **2**(4):761–66.

Wilson SAK. (1941) *Neurology*. Baltimore: Williams & Wilkins Co., Vol. 1:327.

13
Compression neuropathies of the upper extremities in athletes

Robert J. Spinner and Peter C. Amadio

Introduction

Recreational and professional athletes alike develop nerve compression syndromes. While large epidemiologic studies are not available, Hirasawa and Sakakida (1983) identified sports related neural lesions in 66 (5.7%) of 1167 total patients with nerve injuries collected over an 18-year period. In their experience, the brachial plexus followed by radial, ulnar, axillary, median and digital nerves were affected the most frequently in the upper extremity. These injuries were associated predominantly with mountain climbing, gymnastics and baseball, which also are some of the favorite sports in Japan. These data, while useful, are not directly comparable owing to the disproportionate popularity of mountain climbing in Japan.

Clinical studies have revealed certain predispositions. Up to 30% of volleyball players may have manifestations of suprascapular neuropathy (Holzgraefe et al., 1994) or bicyclists of wrist-level median or ulnar nerve sensory symptoms (Weiss, 1985). The association of ulnar neuropathy at the elbow in throwing athletes has led to research which has clarified anatomic relationships about the medial elbow. The fact that volleyball players, swimmers, baseball pitchers, and weightlifters develop various shoulder neural lesions suggests that a thorough understanding of the mechanisms behind a specific athlete's technique may provide a common denominator to the pattern of neural injuries.

Neural injuries occur via different mechanisms (compression, traction, friction). They may result from direct acute trauma or chronic microtrauma.

Excessive physiologic demands of soft tissues and nerves likely occur due to excessive use ('overuse') of repetitive forceful motions in awkward postures, or 'misuse' using improper technique, poor condition or faulty equipment. Certainly variant anatomy, whether congenital (Figure 13.1) or acquired, also predisposes individuals to compression, either unilaterally or bilaterally.

In many cases, these neural lesions represent serious, potentially career ending injuries. Early diagnosis of the neural lesion is important to optimize results. Evaluation is based on a thorough history and detailed physical examination. Confirmation can be achieved with adjuvant

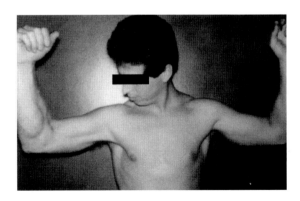

Figure 13.1

This weightlifter had intermittent ulnar nerve symptoms which were caused by infraclavicular compression by a chondroepitrochlearis muscle (a variant axillary arch muscle). Reprinted with permission (Spinner RJ, Carmichael SW, Spinner M (1991). Infraclavicular ulnar nerve entrapment due to a chondroepitrochlearis muscle. *J Hand Surg* **16B**:315–17.

radiographic and/or electrodiagnostic studies (Wilbourn, 1990). The differential diagnosis must always exclude other musculoskeletal disorders and other neurologic localizations – be it other peripheral sites (more proximally or distally) or central sites. Non-operative treatment should include a combination of a trial of rest from the activity and non-steroidal anti-inflammatory agents. Splints and physical therapy should be part of the regimen along with local steroid injection, when appropriate. Surgery is indicated when non-operative therapy has failed to improve symptoms, or clinical or electrical findings within 3–6 months. Refined technique along with improved conditioning and strengthening exercises may be prophylactic measures.

This chapter reviews by anatomic region the most common athletic nerve compression syndromes.

Neck

Thoracic outlet syndrome

Thoracic outlet syndrome represents a spectrum of controversial neurovascular compression syndromes dealing with the brachial plexus (usually the lower trunk) or the subclavian artery and vein. The site of compression can be in the interscalene triangle, the costoclavicular interval or in the subcoracoid space. Thoracic outlet syndrome is relatively rare in athletes. It has been recognized in swimmers, American football quarterbacks, tennis players and baseball pitchers (Karas, 1990; Strukel and Garrick, 1978). Most authors have associated the depressed shoulder girdle with the production of thoracic outlet symptoms. A hypertrophied pectoralis minor has also been identified.

Symptomatic thoracic outlet syndrome is a clinical diagnosis that is based on objective symptoms without confirmatory clinical, electrical or radiographic abnormalities. Typical neurologic symptoms of thoracic outlet syndrome include: neck and shoulder pain which may radiate to the hand, sensory disturbance (numbness, paresthesias), usually in the medial forearm and ulnar aspect of the hand, and hand cramping and fatigability. In this group of patients, neurologic examination is usually normal. Examination should include a combination of various maneuvers including: Adson's test, Wright's

maneuver, costoclavicular maneuver, and Tinel's test; however, one must interpret these cautiously, since the majority of normal asymptomatic individuals will have one or more abnormal tests when performing several tests. Radiographs typically do not reveal cervical ribs, elongated transverse processes or exuberant clavicular calls. Electrodiagnostic studies are typically normal.

In contrast, true neurologic thoracic outlet syndrome occurs when subjective complaints, objective, electrodiagnostic and radiographic findings all are consistent with a diagnosis of thoracic outlet syndrome. Neurogenic thoracic outlet syndrome has been reported in two young athletes, attributed to a cervical rib (Rayan, 1988).

Thoracic outlet symptoms typically improve with physical activity, postural exercises and rehabilitation.

Shoulder

Suprascapular nerve

The suprascapular nerve is vulnerable to injury in athletes (Figure 13.2), especially overhead

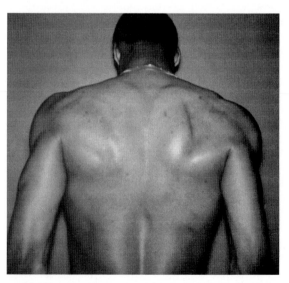

Figure 13.2

This professional baseball pitcher had a right suprascapular nerve lesion. Note the atrophy of the supraspinatus and infraspinatus muscles.

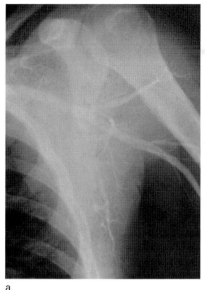
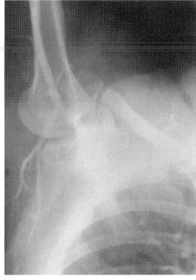

a   b

Figure 13.3

(a) This arteriogram demonstrates the presence of a patent posterior humeral circumflex artery with the arm at neutral. (b) The artery is occluded with the arm fully abducted.

volleyball players and weightlifters; however, it also has been reported in tennis players, pitchers, parasailers, boxers, wrestlers, and handball players (Antoniadis et al., 1996). Mechanisms have included: entrapment at the superior transverse ligament, spinoglenoid ligament, and traction injuries of the nerve at fixed sites against the scapula with forceful shoulder movements from repetitive microtrauma.

Compression of the suprascapular nerve can occur at the suprascapular notch by the superior transverse ligament. In this location, it typically gives rise to weakness of both the supraspinatus and the infraspinatus. Patients usually have posterior shoulder pain, and weakness in abduction and external rotation. There is no cutaneous sensory abnormality.

Compression of the suprascapular nerve more distally at the spinoglenoid notch can also occur. There the suprascapular nerve passes under a spinoglenoid ligament (present in 87% of men and 50% of women (Kaspi et al., 1988)) which can be the site of compression. Compression of the suprascapular nerve at this distal site results in isolated infraspinatus atrophy and these patients have weakness in external rotation only. Pain is an inconstant finding and should raise suspicion of an underlying shoulder pathology. This clinical entity is particularly common in volleyball players (Ferretti et al., 1987; Wang and Koehler, 1996). Up to 33% of high-performance volleyball

players have atrophy of the infraspinatus (Holzgraefe et al., 1994). Some have suggested a link to a 'floating serve' (Ferretti et al., 1998). This lesion has been associated with SLAP (superior labrum anteroposterior) lesions and MRI can be helpful to discern shoulder pathology or to rule out a ganglion (Zeiss et al., 1993). A period of non-operative therapy is warranted.

Axillary nerve

The axillary nerve innervates the deltoid and the teres minor and provides cutaneous sensation to the arm (Figure 13.3). Patients with axillary nerve lesions may present with decreased abduction and paresthesias in the lateral aspect of the proximal arm. Injury occurs most commonly related to traction following shoulder fracture and/or anterior dislocation, or following direct blow, such as in American football linebackers (Kessler and Uribe, 1994) or hockey or rugby players (Perlmutter and Apruzzese, 1998; Perlmutter et al., 1997).

The quadrilateral space syndrome is a controversial syndrome, first popularized by Cahill in baseball pitchers (Cahill and Palmer, 1983). It has been reported in tennis and volleyball players (Paladini et al., 1996) as well. The axillary nerve (along with the posterior humeral circumflex artery) may be compressed within the quadrilateral space. This space is bounded by the teres minor superiorly, medially by the long head of the triceps, laterally by the humerus and inferiorly by the teres major. Patients with quadrilateral space syndrome may have symptoms of diffuse aching pain in the shoulder and paresthesias in a non-dermatomal distribution. Tenderness, however, can be localized directly to the quadrilateral space. Forward flexion and/or abduction and external rotation aggravate the symptoms. Neurologic examination and electrodiagnostic studies are typically normal. Others have reported axillary motor and sensory abnormalities (McKowen and Voorhies, 1987) in addition to teres minor atrophy detected on MRI (Francel et al., 1991; Linker et al., 1993). Arteriography in these patients reveals an occlusion of the posterior humeral circumflex artery with the arm abducted and externally rotated. The majority of patients do not warrant surgery. Surgical exploration has demonstrated muscle hypertrophy, fibrous bands, and scar as possible causes.

Long thoracic nerve

Isolated serratus anterior paralysis does occur in athletes and may be attributed to direct injury, traction or compression of the nerve (Figure 13.4). Patients may have shoulder pain, notice the inability to push or lift with complete power due to the abnormal scapular movements, or decreased active shoulder motion. Patients may note winging of the scapula. This can be best demonstrated with the arm flexed 90 degrees and the elbow fully extended against a wall. It must be distinguished from winging from trapezius or rhomboid palsies. Trapezial winging is present with resisted arm flexion with the elbow flexed or with crossed adduction testing, but which is not present with the arm flexed and the elbow extended. Rhomboid winging can be appreciated by bracing the shoulders backward as in a military position.

  Serratus anterior palsy has been reported in backpackers (Corkill et al., 1980), swimmers, weightlifters (Stanish and Lamb, 1978), volleyball players (Distefano, 1989). It has also been reported as related to other sports such as mountain climbing (rappeling), tennis, golf, hockey, football, rugby, squash, and boxing

(Packer et al., 1993), shooting, and archery. Mechanisms have included repeated microtrauma (exertion) to muscles of the neck with accelerated upward movements of the arm, such as in volleyball or a forceful jerk of the arm, possibly related to shoulder girdle fatigue (Kauppila, 1993). It may follow acute trauma in sports after missing a ball (golf, tennis) or from exertion such as weightlifting or prolonged cross country skiing or swimming (Vastamaki and Kauppila, 1993); its prognosis is uncertain. Treatment is usually nonoperative and consists of physical therapy. Tendon transfers can be offered late if no clinical or electrical recovery has occurred.

Arm

Radial nerve

High radial nerve compression may occur in athletes (Figure 13.5). It has been described in individuals following strenuous muscular activities and contraction, including weightlifting or tennis (Lotem et al., 1971; Mitsunaga and Nakano, 1988; Prochaska et al., 1993; Streib,

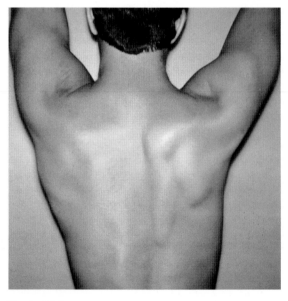

Figure 13.4

This butterfly swimmer had a right long thoracic nerve lesion. The winging of the scapula is evident.

1992). This may also affect arm wrestlers (Ogawa and Ui, 1997) or ball throwers (Bontempo and Trager, 1996), associated with humeral fractures. It has also been related to stretch from the rapid acceleration of throwing, e.g. the windmill pitch in softball (Sinson et al., 1994) or hurling a discus or a stone. Compression usually occurs at the level of the lateral head of the triceps, due to a fibrous arch (Manske, 1977) or anomalous band, but may also occur at the spiral groove. The characteristic pattern of injury produces a wrist and finger and thumb drop. Additional motor loss will include brachioradialis and abductor pollicis longus. Triceps strength is usually intact (these oblique branch(es) are usually more proximal at the level of the axilla). A typical sensory loss occurs in the first dorsal web space as well as the proximal forearm. A variant presentation affected the triceps branch only (Nukada et al., 1996).

Musculocutaneous nerve

Compression of the musculocutaneous nerve in the proximal arm is rare. It may occur at the level where the musculocutaneous nerve (variably) penetrates the coracobrachialis muscle (Kim and Goodrich, 1984; Pecina and Bojanic, 1993), in patients following strenuous exercise and weightlifting (Braddom and Wolfe, 1978). Other neural lesions may follow after frontal blows to the proximal arm or shoulder dislocations. Patients will have biceps and brachialis weakness and sensory loss in the radial aspect of the forearm.

Elbow

Ulnar nerve

Recent papers have studied the biomechanics of overhead throwing (especially the acceleration phase in baseball pitching) and ulnar nerve compression at the elbow in these athletes (Barnes and Tullos, 1978; DelPizzo et al., 1977; Godshall and Hansen, 1971; Hang, 1981; Jobe and Elattrache, 1991; Wojtys et al., 1986). Ulnar nerve compression at the elbow also affects javelin throwers, weightlifters (Dangles and Bilos, 1980), wheelchair athletes, and athletes

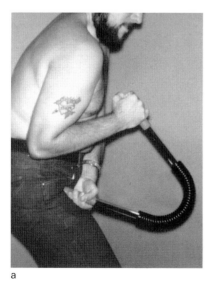
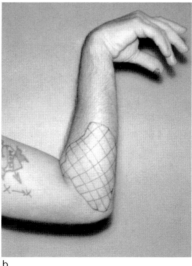
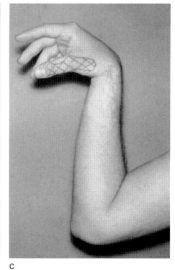

a   b   c

Figure 13.5

(a) This policeman developed a high radial nerve palsy following a period of intense weightlifting. (b) The 'X' demonstrates the site of percussion tenderness. A wrist and finger drop is demonstrated along with the sensory abnormality in the proximal forearm. (c) The area of sensory disturbance in the thumb can be seen.

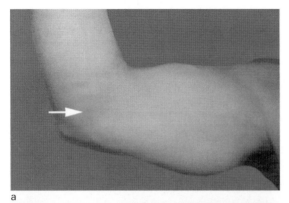

a

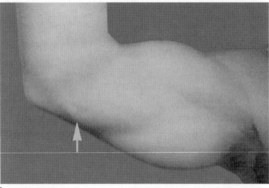

b

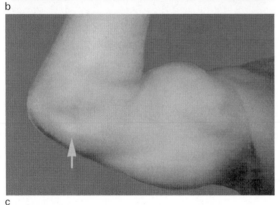

c

Figure 13.6

This recreational weightlifter had persistent elbow pain and snapping after two previous ulnar nerve operations and evaluation by eight different surgeons. The correct diagnosis of snapping of the medial portion of the triceps can be made on observation of elbow flexion.
(a) The previous elbow incision can be seen (arrow); (b) the prominent medial triceps can be seen posterior to the medial epicondyle (arrow) with the elbow flexed 90 degrees; (c) with full elbow flexion, the triceps has dislocated (snapped) over the medial epicondyle (arrow).

involved in racquet sports. Arm wrestlers may develop ulnar nerve compression following medial epicondylar fractures (Figure 13.6).

Patients with ulnar nerve compression at the elbow may present with medial elbow pain, sensory symptoms in the ulnar aspect of the hand and weakness in muscles innervated with the ulnar nerve. Findings typically reveal sensory abnormalities both in the volar and dorsal zones of the ulnar one-and-a-half digits and the palm of the hand, and motor weakness may affect the flexor carpi ulnaris, flexor digitorum profundus to the little and ring fingers, hypothenar muscles, interossei, ulnar innervated lumbricals, and the adductor pollicis. Patients may have percussion tenderness at a point along the course of the ulnar nerve and a positive elbow flexion test.

Ulnar nerve symptoms may occur from static compression at sites in and around the cubital tunnel, including the cubital tunnel retinaculum, the flexor carpi ulnaris or even the variant anconeus epitrochlearis. Dynamic compression related to increased pressure within the cubital tunnel with elbow flexion may develop from impingement by the triceps against the nerve; this might be exacerbated in patients with hypertrophied triceps. In addition, ulnar nerve irritation coexists in as many as 40% of cases of medial collateral ligament laxity or with medial epicondylitis. Patients with ulnar nerve subluxation and dislocation might be predisposed to neuropathy. Secondary changes resulting in calcifications, arthritic spurs, or cubitus varus or cubitus valgus deformities might predispose the nerve to other injury. Baseball pitchers, who as a group have increased valgus and forearm hypertrophy, are predisposed to degenerative changes and susceptible to medial collateral ligament injuries; in them, many risk factors for the development of ulnar nerve compression may coexist simultaneously.

Snapping of a portion of the medial head of the triceps frequently occurs in association with ulnar nerve dislocation and ulnar nerve symptoms (Spinner and Goldner, 1998). This entity has been seen in baseball players, rock climbers, swimmers, and weightlifters, usually associated with hypertrophy of the medial triceps.

The best surgical treatment for athletes is still undecided: some favor subcutaneous transposition (Rettig and Ebben, 1993); others, submuscular transposition.

Musculocutaneous nerve (lateral cutaneous nerve)

Compression of the lateral cutaneous nerve of the forearm (the terminal sensory branch of the musculocutaneous nerve) may occur at the elbow level. Patients may present with forearm pain or sensory abnormalities in the radial aspect of the distal arm. Tenderness can be localized to the region where the nerve pierces the deep fascia of the arm lateral to the bicipital tendon. It has been associated with elbow extension and forearm pronation or resisted elbow flexion. It has been reported in tennis (Bassett and Nunley, 1982) and racquetball players (Felsenthal et al., 1984), basketball players, lifters, throwers, and swimmers. Splinting may be helpful in providing symptomatic relief. Local lidocaine injection can relieve symptoms and confirm the diagnosis. Surgical decompression and partial tenotomy may be necessary for persistent symptoms.

Median nerve

The *pronator syndrome* is a pain syndrome (localized in the volar forearm), which can be accompanied by median nerve sensory complaints in the digits and mild weakness in the hand. It has been reported in three pathologic conditions: a (thickened) lacertus fibrosus, a fibrous band within the pronator teres, and a tight sublimis arch (flexor digitorum superficialis). Specific testing maneuvers may help localize the site including resisted pronation of the extended elbow (pronator teres); resisted supination to the flexed elbow (lacertus fibrosus); resisted flexion of the long finger proximal interphalangeal joint (flexor digitorum superficialis). Compression has been described in weightlifters and baseball pitchers and has also been related to hypertrophy of the forearm musculature (Barnes and Tullos, 1978) or forcibly pronating the forearm.

Anterior interosseous nerve syndrome

Compression of the anterior interosseous nerve branch resulting in motor deficit occurs more frequently than does the pronator syndrome. Anterior interosseous nerve syndrome produces weakness in the flexor pollicis longus, flexor digitorum profundus of the index and/or middle fingers, and the pronator quadratus; sensation is normal. A square pinch attitude is characteristic when performing the 'O' sign. Anterior interosseous nerve syndrome typically occurs owing to compression by the ulnar head of the pronator teres in the proximal forearm, but one report has associated it following extrinsic compression by a forearm band used for treatment of lateral epicondylitis (Enzenauer and Nordstrom, 1991). It must be distinguished from idiopathic neuritis, commonly affecting the anterior interosseous nerve. It has been reported in tennis players.

Posterior interosseous nerve

Compression of the posterior interosseous nerve may present as a motor deficit or as a pain syndrome (radial tunnel syndrome). Most common compression sites include fibrous bands related to the radiocapitellar joint, extensor carpi radialis brevis edge, arcade of Frohse, and supinator muscle.

Patients with posterior interosseous nerve syndrome present with finger drop and elbow pain; wrist dorsiflexion usually occurs in a radial direction due to non-functioning of the extensor carpi ulnaris; sensation is intact. This syndrome has been seen in a Frisbee thrower (Fraim and Peters, 1979).

Refractory or resistant tennis (Lister et al., 1979; Roles and Maudsley, 1972) is seen in racquet players, weightlifters, swimmers, and in throwing athletes. It may result from repetitive pronation and supination or eccentric contraction of the forearm musculature. Differentiating resistant tennis elbow from radial tunnel syndrome is not always easy, and the two may co-exist. In radial tunnel, the maximal point of tenderness is over the posterior interosseous nerve rather than that lateral epicondyle. Patients may have pain with resisted forearm supination with the elbow at 90°. Electrical studies usually are not helpful. Lidocaine injection can relieve symptoms, as can splinting.

Wrist

Superficial radial nerve

The superficial radial nerve may be compressed between the brachioradialis muscle and the extensor carpi radialis longus (Dellon and Mackinnon, 1986) or more distally near the styloid process. Athletes who perform repetitive pronation/supination movements may be affected with the former, while a wrist band or a racquetball strap may produce an extrinsic neuropathy (Rettig, 1990). Patients present with pain and dysesthesias over the dorso-radial aspect of the hand and thumb. They usually have percussion tenderness and a false positive Finkelstein test. Non-operative therapy is usually effective. Splinting in supination may be necessary.

Distal posterior interosseous nerve

Some have attributed dorsal wrist pain to distal posterior interosseous nerve impingement, with or without an associated dorsal ganglion. They have found perineural fibrosis of the distal posterior interosseous nerve secondary to repetitive trauma at the wrist. This has been linked to repetitive wrist dorsiflexion in gymnasts (Aulicino, 1990).

Carpal tunnel syndrome

Median nerve compression by the transverse carpal ligament can occur in athletes (Rettig, 1990). Patients present with wrist pain sometimes radiating proximally or distally, in combination with sensory abnormalities in the radial three-and-half digits and hand weakness. Symptoms may be aggravated with activity or at night. Examination may reveal a positive percussion test at the wrist, positive Phalen's test, diminished 2-point discrimination in the radial three-and-a-half digits, and decreased palmar, tip pinch or both. Weakness in median innervated hand muscles may be seen; thenar atrophy is typically a late finding. Electrodiagnostic studies are usually confirmatory. Median nerve compression at the wrist has been reported in athletes who perform repetitive gripping or sustained wrist hyperextension/hyperflexion or who are exposed to vibration. These include throwers, rowers, canoers, golfers (Murrey and Cooney, 1996), cyclists, bodybuilders, swimmers, motorcross riders, climbers, and wheelchair athletes (Burnham and Steadward, 1994). It may also result from direct trauma to the volar wrist or from associated tenosynovitis of the flexor tendons. Splinting and a rest from the exacerbating activity are often helpful. Some advocate a local steroid injection. Surgical decompression may be necessary for persistent symptoms or neurologic deficit.

Ulnar nerve

The ulnar nerve is vulnerable to injury within Guyon's space in the wrist in athletes. The relationship of the ulnar nerve to the hook of the hamate and the pisiform in addition to the lack of palmar fascia make the nerve particularly susceptible. Injuries may affect the ulnar nerve itself, its deep (motor), or superficial (sensory) branches. It has been reported on extensively in cycling in which some prevalence studies have been performed. For example, Weiss (1985) found palm numbness in 32% of riders in an 8-day 500 mile bicycle tour ('cyclist's palsy or 'handlebar neuropathy') (Converse, 1979; Eckman et al., 1975; Hoyt, 1976; Jackson, 1989; Kulund and Brubaker, 1978; Noth et al., 1980; Richmond, 1994; Smail, 1975). It also occurs in racquet sports, particularly where there is repetitive trauma/forceful sustained grip/pressure on the hands/palms on handlebars. Patients present with hypothenar pain, weakness in the hand and sensory abnormalities in the palm and the ring and little fingers. It may also occur with fractures of the pisiform or hamate. Cyclists should wear properly padded gloves, use padded handlebars, change hand positions frequently and avoid prolonged grasping of dropped handlebars. Vibration may also play a factor. Modified technique and rest is critical. Ulnar nerve compression may be associated with ulnar artery aneurysms, hook of hamate fractures or racquet player's pisiform. It may also occur from multiply sustained blunt impact such as in handball players, martial artists, or gymnasts.

Hand

Palmar digital nerve

A 16-year-old cheerleader was reported to have numbness and tingling involving a portion of the middle and ring fingers secondary to repeated trauma to her palm from clapping and cartwheels (Shields and Jacobs, 1986). Symptoms improved with restricted activity.

Digital nerve

Bowler's thumb refers to perineural fibrosis of the ulnar digital nerve of the thumb. This was given the name 'bowler's thumb' (Dobyns et al., 1972) because of the pattern of injury resulting in a neuroma from pressure from the edge of the largest hole in the bowling ball. Other fingers may be compressed in bowling (Manstein and Lister, 1982). Similar injuries to digital nerves have been reported in other athletes including baseball batters (Belsky and Millender, 1980), tennis players (Naso, 1984), archery (Rayan, 1992) caused by compression against the bat, the racquet handle or the bow. Trauma to a digital nerve may give rise to localized pain, paresthesias and sensory disturbance and difficulty grasping. Percussion tenderness may be observed. Often skin changes including callus or atrophy may help localize the lesion. This is usually due to external trauma from acute or chronic compression to parts of the fingers. Symptomatic relief may be obtained from a molded plastic thumb guard or decreasing the depth of insertion of the thumb. Surgical decompression with or without digital nerve transposition and local muscle flap coverage can be performed.

References

Antoniadis G, Richter HP, Rath S, Braun V, Moese G. (1996) Suprascapular nerve entrapment: experience with 28 cases. *J Neurosurg* **85**:1020–5.

Aulicino PL. (1990) Neurovascular injuries in the hands of athletes. *Hand Clin* **6**:455–66.

Barnes DA, Tullos HS. (1978) An analysis of 100 symptomatic baseball players. *Am J Sports Med* **6**:62–7.

Bassett FH, Nunley JA. (1982) Compression of the musculocutaneous nerve at the elbow. *J Bone Joint Surg* **64**:1050–2.

Belsky M, Millender LH. (1980) Bowler's thumb in a baseball player. *Orthopedics* **3**:122–3.

Bontempo E, Trager SL (1996) Ball thrower's fracture of the humerus associated with radial nerve palsy. *Orthopedics* **19**:537–40.

Braddom RL, Wolfe C. (1978) Musculocutaneous nerve injury after heavy exercise. *Arch Phys Med Rehabil* **59**:290–3.

Burnham RS, Steadward R. (1994) Upper extremity peripheral nerve entrapments among wheelchair athletes: prevalence, location and risk factor. *Arch Phys Med Rehabil* **75**:519–24.

Cahill BR, Palmer RE. (1983) Quadrilateral space syndrome. *J Hand Surg* **8**:65–9.

Converse TA. (1979) Cyclist palsy (letter). *N Engl J Med* **301**:1397–8.

Corkill G, Lieberman JS, Raylor RG. (1980) Pack palsy in backpackers. *West J Med* **132**:569–72.

Dangles CJ, Bilos ZJ (1980) Ulner neuritis in a world champion weightlifter. *Am J Sports Med* **8**:443–5.

Dellon AL, Mackinnon SE. (1986) Radial sensory nerve entrapment in the forearm. *J Hand Surg* **11A**:199–205.

DelPizzo W, Jobe FW, Norwood L. (1977) Ulnar nerve entrapment syndrome in baseball players. *Am J Sports Med* **5**:182–5.

Distefano S. (1989) Neuropathy due to entrapment of the long thoracic nerve. A case report. *Ital J Orthop Traumatol* **15**:259–62.

Dobyns JH, O'Brien ET, Linscheid RL, Farrow GM. (1972) Bowler's thumb: diagnosis and treatment. A review of seventeen cases. *J Bone Joint Surg* **54A**:751–5.

Eckman PB, Perlstein G, Altrocci PH. (1975) Ulnar neuropathy in bicycle riders. *Arch Neurol* **32**:130–1.

Enzenauer RJ, Nordstrom DM. (1991) Anterior interosseous nerve syndrome associated with forearm band treatment of lateral epicondylitis. *Orthopedics* **14**:788–90.

Felsenthal G, Mandell DL, Reischer MA, Mach RH. (1984) Forearm pain secondary to compression syndrome of the lateral cutaneous nerve of the forearm. *Arch Phys Med Rehabil* **65**:139–41.

Ferretti A, Cerullo G, Russo G. (1987) Suprascapular neuropathy in volleyball players. *J Bone Joint Surg* **69A**:260–3.

Ferretti A, DeCarli A, Fontana M. (1998) Injury of the suprascapular nerve at the spinoglenoid notch. The natural history of infraspinatus atrophy in volleyball players. *Am J Sports Med* **26**:759–63.

Fraim CJ, Peters BH. (1979) Unusual cause of nerve entrapment. *J Am Med Assoc* **242**:2557–8.

Francel TJ, Dellon AL, Campbell JN. (1991) Quadrilateral space syndrome: operative decompression technique. *Plast Reconstr Surg* **87**:911–16.

Godshall RW, Hansen CA. (1971) Traumatic ulnar neuropathy in adolescent baseball pitchers. *J Bone Joint Surg* **53A**:359–61.

Hang YS. (1981) Tardy ulnar neuritis in a Little League baseball player. *Am J Sports Med* **9**:244–6.

Hirasawa Y, Sakakida K. (1983) Sports and peripheral nerve injury. *Am J Sports Med* **11**:420–6.

Holzgraefe M, Kukowski B, Eggert S. (1994) Prevalence of latent and manifest suprascapular neuropathy in high-performance volleyball players. *Br J Sports Med* **28**:177–9.

Hoyt CS. (1976) Ulnar neuropathy in bicycle riders (editorial). *Arch Neurol* **32**:372.

Jackson DL. (1989) Electrodiagnostic studies of median and ulnar nerves in cyclists. *Phys Sports Med* **17**:137–48.

Jobe FW, Elattrache NS. (1991) Diagnosis and treatment of ulnar collateral ligament injuries in athletes. In: *The elbow and its disorders*. Morrey BF, ed. Philadelphia, PA: WB Saunders: 566–72.

Karas SE. (1990) Thoracic outlet syndrome. *Clin Sports Med* **9**:297–310.

Kaspi A, Yanai J, Pick CG, Mann G. (1988) Entrapment of the distal suprascapular nerve. An anatomical study. *Int Orthop* **12**:273–5.

Kauppila LI. (1993) The long thoracic nerve: possible mechanisms of injury based on autopsy study. *J Shoulder Elbow Surg* **2**:244–8.

Kessler KJ, Uribe JW. (1994) Complete isolated axillary nerve palsy in college and professional football players: a report of six cases. *Clin J Sports Med* **4**:272–4.

Kim SM, Goodrich JA. (1984) Isolated proximal musculocutaneous nerve palsy: Case report. *Arch Phys Med Rehabil* **65**:735–6.

Kulund DN, Brubaker C. (1978) Injuries in the bike centennial tour. *Phys Sports Med* **6**:74–8.

Linker CS, Helms CA, Fritz RC. (1993) Quadrilateral space syndrome: findings at MR imaging. *Radiology* **188**:675–6.

Lister GD, Belsole RB, Kleinert HE. (1979) The radial tunnel syndrome. *J Hand Surg* **4**:52–9.

Lotem M, Fried A, Levy M, Solzi P, Najenson T, Nathan H. (1971) Radial palsy following muscular effort. *J Bone Joint Surg* **53B**:500–6.

Manske PR. (1977) Compression of the radial nerve by the triceps muscle. *J Bone Joint Surg* **59A**:835–6.

Manstein CH, Lister GD. (1982) Bowler's finger. *J Hand Surg* **7**:631.

McKowen HC, Voorhies RM. (1987) Axillary nerve entrapment in the quadrilateral space: a case report. *J Neurosurg* **66**:932–4.

Mitsunaga NM, Nakano K. (1988) High radial nerve palsy following strenuous muscular activity. A case report. *Clin Orthop* **234**:39–42.

Murrey PM, Cooney WP (1996) Golf-induced injuries of the wrist. *Clin Sports Med* **15**:85–109.

Naso SJ. (1984) Compression of the digital nerve: a new entity in tennis players. *Orthop Rev* **13**:47.

Noth J, Dietz V, Mauritz KH. (1980) Cyclist's palsy. *J Neurol Sci* **46**:111–16.

Nukada H, Taylor PL, August SD. (1996) Isolated triceps weakness in exercise-induced radial neuropathy. *J Sports Med Phys Fitness* **36**:287–90.

Ogawa K, Ui M. (1997) Humeral shaft fracture sustained during arm wrestling: Report on 30 cases and review of the literature. *J Trauma* **422**:243–6.

Packer GJ, McLatchie GR, Bowden W. (1993) Scapula winging in a sports clinic. *Br J Sports Med* **27**:90–1.

Paladini D, Dellantonio R, Cinti A, Angeleri F. (1996) Axillary neuropathy in volleyball players: Report of two cases and literature review. *J Neurol Neurosurg Psychiatry* **60**:345–47.

Pecina M, Bojanic I. (1993) Musculocutaneous nerve entrapment in the upper arm. *Int Orthop* **17**:232–4.

Perlmutter GS, Apruzzese W. (1998) Axillary nerve injuries in contact sports. *Sports Med* **26**:351–61.

Perlmutter GS, Leffert RD, Zarins B. (1997) Direct injury to the axillary nerve in athletes playing contact sports. *Am J Sports Med* **25**:65–8.

Prochaska V, Crosby LA, Murphy RP. (1993) High radial nerve palsy in a tennis player. *Orthop Rev* **22**:90–2.

Rayan GM. (1988) Lower trunk brachial plexus compression neuropathy due to cervical rib in young athletes. *Am J Sports Med* **16**:77–9.

Rayan GM. (1992) Archery-related injuries of the hand, forearm and elbow. *South Med J* **85**:961–4.

Rettig AC. (1990) Neurovascular injuries in the wrist and hands of athletes. *Clin Sports Med* **9**:389–417.

Rettig AC, Ebben JR. (1993) Anterior subcutaneous transfer of the ulnar nerve in the athlete. *Am J Sports Med* **21**:836–40.

Richmond DR. (1994) Handlebar problems in bicycling. *Clin Sports Med* **13**:165–73.

Roles NC, Maudsley RH. (1972) Radial tunnel syndrome: resistant tennis elbow as a nerve entrapment. *J Bone Joint Surg* **54B**:499–508.

Shields RW, Jacobs IB. (1986) Medial palmar digital neuropathy in a cheerleader. *Arch Phys Med Rehabil* **67**:824–6.

Sinson G, Zager EL, Kline DG. (1994) Windmill pitcher's radial neuropathy. *Neurosurgery* **34**:1087–9.

Smail DF. (1975) Handlebar palsy (letter). *N Engl J Med* **292**:322.

Spinner RJ, Goldner RD. (1998) Snapping of the medial head of the triceps and recurrent dislocation of the ulnar nerve. Anatomic and dynamic factors. *J Bone Joint Surg* **80A**:239–47.

Stanish WD, Lamb H. (1978) Isolated paralysis of the serratus anterior muscle: A weight training injury: case report. *Am J Sports Med* **6**:385–6.

Streib E. (1992) Upper radial nerve palsy after muscular effort: report of three cases. *Neurology* **42**:1632–4.

Strukel RJ, Garrick J. (1978) Thoracic outlet compression in athletes: a report of 4 cases. *Am J Sports Med* **6**:35–9.

Vastamaki M, Kauppila LI. (1993) Etiologic factors in isolated paralysis of the serratus anterior muscle: a report of 197 cases. *J Shoulder Elbow Surg* **2**:240–3.

Wang DH, Koehler SM. (1996) Isolated infraspinatus atrophy in a collegiate volleyball player. *Clin J Sports Med* **6**:255–8.

Weiss BD. (1985) Nontraumatic injuries in amateur long distance bicyclists. *Am J Sports Med* **13**:187–92.

Wilbourn AJ. (1990) Electrodiagnostic testing of neurologic injuries in athletes. *Clin Sports Med* **9**:229–45.

Wojtys EM, Smith PA, Hankin FM. (1986) A cause of ulnar neuropathy in a baseball pitcher. A case report. *Am J Sports Med* **14**:422–4.

Zeiss J, Woldenberg LS, Saddemi SR, Ebraheim NA. (1993) MRI of suprascapular neuropathy in a weightlifter. *J Comp Assis Tomog* **17**:303–8.

14
Musicians

Ian Winspur

Introduction

Nerve entrapment syndromes (NES) are some of the most frequently diagnosed and treated non-emergency conditions in the upper limb. A recent report confirms just how frequently the surgical release of the carpal tunnel is performed (Keller et al., 1998). 'Repetitive strain', 'cumulative trauma' and long periods of static positioning in unnatural positions (Mackinnon, 1992) have all been incriminated in the production of NES. Surprising, therefore, is the relative infrequency of NES in musicians compared with the general public, particularly when one considers the long hours spent in a highly repetitive activity in fixed abnormal static positions.

Subtle changes in sensibility in a digit or very subtle loss of motor power will have devastating effects on a musician's performance. Therefore the musician will have cried for help at a very early point when diagnosis is difficult and long before the classical triad of pain, paraesthesia and paralysis will have occurred. Arm pain is a not uncommon symptom in musicians that is not related to specific organic disease or NES and similarly transient paraesthiae (Lambert, 1992). When these two symptoms coincide it is only too easy for the physician to make a diagnosis of NES incorrectly. Hence a careful systematic, logical and thorough approach must be made to these difficult cases before a diagnosis of NES is made (Amadio, 1998). In the next pages I hope to provide a few pointers and guidelines to the diagnosis and treatment of NES in this special group of patients.

Incidence

The incidence of NES in a given population of musicians seems to vary from clinic to clinic. This does seem partially to relate to the subspecialty umbrella under which these clinics run. Hence in the Harvard series (neurology) (Hochberg et al., 1988) the incidence is 15%; in the Mayo Clinic (orthopaedic) (Amadio and Russotti, 1990) 22.5%; the Cleveland Clinic (neurology) (Lederman, 1994) 35%; in the musicians' clinics in London (rheumatology) 2.7% of a total of 617 patients presenting, or 6.8% of those with diagnoses of a specific rheumatologic or orthopaedic condition (Table 14.1) (Wynn Parry, 1998).

Table 14.1 Upper limb problems of musicians (n=617)

Clear diagnosis	257	42%
Symptomatic hypermobility syndrome	17	
True tenosynovitis	38	
Rotator cuff/frozen shoulder	39	
Old injury	68	
Osteoarthritis	26	
Thoracic outlet syndrome	14	
Rheumatoid arthritis	8	
Low back pain	23	
Ganglion	13	
Carpal tunnel syndrome	3	
Tennis elbow	8	
Technical causes	246	40%
Emotional/psychological causes	114	18%

Reproduced with permission from Wynn Parry CB. (1998) The musician's hand and arm pain. In: Winspur I, Wynn Parry CB (eds) *The musician's hand: a clinical guide*. London: Martin Dunitz Ltd: 7.

Among these series there is also a wide varia-tion in the relative incidence of specific entrap-ments. However, by far and away the most common diagnoses are Carpal Tunnel Syndrome (CTS) and Thoracic Outlet Syndrome (TOS): in the Harvard series CTS = 60%, in the Mayo series CTS = 57%, TOS = 26%; in the Cleveland series CTS = 21% and TOS = 26%; in the most recent London series CTS = 25% and TOS = 75%. Also Cubital Tunnel Syndrome (CubTS) was relatively common in the Cleveland series but was uncommon in the other three. In a small personal series of 44 profes-sional musicians undergoing surgery (Table 14.2), NES represented 22% of these cases. No patients in the London series required surgery for TOS. Clearly from a surgical point of view, CTS is much the most common NES in musicians. However, one should not rush the surgery in musicians (Trouli and Reisses, 1994) and the indications for surgery, discussed later in this chapter, should in fact be much stricter than in the general population.

Presentation of NES

Musicians will present long before the triad of pain, paraesthesia and motor or sensory loss have developed. Indeed a miniscule fall-off in perfor-mance may render a professional musician incapable of playing. Distracting intermittent paraesthesia itself or isolated discomfort before any other symptom or sign manifests may also produce damaging fall-off in musical performance.

Table 14.2 Instruments and medical conditions in 44 professional musicians undergoing surgery over a 15-year period

Medical condition	No. of patients (%)
Trauma/post-traumatic	10 (23)
Dupuytren's contracture	10 (23)
Swellings	9 (22)
Carpal tunnel syndrome	8 (1 bilateral) (21)
Arthrodesis	3
Cubital tunnel syndrome	3
Synovitis	1
Instrument	
Piano	21 (48)
String	12 (27)
Woodwind/reed	5 (11)
Guitar	4
Brass	1
Percussion	1

Pain

There are many causes of arm pain in musicians (Lambert, 1992). 60% of those complaining have no physical signs of a recognized orthopaedic, rheumatologic or neurologic disease (Wynn Parry, 1994). They are suffering from muscular fatigue usually related to poor playing technique, poor posture, a mismatch with their instrument or psychological or emotional stress. Emotional and psychological problems in musicians can present as aches and pains and even as more localized symptoms of discomfort with intermit-tent parasthesiae. There are plenty of factors in a musician's life, notwithstanding the normal stresses of daily life, to produce such effects: loneliness and isolation in childhood from inten-sive hours of practice; overdemanding parents and teachers; the intense competition and fear of failure at college or music school; financial and professional worries from the vagaries of a career in music; difficult relationships with musical colleagues and conductors; anxieties from ageing and perceived declining perfor-mance. Musicians will surprisingly readily accept the non-physical basis of their problems and it is seldom necessary to refer them for formal psychological or psychiatric treatment; however, the advice and help from a trusted counsellor in relaxation or coping strategies may be invalu-able, particularly if the therapist involved has musical knowledge and experience. Sometimes musicians may even also suffer the symptoms of transitory paraesthesia in a specific area or areas. Obviously NES must be considered in the differential diagnosis, but unless clear, unequivo-cal constant physical signs and, in the case of CTS or CubTS nerve conduction testing is abnor-mal, a diagnosis of NES should not be made.

Musicians with aching tired arms from long periods in static positions will benefit from physiotherapeutic regimes stretching proximal muscle groups. The apparent 'release' of nerves is coincidental. Great emphasis is placed, certainly by physiotherapists and others, on the hypothesis of 'adverse neural tension'. In musicians (and office secretaries who develop tight tense muscles in the neck and around the shoulders and elbow) with diffuse arm pain and intermittent paraesthesia in mostly non-anatomi-cal distributions, it provides a framework for effective physiotherapy regimes for much

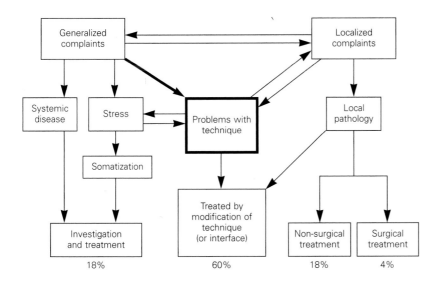

Figure 14.1

The complex interrelationships in the musicians of generalized and localized symptoms and of generalized and localized pathology versus technical factors. Similar complex relationships exist between the need for adjustment of instrument or technique versus medical or surgical care. (Reproduced with permission from Winspur I, Wynn Parry CB. (1997) The musician's hand. *J Hand Surg* **22B**:433–40.)

myo-fascial' pain. However, even accepting that peripheral nerves need some modest amount of free gliding (Wilgis and Murphy, 1986), the hypothesis of neural tension remains controversial. Provocative testing in these tired arms reproducing symptoms should not be taken as confirmation of a proximal nerve entrapment.

Pain may be the only presenting symptom in NES, particularly when a 'pure' motor nerve is involved. This is typically the case in Radial Tunnel Syndrome (RadTS) (see Chapter 10) when the symptoms may be associated with, or mimic, tennis elbow (TE). Also early CubTS particularly in the left fingering hand of string instrumentalists may present in the early stages simply as pain around the inner aspect of the elbow, down the inner aspect of the forearm and into the ulnar two digits. TOS may present only as pain referred down the same area. But arm pain in musicians may be the result of, rather than the presenting symptom of, a localized process distally, unbalancing the musician while playing. Or indeed, generalized arm pain in itself may unbalance the musician and produce focal symptoms distally (Figure 14.1) and produce abnormal local loading and local symptoms (suggestive of distal NES). A clear differentiation can only be made after a thorough history and examination of the patient

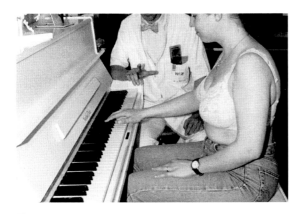

Figure 14.2

Careful examination of the patient with outer garments removed and while playing. Note the presence of the piano in the musician's clinic – an unusual luxury. (Courtesy of Dr A.B.M. Rietveld.)

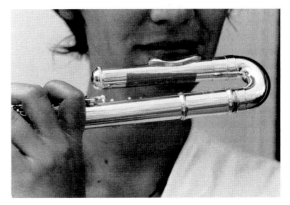

Figure 14.3

Curved mouthpiece on a flute, lowering the right shoulder and reducing the stretch on the right arm for musicians with short arms. (Courtesy of All Flutes Plus, London.)

with outer garments removed and playing (Figure 14.2) has been made. This is tedious and time-consuming and disruptive in a busy clinic. In the case of pianists, where their instrument is not transportable, it may even necessitate a visit to the patient's home or local piano showroom. It may also require consultation with the patient's music teacher or a musically knowledgeable therapist to identify the flaws in the technique or the mismatch between the patient and the instrument. If a local cause is identified, the solution may lie again in modification of technique or indeed adaptation or modification of the instrument (Figure 14.3). In the unusual circumstance of generalized or systemic illness being identified, appropriate medical treatment must be given. If no such condition can be found (60% of cases), then physiotherapy and adjustment of technique and possibly the instrument must be utilized.

Paraesthesia

Paraesthesia in musicians is a confusing symptom. It does not necessarily mean nerve compression. For an episode of slight conduction upset can produce these symptoms, when no true compression exists (see CTS). Fleeting paraesthesia, often seen in musicians with tired, tense muscles, without a specific constant anatomical distribution rules out a NES. Transient paraesthesia with a definite defined anatomical distribution within the territory of a specific peripheral nerve should make one suspicious of NES but again, in most cases, this phenomenon is not related to a specific site of compression. Constant classical paraesthesia in a defined anatomical area, many times nocturnal, should provide a high index of suspicion. It

is most important, however, to realize in the musician patient, all that tingles is not necessarily a compressed nerve.

Motor and sensory loss

A musician will have presented usually long before true neurological deficit (sensory or motor) has developed. Obviously were these signs to be present in a given patient, the diagnosis becomes much more straightforward. But clumsiness may be the first symptom of subtle motor loss (e.g. slight weakness of flexor digitorum V in CubTS). It is also one of the early symptoms of a developing focal dystonia and the physician should be alert to this. Comprehensive history, examination and evaluation, including EMGs and nerve conduction testing may be necessary to untangle these difficult cases.

Sensory loss is not compatible with playing at a high level, therefore musicians will present generally when paraesthesia (a feeling of numbness) rather than measurable sensory loss has developed. Mapping by light touch is usually satisfactory to clinically identify areas of sensory loss. Measurement of vibration or pressure thresholds is much more accurate and may be required to reveal very early sensory changes. When a digital nerve is compressed, a hemi-digital sensory diminution must be identifiable before the diagnosis of NES can be made. Changes in two-point discrimination occur at a later stage.

Role of nerve conduction tests (NCTs) in musicians

One should have developed a high index of suspicion for NES from the history, careful examination

Table 14.3 Differential diagnosis of carpal tunnel syndrome in musicians

	Daytime symptoms	Nocturnal symptoms	Phalen's	Tinel's	Swelling	NCT
CTS	0	+	+	+	0	+
Acute positional	+	0	+	0	0	0
FTS	+	0	*	0	+	0

*Phalen's manoeuvre (forced flexion of the wrist) produces marked discomfort in patients with FTS of the finger flexors at the wrist, which in itself is a useful clinical sign.
Reproduced with permission from Winspur I. (1998) Nerve compression syndromes. In: Winspur I, Wynn Parry CB (eds) *The musician's hand: a clinical guide.* London: Martin Dunitz Ltd: 90.

and observation of the patient while playing. NCT, however, is a most useful diagnostic tool when dealing with musicians particularly in the syndromes where direct measurement is easily achieved and is accurate (CTS, CubTS) (Table 14.3). In these situations the diagnosis of NES should not be made if NCT testing is normal, and there should be no question of surgical release (even accepting the fallibility of NCTs in early compression) unless NCTs are positive. NCTs have proved of little value in the diagnosis of TOS (Lederman, 1994). MRI angiography appears to be the most accurate in the diagnosis of specific mechanical sources of TOS. NCTs are not accurate in radial tunnel syndrome (Lawrence et al., 1995). They can, however, be of value in distal ulnar entrapments and are of particular help in trying to differentiate between CubTS and TOS, or CubTS and cervical radiculopathy, the presenting symptoms of which may be very similar.

Indications for surgery for NES in musicians

Surgical indications in the musician patient vary from the general population; sometimes the indications need to be relaxed, as in trauma; sometimes modified, as in Dupuytren's contracture; sometimes very much stricter, as in NES (Winspur, 1998). In general, surgery should not be contemplated unless there is concrete objective evidence of nerve compression and, if the syndrome is amenable to investigation, positive NCTs. And in those conditions which are not amenable, until a long trial of conservative care, including physiotherapy, adjustment of technique and modification of the instrument have all been attempted, no surgery should be considered. Nowhere is this seen more than in TOS and RadTS. However, in clear-cut clinical cases, with abnormal NCTs, surgical release can prove as beneficial to the musician as to the non-musician and they will normally recover swiftly.

Carpal tunnel syndrome (CTS) in musicians

CTS is the commonest compression neuropathy seen both in the general population and in musicians. It is also the commonest misdiagnosis and incorrect label applied to musicians with arm and hand pain, tingling and numbness. It is therefore worth considering the condition in some detail. CTS refers to compression of the median nerve at the wrist as it lies within the carpal tunnel producing a specific set of symptoms and signs (see Chapter 8). The compression may occur because the rigid tunnel formed by the carpal bones and roofed by the strong rigid transverse carpal ligament is too tight, or because the volume of tissue within the tunnel is too great. The median nerve lying directly under the flexor retinaculum is subject to compression by the ligament – many times at its proximal or distal edge – and symptoms and signs of median nerve compression develop. It has been shown, however, that when the wrist is hyperflexed, the volume of the canal is reduced and the nerve can be physically compressed (Gelberman et al., 1981). This is an important phenomenon when dealing with musicians, particularly guitarists. It is also the basis of the diagnostic provocative test, Phalen's test (Figure 14.4).

Symptoms and signs

Compression of the median nerve at the wrist produces paraesthesias in the median distribution, nocturnal pain and aching in the upper arm and

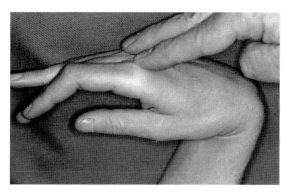

Figure 14.4

Phalen's test. Forced flexion of the wrist should be painless but will produce paraesthesia in under 60 seconds in patients with CTS. In patients with FTS the manoeuvre is immediately uncomfortable. (Reproduced with permission from Winspur I. (1998) Nerve compression syndromes. In: Winspur I, Wynn Parry CB (eds) *The musician's hand: a clinical guide*. London: Martin Dunitz Ltd: 89.

shoulder, sensory disturbance in the median distribution in the fingers (not including the palm) and motor loss causing weakness and wasting of the thenar muscles. Sensory and motor loss are late signs and therefore are not commonly seen in musicians. Indeed the commonest presentation in musicians is of nocturnal dysaesthesia or slightly altered feeling in the fingers in association with nocturnal arm and shoulder aching. The clinical signs of CTS are sensory alteration clearly limited to the distribution of the median nerve distally, thenar muscle wasting and loss of powerful thumb rotation, a positive Tinel's sign over the median nerve at the wrist and positive provocative testing with the wrist hyperflexed, producing paraesthesia and numbness within 60 seconds (see Figure 14.4). At least two of the cardinal symptoms and two of the cardinal signs should be present before a clinical diagnosis can be made. If nocturnal symptoms are not present then we should be very sceptical of the diagnosis.

Differential diagnosis

The differential diagnosis obviously includes all possible causes of median motor and sensory neuropathy, both proximally and distally. General and systemic causes of a peripheral polyneuropathy also have to be ruled out. More proximal compression of the median nerve either in the mid-forearm (pronator syndrome) or of the more proximal nerve trunks and nerve roots must also be excluded. Tumours and swellings within the carpal tunnel must also be ruled out and in this regard, when dealing with musicians, non-specific flexor tenosynovitis of the flexor tendons at the wrist and within the carpal tunnel is by far and away the commonest cause of transient symptoms in the median distribution. This is specifically seen in violinists in the left hand and in keyboard players and pianists in both hands. In fact, in practical terms, the differential diagnosis of CTS in musicians falls into three subgroups:

• Classical idiopathic CTS
• Acute positional CTS
• Flexor tenosynovitis of the wrist.

The principal differentiating features of these conditions are shown in Table 14.3.
In summary, the critical factors differentiating

true median nerve compression at the wrist (i.e. CTS) from acute positional median nerve irritation and flexor tenosynovitis of the wrist without true compression are the presence of nocturnal symptoms and the presence of slowing of nerve conduction. Hence, in dealing with a musician in which the clinical diagnosis cannot be firmly made, nerve conduction testing is a necessary diagnostic step.

Acute positional CTS

This condition should be suspected in all guitarists presenting with symptoms of median nerve irritation at the wrist. However, the history will be subtly different in as much as the patient will complain of paraesthesia and numbness in the median distribution when playing and shortly after playing. They will not complain of symptoms when resting, nor will they complain of nocturnal symptoms. The clinical examination will be entirely normal, apart from a positive Phalen's test. When observing the guitarist playing, it will be noted how rotated he or she is holding the instrument and how hyperflexed either wrist may be during playing (Figure 14.5). Many guitarists are self-taught and this poor positioning of the instrument may be deliberate mimicking of a musical idol who is also mishandling the guitar. Also the wide-necked twelve-string guitar tends to encourage this malpositioning of the left wrist. The treatment of the condition in guitarists obviously requires modification of technique with possibly a change to an instrument with a narrower neck. This should be supervised by a suitable guitar teacher. These patients fare badly following unnecessary surgical releases.

Flexor tenosynovitis of the wrist

Keyboard players present complaining of numbness in the median innervated fingers, usually occurring while playing or shortly after playing. Violinists also will present with similar complaints, but usually in the left hand and usually following periods of intensive playing with vibrato. The long and ring flexor tendons

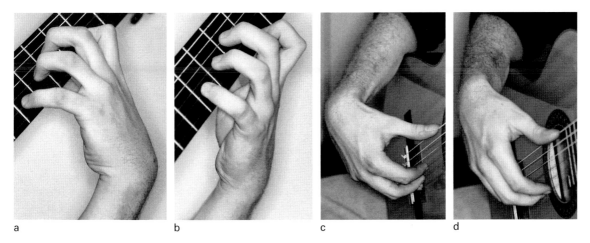

a   b   c   d

Figure 14.5

Incorrect wrist positioning when playing the guitar which may produce carpal tunnel-like symptoms: (a) left hand – incorrect; (b) left hand – correct; (c) right hand – incorrect; (d) right hand – correct.

are the ones usually involved and are tender and swollen. On careful questioning it usually emerges that these symptoms follow a period of intense practice, prolonged practice of unfamiliar difficult pieces or prolonged performance. When the symptoms are at their worst, the patients may complain of occasional nocturnal symptoms, but nocturnal symptoms do not predominate. The symptoms are not present when the musician has a break from playing, while on holiday or limits playing. Examination will show boggy swelling at the wrist also involving commonly the flexor tendons to the long and ring fingers. These tendons will usually be swollen, nodular and tender. There will be a lack of specific findings in relation to the median nerve at the wrist and Phalen's manoeuvre will produce discomfort but no paraesthesia. Nerve conduction testing will be normal. The patient has flexor tenosynovitis, a transient swelling of the wrist tenosynovium which is causing temporary dysfunction and conduction delay in the adjacent median nerve from oedema rather than from true sustained pressure. This same classical picture can be seen in violinists when playing complex pieces requiring excessive vibrato. The treatment for flexor tenosynovitis of the wrist is conservative and most certainly non-surgical, even if neurological symptoms seem to predominate. A reduction (not a cessation) in playing and critical analysis of technique and instrument

– particularly the weight of the piano action – is obligatory. Oral anti-inflammatory medicine will help. Injection of non-absorbable steroids into the carpal canal (Frederick et al., 1992; Minanikawa et al., 1992), with careful avoidance of direct injury to the median nerve can be of great value with rapid onset of action and relief of symptoms (Figure 14.6) (Tavares and Giddens 1996; Frederick et al., 1992). Surgery is not indicated unless NCT is abnormal and surgery, even when indicated, gives dismal results and should only be considered as a last resort.

Classical CTS

In musicians with early symptoms of the disease, relief can many times be achieved using night splints or anti-inflammatory medicine and some modification in playing. Believers also swear by the benefits of large doses of oral vitamin B_6 and acupuncture. However, when the condition is well established, and NCTs are positive, surgical decompression is usually required to provide permanent relief. The fact that the patient is a musician should be no contraindication. The standard surgical techniques should be used. Clear visualization of the median nerve is imperative, and therefore the open technique using a palmar incision is to be recommended in musicians rather than the endoscopic techniques,

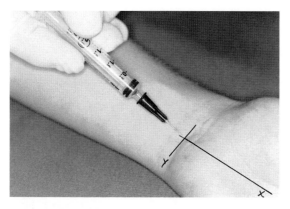

Figure 14.6

Carpal tunnel injection: this is the safe technique, avoiding any risk of direct injury to the median nerve. Note the short needle. Axis Y = 1 cm proximal to the wrist crease; axis X = extension of mid-line of ring finger. If the needle is positioned too far ulnarward, direct injury to the ulnar nerve may occur. (Minamikawa Y, et al. (1992) Tenosynovial injection for carpal tunnel syndrome. *J Hand Surg* **17A**:178–81; reproduced with permission from Winspur I. (1998) Nerve compression syndromes. In: Winspur I, Wynn Parry CB (eds) *The musician's hand: a clinical guide*. London: Martin Dunitz Ltd: 92.)

where there is a slightly increased chance of serious nerve injury (Evans, 1994; Lewis, 1995). The incisions should not cross the wrist crease unless formal exploration of the distal forearm is required. Postoperatively the wrist should be splinted in slight extension for a few days to minimize the chance of postoperative bowstringing or disloca-tion of the flexor tendons, a disaster in a musician. Gentle finger exercises and light playing for short periods is started immediately postoperative eleva-tion ceases – usually at 36 hours. Removable wrist splintage with the wrist in slight extension is started at 5 days, when practice playing can be resumed, but full sustained wrist flexion is not allowed till 10–12 days following surgery. The results of surgery can be expected to be as dramat-ically effective as those in the general population and this has been confirmed in published series in musicians (Lederman, 1994; Winspur and Wynn Parry, 1997). In our experience, all patients have returned to full playing rapidly with the exception of one who, while clearly suffering CTS, as shown by positive NCT, also proved to have a double-crush lesion with C-6, -7 and -8 radiculopathy, also requiring surgical decompression. Indeed the

commonest cause of failure following carpal tunnel release in musicians is incorrect diagnosis, once again confirming the importance of making a very accurate diagnosis and not labelling just any distal neuropathy as 'carpal tunnel syndrome'.

Cubital tunnel syndrome (CubTS)

As with nerve compression syndromes in general, given that so many musicians, particularly string players, have to spend so many hours in static positions with their elbows flexed beyond 90 degrees, CubTS is surprisingly uncommon. The incidence in a series from a larger musicians' clinic was given earlier in this chapter. From a personal series of 43 professional musicians undergoing surgery (Table 14.2), three suffered CubTS and 6 CTS (1 bilateral). Two of these CubTS cases involved the left elbow of string players (1 viola and 1 cello) and were probably related to minor anatomical abnormalities compounded by long periods of fixed flexion of the left elbow. The third case involved a pianist, but the CubTS was secondary to a long period of elbow flexion while undergoing emergency neurosurgery.

The diagnosis of CubTS in musicians can be difficult because the very early complaints may only be of arm pain (usually down the inner border of the arm and forearm) with some subtle loss of control in the little finger. Testing the power of the long flexor to the little finger is a useful clinical guide as subtle weakness may be discernable at an early point. Local signs on the ulnar nerve at the elbow (tenderness, paraesthe-sia with palpation and a Tinel's sign) may also aid the diagnosis. The differential diagnosis must include the general causes of arm and elbow pain and other causes of transient paraesthesia in musicians. It must also include proximal and distal causes of ulnar neuropathy and TOS. The critical diagnostic test is NCT. Indeed in a musician a positive test is required before the diagnosis can be confirmed. Surgical decompres-sion should not even be contemplated without a positive nerve conduction test. A focal dystonia, presenting as clumsiness or disobedience of the little or ring finger can easily be mistaken for early CubTS and it is a disaster for these patients to have surgical exploration of the ulnar nerve

(Wynn Parry, 1998). Distal entrapment of the ulnar nerve in Guyon's canal or deeply in the palm or associated with fractured hook of hammate is rare but not unknown in musicians (Wainapel and Cole, 1988).

When faced with a musician with CubTS, an initial exploration into compounding factors is well worthwhile. Long periods on the telephone with the elbows bent, driving for long periods with the seat too close to the steering wheel or with the elbow out of the window, or periods of falling asleep or catnapping with the elbow bent are all too familiar, even among top-ranking musicians. The remedy in these cases comes easily to hand. If all adjustments, including night-time resting splints with the elbow extended, have been made and the musician is still symptomatic, or more importantly developing motor loss, albeit slight, one must seriously consider surgical decompression.

The ideal technique in general for decompression of the ulnar nerve is still debated. Based on the principle that the musician should be able to return to playing at the earliest possible moment, the most simple decompression would seem logical. However, the string players spend such long periods with the elbow bent that it is illogical not to transpose the nerve (Lundborg, 1992). Additionally, there does seem to be an increased incidence of recurrence following simple decompression, possibly related to interference in nerve gliding. Therefore, we have used decompression and anterior subcutaneous transposition on musicians with some success in three cases. Although the numbers are very small, all treated cases returned to full playing 8 weeks after surgery.

Radial nerve compression

Radial nerve entrapment (RadTS) in the proximal forearm is an acknowledged cause of atypical or chronic tennis elbow. RadTS can also co-exist with tennis elbow. It may present, however, simply as arm pain associated with intermittent paraesthesia in the distribution of the superficial radial nerve. This scenario is seen not uncommonly in musicians complaining of arm pain. The diagnosis is confirmed by the deep tenderness over the radial nerve in the flexor muscle

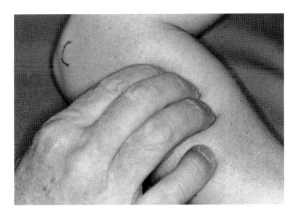

Figure 14.7

Testing for radial nerve tenderness (lateral epicondyl marked). Comparison with the non-involved side should always be made as this test can be uncomfortable even in normal arms. (Reproduced with permission from Winspur I. (1998) Nerve compression syndromes. In: Winspur I, Wynn Parry CB (eds) *The musician's hand: a clinical guide*. London: Martin Dunitz Ltd: 96.)

mass (Figure 14.7). Provocative testing (see Chapter 12) may also help in making the diagnosis. Motor loss and weakness is usually not present and nerve conduction testing is of no value (Lawrence et al., 1995). If the symptoms persist for more than 6–9 months then consideration should be given to surgical release. The results in non-musicians have been gratifying but in 15 years working with musicians I have never had to surgically release the radial nerve or one of its branches.

Compression on the posterior interosseous branch of the radial nerve causes pain and paralysis. However, this is very uncommon in musicians, although a group of young violinists have been described (Maffulli and Maffulli, 1991) with transitory weakness of the finger extensors and some forearm discomfort while playing secondary to posterior interosseous nerve irritation. Chronic tennis elbow unfortunately is seen in some older musicians associated with signs of radial tunnel syndrome. This is in fact a grave situation in musicians and I have known of two who have been forced to retire from professional careers. I have never had the opportunity to surgically release tennis elbow and radial tunnel simultaneously in a musician, although this combination has given dramatic results in the non-musical patient

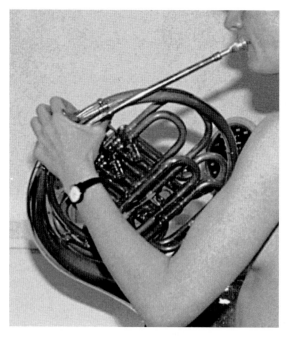

Figure 14.8

The left thumb of a French horn player subject to the same trauma as the right thumb of ten-pin bowlers.

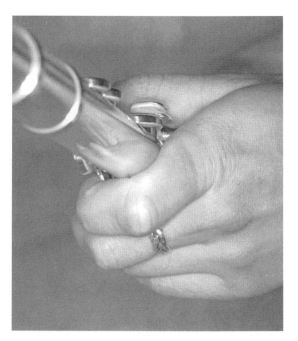

Figure 14.9

Position of left index finger on a flute. The hyperextension of the metacarpophalangeal joint places the radial digital nerve vulnerable to direct injury from the weight of the instrument. (Courtesy of All Flutes Plus, London.)

(Crawford, 1984). I fear, given the unpredictabililty of the surgical release for tennis elbow, that a musician is unlikely to return to full professional playing following this type of surgery.

Digital nerve compression

The commonest site of digital nerve compression (DNC) in the human is in the foot, producing the well recognized painful Morton's neuroma. A similar lesion is recognized in the thumb of ten-pin bowlers – Bowler's thumb (Dobyns et al., 1972). In this lesion, the radial digital nerve of the bowler's dominant thumb is repeatedly compressed against the rigid edge of the thumb holding the bowling ball and a painful neuroma develops with concomitant hemidigital sensory disturbance. A very similar lesion has been described in the left thumb of French horn players (Figure 14.8). Other such lesions have also been described in musicians; 'flautist's

finger' when the radial digital nerve of the left index finger is exposed to pressure over the metacarpophalangeal joint in the hyperextended position of the finger while supporting the flute (Figure 14.9); 'violinist's finger' reported in the left index finger of hypermobile violinists (Patrone, 1989); 'harpist's and cellist's finger' due to painful digital neuromas in the pulp from excess direct pressure on the small terminal branches of the digital nerve. And judging by the number of the string instrumentalists who use protective self-adhesive dressings on their finger tips both in practice and in performance, these lesions are more common than acknowledged.

The treatment of these conditions is either the cessation of playing (or bowling) which is usually neither acceptable nor practical, or more practically, an adjustment of the interface between the musician and the instrument. In the case of cellists with the finger tip neuromas or the hypermobile violinists this may require modification of the musician's technique. The cellist, harpist or guitarist should be encouraged to reduce the pressure applied to the strings, and in some cases the type of string used or the string tension should be altered. The hypermobile violinist should be protected by an extension blocking splint (Patrone et al., 1989). In the case of the flautists, a modified flute support is available where the weight of the instrument is taken on the thumb index web rather than directly over the hyperextended base of the index finger (Figure 14.10). This allows the index finger to be slightly repositioned so taking additional tension off the traumatized digital nerve. The French horn player's thumb will benefit from a re-engineering of the thumb ring to make it broader and better contoured. In refractory cases, if adjustments have been made, steroid injection adjacent to the neuroma seems to be beneficial and speeds resolution. The suggested surgical treatments by exploration and transposition of the nerve under some adjacent protective structure are seldom indicated.

However, one unusual but certainly recognized cause of painful pulp neuroma – Pacinian corpuscle hyperplasia (Dobyns, 1992) – which is probably more common in the players of plucked string instruments than is realized can only be treated by surgical excision. This should only be performed in extremis. It should be performed through a tiny direct longitudinal incision. The small scar should not be troublesome but the residual area of numbness may be.

Thoracic outlet syndrome in musicians

A common presenting symptom among musicians is pain spreading down the inner aspect of the arm with paraesthesia in the ring and forefinger, clumsiness and difficulty playing. Lifting and carrying causes pain and abduction of the arm may cause pain (Wynn Parry, 1997). Classical clinical findings of true sensory loss, motor loss and intrinsic muscle wasting are not present. This clinical scenario is more common in those musicians who are tall and thin and have long sloping shoulders. It is often associated with playing of one of the heavier instruments. Ledermann, whose series for the Cleveland Clinic includes the highest number of TOS cases, has coined the phrase 'clinical TOS', and this is apt. For these patients seem clinically to have TOS, although the only objective findings are muscle tenderness around the neck and shoulders, deep tenderness in the root of the neck and the posterior triangle (a reliable clinical sign) and occasional provocative testing by the 'overhead test' (Wynn Parry, 1998). The classical signs and X-ray changes of a cervical rib narrowing of the subclavian/brachial artery or vein, and a positive Adson's tests are seldom present and in this regard purists would not consider the

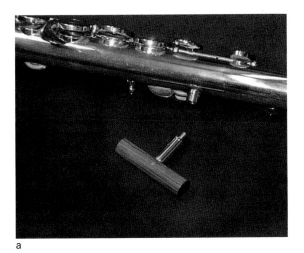

a

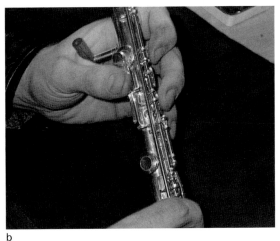

b

Figure 14.10

(a) Flute support to ease pressure on the radial digital nerve in the left index finger; (b) and allow repositioning of the index metacarpophalangeal joint. (Courtesy of All Flutes Plus, London.)

patient to have the ill-defined condition of TOS. The most satisfactory investigation to rule out a static or anatomical cause is high resolution MRI angiography. This will usually be normal. NCT is of no value (Lederman, 1994). Most of these patients will respond to conservative care (Ledermann, 1994; Wynn Parry, 1998). The first line of attack should be an analysis of the musical interface. Patients playing heavy instruments with neck straps should be changed to other types of support (Figure 14.11). Violinists with long thin necks should be advised on raised chin and shoulder supports (Figure 14.12). Flautists with short arms and difficulty with arm and neck position should consider a curved mouthpiece on the flute (see Figure 14.3). Musicians who are playing with incorrect techniques should be assessed by a skilled teacher and instructed in Alexander and Feldenkreis techniques. Physiotherapy to the neck and shoulder girdles can be extremely beneficial, but it has to be supervised by a skilled and sympathetic therapist for a given set of exercises may benefit one patient and severely aggravate the next.

Much has been made of the surgical treatment of TOS (Roos, 1986). Indeed success has been claimed in the treatment of musicians by surgery. Lederman supports satisfactory results from surgery in 2 of 45 patients with the diagnosis of TOS. But other experienced surgeons are alert to the dangers associated with these operations (Leffert, 1991) and have pointed to the fact that most musicians will improve without surgery. Indeed in his most recent review (Wynn Parry 1998) all cases of TOS were treated conservatively and all recovered completely.

Focal dystonia

No discussion of nerve compression syndromes in musicians would be complete without mention of focal dystonia (writer's cramp). Although of central origin, it must be considered in the context of peripheral nerve entrapment in musicians for a number of reasons; it is unfortunately not an uncommon neurological disorder in the musician population (Lederman, 1994); it often mimics a peripheral compression neuropathy and is frequently incorrectly diagnosed as such (Hochberg et al., 1990); it has been associated in some series with electrophysiologically

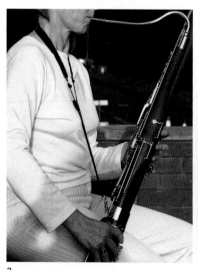 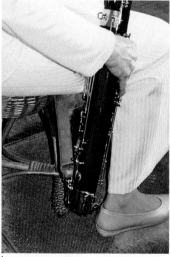 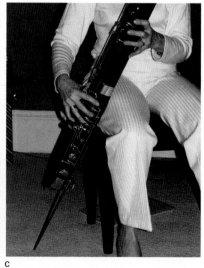

a   b   c

Figure 14.11

Devices to support the weight of a heavy bassoon and unload the right shoulder girdle: (a) next strap – simple but unsuitable for musicians with cervical spondylosis; (b) chair strap; (c) spike – also available in extended form for oboes and heavy saxophones. (Courtesy Dr J. Riley.)

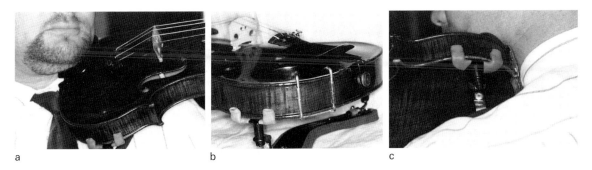

a   b   c

Figure 14.12

(a) Use of a chin support (common) and; (b) adjustable shoulder support (uncommon) to allow improved positioning of the neck; (c) left shoulder girdle in violinists and viola players with longer necks. (Courtesy of Guivier & Co. London.)

proven CubTS (Charness et al., 1996); incorrect surgical treatment when no surgical condition exists causes additional complications and worsens an already poor prognosis.

Focal dystonia presents in musicians as a painless disobedience of a digit or multiple digits when playing (Wynn Parry, 1998). It not infrequently involves the little and ring fingers. It mimics triggering or the slight clawing of a mild ulnar palsy. It usually occurs after the musician has been playing for 20 years. In the early stages it only occurs when playing and not when using the hand for similar but unrelated activity, i.e. typing.

As the condition progresses, it may involve additional fingers, may occur when contemplating playing before actual fingering has commenced, and in the later stages the interesting 'mirror effect' – disobedience of the equivalent fingers in the contralateral hand when the instrument is handled in reverse – may develop.

The condition should be diagnosed by exclusion after suspicion has been aroused. A thorough neurological evaluation including, when appropriate, MRI scanning, should be performed to exclude a central lesion such as meningioma. Nerve entrapments peripherally should be specifically sought and nerve conduction testing used in excluding these, particularly CubTS.

The condition is refractory to treatment particularly if well established or additionally confused by ill-advised surgery. Botulinum toxin has not been effective in musicians and has been abandoned by most experienced workers in the field (Lederman, 1994). When associated with an electrophysiologically proven nerve entrapment,

surgical release of the involved nerve does not seem to have a material effect on the dystonia. The most encouraging results have been obtained from utilizing combined regimes of physiotherapy and motor re-learning techniques, concentrating on posture and the understanding of movement and the movements of playing (Tubiana, 1998). The results, however, are not good and the condition remains frustratingly difficult to treat.

Results of surgery for NES in musicians

Surgery on musicians' hands in general has been regarded with scepticism (Branfonbrener, 1991). Certainly if the diagnosis is incorrect, vast amounts of additional damage can be done by inappropriate surgery. Nowhere is this more clearly seen than in a misdiagnosed case of focal dystonia. Tragedy can also occur when the carpal tunnel is surgically released on a patient with non-specific flexor tenosynovitis and conduction disturbance but no true nerve compression. However, the successful role of surgery in other conditions has been demonstrated (Winspur, 1998) and nowhere is this more clearly seen than in the treatment of idiopathic CTS.

Lederman describes 16 patients with excellent results following carpal tunnel release (CTR). An additional 18 patients who were treated conservatively fared less well. Our experience (Table 14.4) consists of 7 cases of professional musicians (one bilateral). All 7 patients made a complete recovery from CTR and all returned to full-time playing 6 weeks after surgery. There was one failure which proved to be an error in diagnosis for although appearing to have CTS by positive NCT, in fact there was co-existing proximal severe cervical radiculopathy. This patient to date has not returned to full playing. Our small series of 3 cases of professional musicians undergoing surgical treatment for CubTS by release and subcutaneous transposition had similarly been successful. All have returned to full-time playing and have been symptomatically improved but not completely 'cured'. The results of surgery in TOS are difficult to assess because the strict criteria for the diagnosis have not been laid down. However, Roos reports success in musicians following surgery as does Lederman as previously mentioned.

In conclusion NES do occur in musicians but not as frequently as one would expect. The diagnosis must be very precise and ideally confirmed by NCT. Many patients will respond to conservative care which in the musician may require analysis of their playing and modification of their instruments, instrumental supports or technique. However, given a clear confirmed diagnosis, particularly in the most common condition, idiopathic CTS, surgical release can prove dramatic and be as successful as in the general population.

References

Amadio PC, Russotti G. (1990) Evaluation and treatment of hand and wrist disorders in musicians. *Hand Clin* **6**:405–16.

Amadio PC. (1998) Surgical evaluation: Avoidance of pitfalls. In: Winspur I, Wynn Parry CB, eds. *The musician's hand: a clinical guide*. London: Martin Dunitz: 37–40.

Branfonbrener A. (1991) A special treatment for musicians? Some specific hazards of elective surgery. *Med Probl Perf Artists* **6**:37–8.

Charness ME, Ross MH, Shefner J. (1996) Ulnar neuropathy and dystonic flexion of the 4th and 5th digits: clinical correlation in musicians. *Muscle Nerve* **19**:431–7.

Crawford GP. (1984) Radial tunnel syndrome. *J Hand Surg* **9A**:451–2.

Dobyns JH, O'Brien E, Linscheid R, et al. (1972) Bowler's thumb: diagnosis and treatment. *J Bone Joint Surg* **54A**:751–5.

Dobyns J. (1992) Digital nerve compression. *Hand Clin* **8**:359–67.

Evans D. (1994) Endoscopic carpal tunnel release the hand doctor's dilemma. *J Hand Surg* **198**:3–5.

Table 14.4 Results in 42 professional musicians[a] by operation (1 lost to follow-up, 1 failure[b])

Medical condition	No. of patients	Time off instrument (weeks)	Time to full playing (weeks)
Trauma/post-traumatic	10	5.5	9
Dupuytren's contracture	10	2.1	5.2
Swellings	9	1	4
Carpal tunnel syndrome	7 (1 bilateral)	2	6
Arthrodesis	3	3.	13
Cubital tunnel syndrome	3	4	8
Instrument			
Piano	19	3.9	7.4
String	12	2.5	6.4
Woodwind/reed	5	2.5	5.5
Guitar	4	2	5
Percussion	1	1	2
Brass	1	2	6

[a]Follow-up 3 months–2 years.
[b]One carpal tunnel syndrome release subsequently shown to have co-existing cervical root compression failed to return to full playing.

Frederick HA, Carter P, Littler JW. (1992) Tenosynovial injection for carpal tunnel syndrome. *J Hand Surg* **17A**:645–7.

Gelberman R, Hergenroeder PT, Hargens AR, et al. (1981) The carpal tunnel syndrome. A study of carpal tunnel pressures. *J Bone Joint Surg* **63A**:680–3.

Hochberg FH, Leffert RD, Heller MD, Merriman L. (1983) Hand difficulties among musicians. *J Am Med Assoc* **249**:1869–72.

Hochberg FN, Harris SU, Blattert TR. (1990) Occupational hand cramps: professional disorders of motor control. *Hand Clin* **6**:417–28.

Keller RB, Largay A-M, Soule D, Manchester ME, Katz J. (1998) Maine carpal tunnel study: small area variation. *J Hand Surg* **23A**:692–7.

Lambert MC. (1992) Hand and upper limb problems of instrumental musicians. *Br J Rheumatol* **31**:265–71.

Lawrence T, Mobbs P, Fortems Y, et al. (1995) Radial tunnel syndrome. *J Hand Surg* **20B**:454–9.

Lederman R. (1994) Neuromuscular problems in the performing arts. *Muscle Nerve* **17**:569–77.

Leffert RD. (1991) Thoracic outlet syndrome. In: Tubiana R, ed. *The Hand*, Vol 4, Philadelphia, PA: WB Saunders: 243–51.

Lewis DS. (1995) Progress? At what price? *J Hand Surg* **20A**:172.

Lundborg G. (1992) Editorial. Surgical treatment of ulnar nerve entrapment at the elbow. *J Hand Surg* **17B**:245–7.

Mackinnon SE. (1992) Double and multiple crush syndromes. *Hand Clin* **8**:369–95.

Maffulli N, Maffulli F. (1991) Transient entrapment neuropathy of the posterior interosseous nerve in violin players. *J Neurol Neurosurg Psychiatry* **54**:65–7.

Minamikawa Y, Peimer C, Kambe K, Wheeler D, Sherwin F. (1992) Tenosynovial injection for carpal tunnel syndrome. *J Hand Surg* **17A**:178–81.

Patrone N, Hoppman R, Whaley J, Schmidt R (1989) Digital nerve compression in violinists with benign hypermobility. *Med Probl of Perf Artists* **4**:91–4.

Roos DB. (1986) Thoracic outlet syndromes: symptoms diagnosis, anatomy and surgical treatment. *Med Probl Perf Artists* **1**:90–2.

Tavares SP, Giddens GEB. (1996) Nerve injury following steroid injection for carpal tunnel syndromes. *J Hand Surg* **21B**:208–9.

Trouli H, Reisses N. (1994) Carpal tunnel symptoms in pianists. Anxiety for both patient and surgeon. *J Hand Surg* **19B**:(Suppl. II).

Tubiana R. (1998) Dystonia – incidence, classification of severity and results of therapy. In: Winspur I, Wynn Parry CB, eds. *The musician's hand: a clinical guide*. London: Martin Dunitz Ltd: 164–7.

Wainapel SF, Cole JL. (1988) The not so magic flute; two cases of distal ulnar entrapment. *Med Probl Perf Artists* **3**:63–5.

Wilgis S, Murphy R. (1986) The significance of longitudinal excursion in peripheral nerves. *Hand Clin* **2**:761–8.

Winspur I. (1998) Surgical indications, planning and technique. In: Winspur I, Wynn Parry CB, eds. *The musician's hand: a clinical guide*. London: Martin Dunitz: 41–52.

Winspur I, Wynn Parry CB. (1997) The musician's hand. *J Hand Surg* **22B**:433–40.

Wynn Parry CB. (1994) Musicians suffer a variety of problems. *J Hand Surg* **19B** (suppl 11–12).

Wynn Parry CB. (1998) The musician's hand and arm pain. In: Winspur I, Wynn Parry CB, eds. *The musician's hand: a clinical guide*. London: Martin Dunitz: 5–12.

Wynn Parry CB. (1998) Dystonia. In: Winspur I, Wynn Parry CB, eds. *The musician's hand: a clinical guide*. London: Martin Dunitz: 161–8.

15
The role of the physical therapist

Michel Romain, Anne Brunon, Jean-Claude, Jeanine Laurent and
Rouzard, Yves Allieu

The upper limb is rich in zones where a nerve trunk is likely to undergo compression. This compression is, in general, situated in an anatomic, muscular or osteofibrous outlet whose diameter reduces according to the position of the limb, the degree of the muscular contraction or an abnormal thickening of a constituent structure.

The clinical aspect can vary according to the level of the conflict and the nerve trunks concerned. The first signs are intermittent dysesthesias or paresthesias, often occurring at night and positioned in the zone of the concerned nerve. A lack of treatment gives rise to permanent pain and signs of deficiency appear: hypoesthesia, amyotrophy, and active motion disorders with axonal disruption.

The physical therapist has an important role to play in the treatment of this pathology, by a specific rehabilitation whose aim is to reduce the mechanical conflict, associated with use of pain-relieving physical agents. This treatment will be all the more efficient if begun early, and in all cases before any irreversible axonal lesions occur.

General diagnostic notions

The diagnosis is essentially clinical. The first stage of the examination will consist of locating postural disorders of the cervico-scapular zone or of the upper limb caused by muscular imbalance or by vicious attitudes acquired by active professionals (secretaries, musicians, sportsmen, etc.). These disorders are located by an examination of the position of the trunk, and the position of the shoulders and the upper limbs at rest. If the symptomatology is related to a particular movement or a professional attitude, the patient must reproduce it during the examination.

Palpation of muscular mass, evaluation of muscle strength and measuring the articular range of motion (ROM) bilaterally and comparatively allows identification of contractures, retractions or muscular weakness, which in turn will condition the nature of the physical treatment.

Tests and sensibilization maneuvers aim at reproducing the symptomatology by percussion, compression or stretching the nerve trunks. Tinel's sign, if present, is an excellent means to locate the anatomic seat of the conflict. It is located by cutaneous percussion on the nerve excursion, facing the zones of potential compression. The same test can be done by a manual compression of the nerve during 1 to 2 minutes.

Reproduction of pain by stretching the nerve trunk is of important diagnostic value (Butler, 1991; Totten and Hunter, 1991). The maneuver of global mobilization of the roots of the upper limb is carried out with the patient lying on his back, head inclined and turned to the contralateral side. The shoulder is placed in external abduction-rotation and the wrist in supination and extension. In this position, elbow extension stretches the upper roots of the brachial plexus by intermediary of the median nerve whilst elbow flexion stretches the lower roots of the brachial plexus by intermediary of the ulnar nerve (Figure 15.1). The test is then carried out comparatively with the contralateral side. It

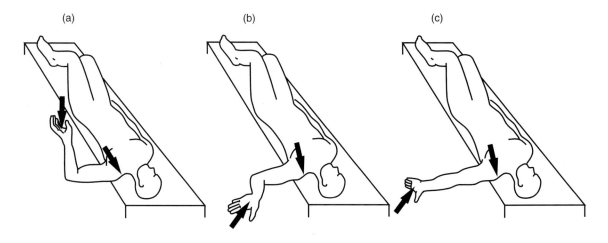

Figure 15.1

Mobilization of the brachial plexus by the median nerve (the arrows indicate the position of the physical therapist's hands and the direction of the mobilization). (a) The head is turned and inclined on the contralateral side. The shoulder is placed in 100° abduction. (b) The shoulder is placed in external rotation and the wrist is placed in supination and extension. (c) The elbow is placed in extension (if the brachial plexus has to be mobilized by the ulnar nerve, the elbow must be placed in flexion).

allows an approximate evaluation of the degree of the conflict according to the ROM necessary to release pain. The more the ROM is reduced, the more serious is the conflict. It is also a good means of controlling the evolution during the course of the treatment.

The 'double crush syndrome' (Upton and McComas, 1973) must be systematically located, because a proximal compression of a nerve makes it less tolerant to a simultaneous distal compression. Table 15.1 recalls the main zones of trunk compressions and the corresponding sensibilization tests.

Examination of the discriminative sensibility could reveal the start of a hypoesthesia thanks to the Weber static test or two-point discrimination test, the Dellon dynamic test or moving two-point discrimination test (Dellon, 1978), the Semmes–Weinstein (Bell-Krotosky, 1990) monofilaments and the vibratory test (Dellon, 1980; Gelberman et al. 1983; Szabo et al., 1984).

Exploration is completed by an electrophysiologic examination of the concerned zone, which allows confirmation of the chronic compression as well as its location. This examination includes the study of motor and sensitive conduction speeds along the nerve excursion, as well as the

study of spontaneous and voluntary activity. The time needed for stimulo-detection contributes largely in detecting early compressions. This examination must be carried out in a comparative manner on the opposite limb and in a sensibilized position.

Rehabilitation

Postural proprioceptive rehabilitation

After having identified the static disorders or the incorrect postures during daily life activities, the physical therapist must make the patient aware of them so that the latter can correct them. The use of a mirror is very useful. These disorders generally concern the cervical spine and the shoulder girdles whose most frequent attitude is: head projected forward, kyphosis of the cervico-dorsal joint with upper cervical compensating hyperlordosis, shoulders in internal rotation.

It is fundamental to find the correct position, because all the exercises will be carried out in this position. In the beginning the patient needs

Table 15.1 Sensibilization tests and maneuvers

Nerve trunks	Compression zones	Sensibilization tests
Radial nerve		
Brachial part	Lotem tunnel	Pressure at lower ¼ of the lateral side of the humerus
Posterior interosseous nerve	Fröhse tunnel or radial tunnel	Supinator pressure Pronation–flexion of the wrist Extension against resistance of the wrist and 3rd finger
Superficial branch (Wartenberg's syndrome)	Fascia between the brachio-radialis and the extensor carpi radialis brevis	Flexion–ulnar deviation of the wrist Percussion of the medial part of the lateral side of the forearm
Ulnar nerve		
At the elbow	Ulnar tunnel	Percussion of the ulnar tunnel Elbow flexion
At the wrist	Guyon's canal	Percussion of Guyon's canal
Median nerve		
Anterior interosseous nerve	Pronator teres	Pressure of the pronator teres Elbow extension and wrist supination Pronation–flexion against resistance of the wrist
At the wrist	Carpal tunnel	Percussion of the carpal tunnel Forced flexion of the wrist (Phalen's test)

tactile references. In a lying-down position the contact of the table will serve as a reference. In a sitting or standing position, either the physical therapist's hand or the vertical plane of a wall will be the reference. Progressively, these references are removed and the patient must adapt his corrected position as often as possible during the day.

This postural correction is facilitated by slow and deep respiratory movements based on thoracic expiration and diaphragmatic inspiration.

If the incorrect posture has continued for some time it may be fixed by a local stiffening of the joint. In this case its correction can be obtained only after stretching by passive mobilization of the scapulo-thoracic, the sterno-clavicular, or the acromio-clavicular joint and of the cervical spine.

Decontracturing maneuvers

Superficial massages stimulate cutaneous receptors and favor the release of tissue infiltrates. Deeper, on the insertions and muscular excursions, they stimulate the musculo-aponeurotic proprioceptive receptors and produce contracture release and sedation of painful reflex points.

Muscular rebalance

The goal is to stretch muscles that are retracted or hypertrophic by overuse and that compress the nerve trunk and to strengthen those that are weak and cause a lack of articular stabilization.

The stretching maneuvers are carried out by a very soft passive mobilization. They must not cause pain so as not to provoke a reactional contraction. Muscular relaxation must be favored by a brief isometric contraction followed by a total relaxation during which the muscle is stretched.

Remusculation is carried out by analytical techniques against manual resistance of the physical therapist. This work must be limited only to the weakened muscles, avoiding spreading contraction to the adjacent muscles so as not to accentuate the imbalance. Progressively the patient is taught to perform these exercises on his own with the help of small barbells, accompanied by breathing exercises.

Mobilization of the nerve trunks

The goal of this mobilization is to restore tolerance of the nerve to traction as well as its mobility, and to avoid or reduce epineural and endoneural adhesions (Butler, 1991). Like in sensibilization maneuvers, the patient is placed in supine position, head turned and inclined to the contralateral side. Progressively and successively the physical therapist places the shoulder in 110° abduction, then in retropulsion followed by external rotation. Next, the wrist is placed in supination and in extension. Lastly, the elbow is either extended, if the median nerve or the upper roots of the brachial plexus have to be mobilized, or flexed, if the ulnar or the lower roots of the brachial plexus have to be mobilized (Figure 15.1). As soon as the patient reports pain, the position is maintained for a few seconds, then the arm is brought back to the rest position. The maneuver is repeated about ten times with a pause between each mobilization.

These nerve trunk mobilization maneuvers are also carried out early after surgical neurolysis so as to favor nerve gliding and thus avoid the formation of new epineural adhesions (Totten and Hunter, 1991).

Physical agents

The efficacy of physical agents on neurologic pain is well known (Allegrante, 1996; Fredoreczyk, 1997) and is highly appreciated by the patients, although their mode of action is not always well known.

Electroanalgesia

Electroanalgesia is a very old pain relieving method, at first used empirically, afterwards codified by the works of Duchenne de Boulogne in 1855. This method was relaunched with interest in the 1970s thanks to a better knowledge of the neurophysiologic mechanisms of nerve conduction and pain messages, which favored the marketing of portable transcutaneous electrical neurostimulation devices (TENS). These devices produce a low frequency current (1 to 1000 Hz) consisting of asymmetric biphasic waves which are better tolerated than polarized currents. The intensity varying from 0 to 250 mA as well as the duration of impulsion from 10 μs to 200 μs are modulated according to the clinical needs and possibilities of the device.

Three modes are mainly used.
* *Conventional mode.* The frequency varies from 50 to 150 Hz with brief impulsions from 30 to 200 μs and weak intensity from 10 to 40 mA. This mode corresponds to the 'gate-control' system (Melzac and Wall, 1965) by activation of class A fibers.
* *Electropunctural mode.* This is a very low frequency current (1 to 5 Hz) and of long duration (150 to 200 μs). Classically the mode of action of these frequencies is related to their effect, stimulating secretion of endogenous opoids: metenkephalin, beta-endorphin (Mayer et al., 1977; Sjölund and Eriksson, 1976). However, several recent works (Freeman et al., 1983; Hansson et al., 1986; O'Brien et al., 1984) oppose this theory.
* *Intense and brief stimulation mode.* The goal is to stimulate only the Aβ myelinated big fibers in such a way, according to the gate-control theory, as to inhibit, at the level of the posterior horn of the spinal cord, the transmission of nociceptive messages, conveyed by the Aδ and C fibers. A stimulation of 150 μs stimulates the three types of fibers. In order to stimulate the Aδ alone, the duration of the stimulus must not exceed 10 μs (Smith and Mott, 1986). Since there exists a linear relation between the duration of electric impulse and the quantity of electricity produced (Weiss law) the strength of the current must be very high, which is uncomfortable for the patient.

Contraindications to electroanalgesia are patients with pace-makers, cutaneous lesions, vascular or infectious irritations, and the presence of osteosynthesis material near the zone to be treated.

Transcutaneous vibratory stimulations

The first publication on the analgesic effect of transcutaneous vibratory stimulations (TVS) concerns a series of patients suffering from dental pain (Otosson et al., 1981). Several works later confirmed the antalgesic action of the vibrations on acute or chronic pain (Lundeberg et al., 1984; Romain et al., 1989; Spicher and Kohut, 1996; Tardy-Gervet et al., 1993). This antalgesic technique, whose best indications seem to be neuropathic pain of neuralgic origin, is recent and still not widespread.

The stimulation is produced by an electro-mechanical device producing a vibration from 5 to 1000 Hz which is applied on the skin facing the pain zone. Frequency and vibratory strength can be adjusted. The most antalgesic frequencies are included between 80 and 200 Hz.

The antalgesic effect of the vibrations does not seem to be related to the release of endogenous opioids because it is not influenced by the injection of naloxone (Guieu et al., 1992; Hansson et al., 1986; Lundeberg, 1985). Therefore most authors agree on the fact that the action of the TVS is a result of a 'gate-control' type of mechanism, but does not use exactly the same type of afferent fibers as the TENS. The efficiency of both techniques seems identical in intensity and duration (Guieu et al., 1990; Lundeberg 1984). If they are used simultaneously, their effect is cumulative (Guieu et al., 1991). When with length of use the TENS becomes inefficient due to the patient's accommodation, the use of TVS remains effective.

Splinting

Splinting does not hold an importance place in the treatment of nerve compressions when there are no motor deficits. However, it can be useful as part of a conservative treatment whose aim is to correct a muscular imbalance or when an important inflammatory factor aggravates the conflict.

Thus, in the thoracic outlet syndrome, where muscular imbalance is common, this method can be temporarily used until the conservative treatment restores muscular imbalance. The best results are reported in patients whose shoulders are low and held far forward (Nakatuschi et al., 1995). This splint lifts the shoulder girdle by an arm-band and strap system which is passed around the two shoulders in the shape of a figure of eight.

Undoubtedly, the carpal tunnel is the best indication for a rest splint. Several studies (Court, 1995; Kruger et al., 1991; Stutzmann et al., 1998) report 67–76% relief in moderate cases in which surgical intervention is still not indicated or has to be delayed. The splint, worn at night, immobilizes the wrist in neutral position, but some authors also immobilize the patient's fingers, slightly flexed, in order to reduce flexor tenosynovitis.

Concluding comment

The therapeutic possibilities of rehabilitation of nerve compressions of the upper limb must not be neglected when they provoke irritative syndromes, especially if they are related to a postural disorder. The role of the physical therapist is to identify the dynamic anatomic causes of the conflict, to correct them and to prevent their recurrence by making the patient aware of the importance of adopting good postural habits. Physical agents such as electrotherapy and vibration certainly find their best indications in these disorders.

References

Allegrante JP. (1996) The role of adjunctive therapy in the management of chronic nonmalignant pain. *Am J Med.* **101(Suppl 1A)**:33S–39S.

Bell-Krotosky JA. (1990) Light touch-deep pressure testing using Semmes–Weinstein monofilaments. In: Hunter JM, Schneider LH, Mackin EJ, Callahan AD, eds. *Rehabilitation of the hand*, 3rd edn. St Louis, MO: CV Mosby: 585–93.

Butler D. (1991) *Mobilization of the nervous system.* Melbourne: Churchill Livingstone.

Court RB. (1995) Splinting for syndromes of CTS during pregnancy. *J Hand Ther* **8**:31–4.

Dellon AL. (1978) The moving two-point discrimination test: clinical evaluation of the quickly adapting fiber/receptor system *J Hand Surg* **3**:474–80.

Dellon AL. (1980) Clinical use of vibratory stimuli to evaluate peripheral nerve injury and compression neuropathy. *Plast Reconstr Surg* **65**:466–76.

Fredorczyk J. (1997) The role of physical agents in modulating pain. *J Hand Ther* **10**:110–21.

Freeman TB, Campbell JN, Long DM. (1983) Naloxone does not affect pain relief induced by electrical stimulation in man. *Pain* **17**:189–95.

Gelberman RH, Szabo RM, Williamson RV, Dimick MP. (1983) Sensibility testing in peripheral-nerve compression syndromes. An experimental study in humans. *J Bone Joint Surg* **65A**:632–8.

Guieu R, Tardy-Gervet MF, Blin O, Pouget J. (1990) Pain relief achieved by transcutaneous electrical nerve stimulation and/or vibratory stimulation in a case of painful legs and moving toes. *Pain* **42**:43–8.

Guieu R, Tardy-Gervet MF, Rou JP. (1991) Analgesic effects of vibration and transcutaneous electrical nerve stimulation applied separately and simultaneously to patients with chronic pain. *Can J Neurol Sci* **18**:113–19.

Guieu R, Tardy-Gervet MF, Giraud P. (1992) Met-enkephalin and beta-endorphin are not involved in the analgesic action transcutaneous vibratory stimulation. *Pain* **48**:83–8.

Hansson P, Ekblom A, Thomsson M, Fjellner B. (1986) Influence of naloxone on relief of acute oro-facial pain by transcutaneous electrical nerve stimulation (TENS) or vibration. *Pain* **24**:323–9.

Kruger VL, Kraft GH, Deitz JC, Ameis A, Polissar L. (1991) Carpal tunnel syndrome: objective measures and splint use *Arch Phys Med Rehabil* **72**:517–20.

Lundeberg T. (1984) The pain suppressive effect of vibratory stimulation and transcutaneous electrical nerve stimulation (TENS) as compared to aspirin. *Brain Res* **5**:201–9.

Lundeberg T. (1985) Naloxone does not reverse the pain-reducing effect of vibratory stimulation. *Acta Anesthesiol Scand* **29**:212–6.

Lundeberg T, Nordemar R, Ottoson D. (1984) Pain alleviation by vibratory stimulation. *Pain* **20**, 25–44.

Mayer DJ, Price DD, Rafil A. (1977) Antagonism of acupuncture analgesia in man by the narcotic antagonist naloxone. *Brain Res* **121**:368–40.

Melzack R, Wall PD. (1965) Pain mechanism: a new theory. *Science* **150**, 971–8.

Nakatsuchi Y, Saito S, Hosaka M, Matsuda S. (1995) Conservative treatment of thoracic outlet syndrome using an orthesis. *J Hand Surg* **20B**:34–9.

O'Brien WJ, Rutan FM, Sanborn C, Omer GE. (1984) Effect of transcutaneous electrical nerve stimulation on human blood beta-endorphin levels. *Phys Ther* **64**:1367–74.

Ottoson D, Ekbloma A, Hansson P. (1981) Vibratory stimulation for the relief of pain of dental origin. *Pain* **10**:37–45.

Romain M, Ginouves P, Durand PA, Riera G, Allieu Y. (1989) La stimulation vibratoire transcutanée en algologie. *Ann Rééd Med Phys* **32**:63–9.

Sjölund B, Eriksson M. (1976) Electro-acupuncture and endogenous morphines. *Lancet* **2**:1085.

Smith PJ, Mott G. (1986) Sensory threshold and conductance testing in nerve injuries. *J Hand Surg* **11**:157–62.

Spicher C, Kohut G. (1996) Rapid relief of a painful, long-standing post-traumatic digital neuroma treated by transcutaneous vibratory stimulation (TVS). *J Hand Ther* **9**:47–51.

Stutzmann S, Buch-Jaeger N, Marin-Braum F, Foucher G. (1998) Syndrome du canal carpien: résultats du traitement conservateur par orthèse de repos nocturne. *La Main* **3**:203–9.

Szabo RM, Gelberman RH, Williamson RV, Dellon AL, Yaru NC, Dimick MP. (1984) Vibratory sensory testing in acute peripheral nerve compression. *J Hand Surg* **9A**:104–9.

Tardy-Gervet MF, Guieu R, Ribot-Ciscar E, Roll JP. (1993) Les vibrations mécaniques transcutanées. Effets antalgiques et mécanismes antinociceptifs. *Rev Neurol* **149**:177–85.

Totten P, Hunter J. (1991) Therapeutic techniques to enhance nerve gliding in thoracic outlet syndrome and carpal tunnel syndrome. *Hand Clin* **7**:505–20.

Upton AR, McComas AJ. (1973) The double-crush in nerve entrapment syndromes. *Lancet* **18**:359–62.

Index